Fundamentals of Clinical Pharmacy Practice

Fundamentals of Clinical Pharmacy Practice

D. Sudheer Kumar
M.Pharm, MBA
Professor, Care College of Phamacy
Warangal, A.P.

Dr. J. Krishnaveni
M.Pharm, Ph.D
Asst. Professor, University College of Pharmaceutical Sciences
Kakatiya University, Warangal, A.P.

Dr. P. Manjula
M.Pharm, Ph.D
Principal, Care College of Pharmacy
Warangal, A.P.

Pharma Med PRESS An Imprint of Pharma Book Syndicate

PharmaMed Press
An imprint of Pharma Book Syndicate
A unit of **BSP Books Pvt., Ltd.**
4-4-309/316, Giriraj Lane,
Sultan Bazar, Hyderabad - 500 095.

Third Reprint 2021

Published by

PharmaMed Press

An imprint of Pharma Book Syndicate

A unit of BSP Books Pvt., Ltd.

4-4-309/316, Giriraj Lane, Sultan Bazar, Hyderabad - 500 095.
Phone: 040-23445600, 23445688; Fax: 91+40-23445611
E-mail: info@pharmamedpress.com
www.pharmamedpress.com/pharmamedpress.net

Printed at

Adithya Offset Process (I) Pvt. Ltd.
Hyderabad.

Price : Rs. 525.00

ISBN : 978-81-910192-7-8 (Paperback)

Dedicated to

My Parents

Late Smt. Dundigalla Padmavathi
Late Sri Dundigalla Vasudeva Rao

Foreword

Prof. Dr. D. Rambhau
Rtd. Professor, Dean,
Principal, University College of
Pharmaceutical Sciences,
Kakatiya University,
Warangal -506009

Presently:
Advisor-NDDS
Natco Pharma Limited, Natco Research Centre
B-13, Industrial Estate, Sanath Nagar, Hyderabad - 500 007
Ph. No: (91) 040-23710575 & (91) 040-23710576,
(91) 040-23812583 (Direct)
Fax: (91) 040-23710578.

A clinical pharmacy book complied by D. Sudheer Kumar, Professor, working at Care College of Pharmacy, Warangal has impressed me a lot. While reading this scientific book, I was attached to not only to its vast content but to the easy style with which it is being written. The Professor is conscious of its readers and hence the book is targeted for a general student who wishes to seek the knowledge of clinical pharmacy. The book is divided into 20 chapters. Each chapter contains a brief introduction, which prepares the student to read the chapter with a specific objective of learning. At the end of chapter there is an outline of the descriptive subject matter which is dealt in the chapter.

I strongly believe that, these days, books are being compiled hurriedly to gain some petty means. In these hard days when pharmacy education is at cross roads, there are a few teachers like D. Sudheer Kumar who felt the need to write books with a sole motive of educating the large community of pharmacy students.

I congratulate and bless him to write many more such books. As a University teacher and researcher for more than three decades, I strongly recommend this book as a text book of clinical pharmacy for undergraduate and postgraduate courses.

Dr. D. Rambhau

Preface

Clinical Pharmacy is a concept emphasizing the safe and appropriate use of drugs in patients. It places the emphasis of drugs on the patient, not on the product. Clinical Pharmacy is concerned with all those services provided by pharmacists in an attempt to provide rational drug therapy that is safe, appropriate and cost effective.

Although Clinical Pharmacy constitutes one of the important aspects of pharmacy profession throughout the world, in our country it has been neglected till recent years. The curriculum is mainly designed to suit the industry needs. The apex bodies regulating the pharmacy profession and also the universities framing the syllabus realized this anomaly in our curriculum and introduced Clinical Pharmacy as one of the subjects at Undergraduate level and as a specialization at Postgraduate level. A new six course is Pharm.D was started recently with complete clinical orientation.

A Pharmacy student is expected to have a thorough knowledge of Clinical Pharmacy, as to how it can be put into practice in actual clinical settings and the various aspects of therapeutics. But in reality the Pharmacist or Pharmacy student has only a vague idea of what Clinical Pharmacy is. Added to this there are not many books on this subject available to the student community. This has prompted me to come up with a book for students which would give them a fair understanding of the fundamental aspects of Clinical Pharmacy. My experiences as a Hospital and Clinical Pharmacist in the western hospital setup, as a community pharmacist in Middle East and in India has come in handy in authoring the present book.

This book contains about 20 chapters dealing with various topics covering the basic aspects of Clinical Pharmacy, Ambulatory Pharmacy, Patient Counseling, Medication History Review, Drug Therapy Monitoring, Therapeutic Drug Monitoring, Drug Utilization Review, Ward Round Participation, Drug Information Services, Drug Interactions, Drug-Drug

Interactions, Drug-Food Interactions, Drug-Lab test Interactions, Medication Misadventures, Medication Errors, Adverse Drug Reactions and Management, Total Parenteral Nutrition, Drugs in Pregnancy and Lactation, Pharmacoeconomics, Technology and Automation, Pharmacoepidemiology, and Clinical laboratory tests.

The contents of the book are not only aimed at fulfilling the curriculum needs but also attempts to give the student a lucid and clear picture of Clinical Pharmacy set up. I hope this book will be useful to the student community at large.

D. Sudheer Kumar

Acknowledgement

I am extremely thankful to my beloved teacher, Prof.D.Rambhau for his foreword and valuable suggestions. I place on record my sincere thanks to Prof.D.R.Krishna, University College of Pharmaceutical Sciences, Kakatiya University, Warangal, AP for reviewing the manuscript. I thank Mr.Subbaiah Ganesh, Asst.Professor, Care College of Pharmacy for his suggestions and proof reading.

I thank Mrs.E. Annapoorna, Care College of Pharmacy for the excellent DTP work.

I also express my thanks to Mr.Anil Shah and his team at M/s PharmaMed Press Hyderabad, for their painstaking efforts in bringing out this edition.

D. Sudheer Kumar

Contents

Chapter 3
Patient Counseling

Chapter 4
Medication History Review

Chapter 5
Ward Round Participation

CHAPTER 6
Monitoring Drug Therapy

CHAPTER 7
Therapeutic Drug Monitoring

CHAPTER 8
Drug Utilization Review

CHAPTER 14

Adverse Drug Reactions and Management

CHAPTER 15

Total Parenteral Nutrition

CHAPTER 18
Pharmacoeconomics

CHAPTER 19
Pharmacoepidemiology

CHAPTER 20
Clinical Laboratory Tests and Their Significance

CHAPTER 1

Introduction to Clinical Pharmacy

Objectives

After reading this chapter, the student should be able to:

- Understand the definition, concept and scope of Clinical Pharmacy
- Identify the basic components of Clinical Pharmacy
- Identify the factors responsible for the development of Clinical Pharmacy
- Recognize the role of Clinical Pharmacist in the health care system
- Understand the concept of Pharmaceutical Care

1.1 Introduction

One of the most dramatic changes affecting pharmaceutical education and the future of pharmaceutical practice is the emerging concept of clinical pharmacy. This concept has emerged in different guises since the late fifties or early sixties, although its roots lie deeply ingrained in many facets of the profession.

Clinical pharmacy includes community practice, hospital practice, and public health. According to one of the authors Dr.Glenn Sperandio "Clinical Pharmacy can be defined as that area which embraces the acquisition and preparation of medications and their distribution to the public". This is an accurate and appropriate description of the activities of the community pharmacist or the hospital pharmacist.

Clinical Pharmacists: Clinical pharmacists care for patients in all health care settings. They often collaborate with physicians and other healthcare professionals. They have extensive education in the biomedical, pharmaceutical, socio-behavioral, and clinical sciences. They are a primary source of scientifically valid information and advice regarding the safe, appropriate, and cost-effective use of medications.

Clinical Pharmacy Practice: Clinical Pharmacy Practice is the discipline of pharmacy which involves developing the professional roles of pharmacists.

Areas of pharmacy practice include disease-state management, clinical interventions (refusal to dispense a drug, recommendation to change and/or add a drug to a patient's pharmacotherapy, dosage adjustments etc.), professional development, pharmaceutical care, extemporaneous pharmaceutical compounding, communication skills, health psychology, patient care, drug abuse prevention, prevention of drug interactions, (including drug-drug interactions or drug-food interactions), prevention or minimization of adverse events, incompatibility, drug discovery and evaluation, detect pharmacotherapy-related problems such as - the patient taking a drug which he/she does not need; the patient taking a drug for a specific disease other than one afflicting the patient; the patient needs a drug for a specific disease, but is not receiving it; the patient is taking a drug underdose, the patient is taking a drug overdose; the patient having an adverse effect to a specific drug; the patient suffering from a drug interaction.

Dictionary definitions of the word "*Clinical*" differ in their complete interpretation of its meaning yet all of them agree that direct contact with a person or persons is basic. Thus, we have clinical medicine, clinical psychology, clinical pharmacology, and clinical investigation – all specifically denoting a professional service or activity involving live human subjects. Certainly, the transfer of a physician's order for medication from pharmacist to patient is a clinical situation. The other health services which a pharmacist performs daily are best described as clinical activities. In this age of specialization, every progressive vocation has specialized divisions. Pharmacy as a profession has been recognized for some time as having these divisions. The name "*Clinical Pharmacy*" identifies one such area.

The Clinical Pharmacy Concept

Development of a new role for the pharmacist came about gradually along with the many social and economic changes related to providing medical care. Since the practice of clinical pharmacy is the direction toward which the profession of pharmacy is traveling, it is appropriate to examine the history of this concept. Use of the term "Clinical Pharmacy" is usually thought of as having developed in the early sixties. Clinical pharmacy as an educational tool was initiated by Professor L.Wait Rising of The University of Washington in 1944, but was disapproved by resolution by both American Association of Colleges of Pharmacy and the American Council of Pharmaceutical Education in 1946. Rising pointed out that clinical experience for academic credit was the keystone of modern education and noted its use in medicine. An attempt was made to rekindle interest in clinical pharmacy by Professor H.W. Youngken Jr. who in 1953 wrote an article entitled " The Washington Experiment – Clinical Pharmacy" published in the *American Journal of Pharmaceutical Education*. However, there was no progress and only from early sixties the concept of clinical pharmacy was reborn and development is now proceeding at a rapid rate. The idea of the new role referred to as "Clinical Pharmacy" evolved in USA sometime in early sixties and all of which emerged as a broad concept by 1969 which connotes all the activities related to the patient (often referred to as a "patient oriented).

During the 1960s, a number of health care and pharmacy leaders in the United States recognized that most pharmacists, working both in community and hospital settings, were overeducated for the actual services they provided and underutilized as health professionals. The traditional role of pharmacists, compounding and preparing drugs had been lost to industry; the pharmacist's current functions centered primarily upon stocking, dispensing, and distributing drugs. During this decade, for a number of reasons, the climate was right to make a major change in pharmacy practice.

Pharmacy educators and practitioners who were concerned about the state of pharmacy practice in the United States and about the many unresolved problems with drug use control (e.g., drug abuse, drug overuse, untoward drug effects), began to press for change in pharmacy practice and education. Greater emphasis was placed on the "clinical" involvement of pharmacists to use their professional knowledge and judgment in making therapeutic decisions or in assisting others in making such decisions. The intent of such changes was to broaden the fundamental purpose of the profession to include greater responsibility for the safe and appropriate use of drugs in society.

Since the 1960s, the concept of clinical pharmacy has evolved to include all those activities of pharmacists which are directed towards the rational use of drugs by patients and other health professionals.

Definitions: Clinical pharmacy is an area of pharmacy practice that, since its inception, has been poorly defined. "Clinical" implies the practice of pharmacy in the presence of patients, whether they are hospitalized or ambulatory outpatients visiting their community pharmacy or neighborhood health care centre. The term does not imply that this practice be confined to the institutional setting. However, the institution is the ideal training ground for the clinical practice of pharmacy because it provides the opportunity to:

- study and observe a multitude of disease states and drug therapy regimens.
- observe on a day-to-day basis patient responses to drug therapy.
- gain access to the patient's medical record.
- communicate directly with patients, physicians, nurses and other health professionals.

- monitor patients on a myriad of drug regimens and detect, observe or minimize drug-drug interactions, drug-food interactions, drug-laboratory test interactions, adverse drug reactions, intravenous admixture incompatibilities and iatrogenic diseases.

The American Association of College of Pharmacy published the following definition for the clinical component of the baccalaureate pharmacy curriculum:

Clinical Pharmacy is that area within the pharmacy curriculum which deals with patient care with emphasis on drug therapy. Clinical pharmacy seeks to develop a patient-oriented attitude. The acquisition of new knowledge is secondary to the attainment of skills in inter-professional and patient communication.

The Committee on Clinical Pharmacy as a specialty prepared the following definition of clinical pharmacy,

Clinical Pharmacy is a health science specialty whose responsibility is to assure the safe and appropriate use of drugs in patients through the application of specialized education and/or structured training. It requires use of judgment in the collection and interpretation of data, patient-specific involvement, and direct interprofessional interactions.

Clinical Pharmacy has been defined as those services provided by pharmacists in an attempt to promote rational drug therapy that is safe, appropriate, and cost-effective.

Clinical Pharmacy is a concept or a philosophy emphasizing the safe and appropriate use of drugs in patients. It places the emphasis of drugs on the patient not on the product and it is achieved only by interacting responsibly with all the health disciplines who are in anyway concerned with drugs.

Abridged definition: *Clinical Pharmacy* can be defined as that area of pharmacy concerned with the science and practice of rational medication use.

Unabridged definition: *Clinical Pharmacy* is a health science discipline in which pharmacists provide patient care that optimizes medication therapy and promotes health, wellness and disease prevention. The practice of clinical pharmacy embraces the philosophy of pharmaceutical care; it blends a caring orientation with specialized therapeutic knowledge, experience, and judgment for the purpose of ensuring optimal patient outcomes. As a discipline clinical pharmacy also has an obligation to contribute to the generation of new knowledge that advances health and quality of life.

Clinical Pharmacists: Clinical Pharmacists care for patients in all health care settings. They possess in-depth knowledge of medications that is integrated with a foundational understanding of the biomedical, pharmaceutical, socio-behavioral, and clinical sciences. To achieve desired therapeutic goals, the clinical pharmacist applies evidence-based therapeutic guidelines, evolving sciences, emerging technologies, and relevant legal, ethical, social, cultural, economic and professional principles. Accordingly, clinical pharmacists assume responsibility and accountability for managing medication therapy in direct patient care settings, whether practicing independently or in consultation/collaboration with other health care professionals. Clinical pharmacist researchers generate, disseminate, and apply new knowledge that contributes to improved health and quality of life.

Within the system of health care, clinical pharmacists are experts in the therapeutic use of medications. They routinely provide medication therapy evaluations and recommendations to patients and health care professionals. Clinical pharmacists are a primary source of scientifically valid information and advice regarding the safe, appropriate, and cost-effective use of medications

A Three-part Definition

The unabridged definition is organized into three sections:

- The discipline of clinical pharmacy;
- The clinical pharmacist; and
- The roles of the clinical pharmacist in the health care system.

The Discipline of Clinical Pharmacy: The concept of *optimizing therapy and promoting health, wellness, and disease prevention* was felt to be essential in highlighting the focus on both pharmacologic and non-pharmacologic strategies for promoting patient health. By noting that clinical pharmacy *embraces the philosophy of pharmaceutical care*, the definition calls attention to the fact that the primary object of practice and research is ultimately the patient. Finally, emphasizing that the discipline relies on *caring values with specialized knowledge, experience, and judgment* underscores the critical importance of the synergy achieved by combining a caring ethos, in-depth therapeutic knowledge, clinical experience, and expert judgment. As a discipline, clinical pharmacy must also be engaged also in research to contribute *to the generation of new knowledge that advances human health and quality of life.*

***The Clinical Pharmacist*:** The statement that clinical pharmacist *cares for patients in all health care settings* emphasizes two points: that clinical pharmacists provide care to their patients (i.e., they don't just "provide clinical services") and that this practice can occur in any practice setting. The clinical pharmacist's application of *evidence* and *evolving* sciences points out that clinical pharmacy is a scientifically rooted discipline; *the application of legal, ethical, social, cultural, and economic principles* serves to remind us that clinical pharmacy practice also takes into account societal factors that extend beyond science. By stating that clinical pharmacists *assume responsibility* and *accountability* for achieving therapeutic goals, the definition makes it clear that they are called upon to be more than consultants. Further, the mention of managing therapy in *direct patient care settings* is particularly important because it reinforces existing definitions of the term "clinical." That is, clinical pharmacists are involved in direct interaction with and observation of the patient. In addition, it is noted that clinical pharmacists practice both *independently and in consultation/collaboration* with other health care professionals, making it clear that they are members of an autonomous profession within their scope of practice and they also function as members of a cooperative health care team. At the conclusion of this paragraph, attention is drawn to the scientific impact of clinical pharmacist researchers by stating that they *generate, disseminate and apply new knowledge that contributes to improved health and quality of life.*

Roles within the Health Care System: By noting that the clinical pharmacist is an *expert in the therapeutic use of medications*, this section indicates that the clinical pharmacist is recognized as providing a unique set of knowledge and skills to the health care system and is therefore qualified to assume the role of "drug therapy expert." In addition, this expertise is used proactively to ensure and advance rational drug therapy, thereby averting many of the medication misadventures that ensue following inappropriate therapeutic decisions made at the point of prescribing. Stating that the clinical pharmacist is *a primary source of scientifically valid information and advice* on the best use of medications emphasizes that the clinical pharmacist serves as an objective, evidence-based source of therapeutic information and recommendations. This expertise extends beyond traditional medications to include nontraditional therapies as well. Finally, indicating that clinical pharmacists *routinely* provide therapeutic evaluations and recommendations underscores the fact that their daily practice involves regular consultation with patients and health care professionals regarding medication therapy evaluations and recommendations.

1.2 Basic Components

Three basic components of the clinical role in the practice of pharmacy are

- Communication • Counseling • Consulting
- ***Communication:*** Pharmacist must have excellent communication skills to serve patients and other health professionals. Many a times the potential for service to patients and other health professionals is not realized simply because of lack of communication. The pharmacist must possess and convey a confidence in his abilities, a willingness to listen, a concern for the patient's well being, and an enthusiasm for contributing to patient care.
- ***Counseling:*** Another primary component of the clinical practice of pharmacy is counseling. Counseling used in the context of pharmacy practice might be defined as the provision of advice on therapeutic matters to patients or members of the health care team. Community pharmacist has the greatest potential and is in a unique position for counseling because of recurring and frequent contact with patients.

An essential component for proper counseling is the maintenance of a patient drug profile that provides the pharmacist with biographic information about the patient and summarizes his complete drug therapy, including over-the-counter medications. By properly utilizing this document and applying his knowledge of pharmacology and pathology, the pharmacist can monitor the patient for possible drug-drug interactions, drug-food interactions, adverse drug reactions etc., and can counsel the patient and /or physician accordingly.

- ***Consulting***: One of the most promising and potentially significant aspects of the clinical practice of pharmacy is consulting. The demand for a source person for detailed drug information will increase as the information explosion continues, medical care becomes more complex, health man power shortage becomes more acute and potential hazards of drug therapy become more evident. That source person, logically, is the pharmacist.

1.3 Scope

The scope of clinical pharmacy encompasses the following areas:

- ***Drug Distribution Systems:*** Although not all pharmacists will work directly in this area, a complete understanding and appreciation of the various drug distribution systems are essential for communication with other health professionals and the public regarding unit–dose packaging, unit-dose systems of distribution and control procedures.
- ***Drug Information:*** The provision of drug information is the foundation of clinical pharmacy practice. The drug information center, which serves as a data bank of pertinent information for utilization by the health professions, can be a tremendous resource. Pharmacists have been involved in the development of the concept of a center for information retrieval and dissemination since its inception, and their continued involvement in and utilization of the drug information center is encouraged.
- ***Drug Utilization:*** The pharmacist has a professional obligation to monitor drug utilization regardless of his locus of practice. He should be mindful of

  (1) drug abuse (2) drug misuse (overdose or underdose) (3) abnormal prescribing patterns (4) duplicated prescriptions (5) drug-drug interactions (6) drug food interactions (7) drug-laboratory test interactions (8) adverse drug reactions (9) intravenous admixture incompatibilities and (10) pathologic conditions of the patient that might predispose him to adverse effects from the prescribed drug therapy.
- ***Drug Evaluation and Selection:*** The pharmacist is a valuable resource person in the selection of drugs for various disease states. In addition, he has the opportunity to provide a unique service in evaluating the formulation of various dosage forms.

This type of information service has brought about a significant improvement in the prescribing and administering of drugs. Drug information and poison information centers have been developed in many areas to organize and coordinate the retrieval, analysis, and dissemination of drug and poison information. Many pharmacists provide drug information while attending medical rounds and at medical staff conferences.

2. ***Obtaining Patient Medication Histories and Using Patient Medication Profiles to Assure Proper Drug Utilization:*** Many hospital pharmacists maintain medication profiles for in-patients as well as for out-patients and use these to assess the appropriateness of drug therapy, screen for proper patient compliance, check for drug sensitivities and interactions, and record other patient data that can affect drug therapy.

   At a minimum, an ambulatory patient profile should contain the following essential information.

   - Patient name
   - Patient address
   - Patient telephone number
   - Patient birth date
   - Previous drug allergies, idiosyncratic reactions and / or other untoward drug effects.
   - Diseases / condition of the patient
   - Previous ineffective therapy
   - Prescription number(s)
   - Date(s) of service
   - Drug product name
   - Dosage form
   - Strength of drug(s) used
   - Quantity dispensed
   - Name of prescriber(s)
   - Identification of pharmacists(s)

   Data maintained as part of an inpatient profile may be modified, depending upon the accessibility of medical records to pharmacists who are actively involved in reviewing new drug orders and monitoring drug response. Additional drug-specific monitoring information (e.g., blood pressure, temperature, pulse, culture and sensitivity, urinary output etc). may be obtained on either ambulatory or in-patient profiles.

3. ***Monitoring Drug Therapy***: Many hospital pharmacists actively monitor individual response to drug therapy for effectiveness, ineffectiveness, adverse drug reactions, toxicity, etc. and if necessary recommend modifications in the patient's drug therapy. Unusual adverse drug reactions detected by pharmacists are often reported in the literature; additionally, many pharmacists participate in the Food and Drug Administration Adverse Reaction Reporting Program. Medication profiles, laboratory data, physical examination data, nurses and physicians progress notes, and even the results of such drug-sensitive diagnostic tests as ECGs and X-rays, are used to monitor drug therapy response.

4. ***Providing Patient Education and Medication Counseling***: Many hospital pharmacists are also involved in providing drug information to patients. They may do this by performing patient discharge medication counseling, outpatient medication counseling, or self-administration drug counseling for inpatients. The desired endpoint of patient drug counseling by pharmacists is improved compliance by patients with prescribed directions for taking their medication, more careful drug usage and storage patterns, greater understanding by patients of their disease and the purpose(s) of the drugs they are taking, and, ultimately, better treatment response. It is often necessary for pharmacists to develop special teaching programs to educate patients about their disease, diet, and drug therapy.

5. ***Providing Disease Screening, Monitoring, and Maintenance Care for Patients with Chronic Diseases:*** Pharmacists are involved in a variety of organized ambulatory care settings in providing disease screening, monitoring, and maintenance care for patients with chronic diseases such as hypertension, diabetes, mental health disorders, angina, congestive heart failure, psoriasis, and others. Most often, the patient's problems are diagnosed and stabilized by a physician, and chronic maintenance care is then provided by the pharmacist. Pharmacists monitor patients for drug compliance, response to therapy, and drug-related problems. If the drug regimen requires adjustment, the pharmacist usually does this according to protocols that have been collaboratively established by pharmacists and physicians.

6. ***Participation in the Management of Emergency Medical Care:*** Pharmacists participate in cardiopulmonary resuscitation teams in many hospitals. Their involvement may include: (a) initiating and maintaining cardiopulmonary resuscitation, (b) providing needed drugs and supplies, (c) providing drug information to the physician-leader of the team, (d) recording CPR events, and (e) setting up and operating equipment.

A number of pharmacists are now serving as clinical toxicology consultants to emergency room physicians and to those responsible for in-patient care of individuals with drug or material poisoning.

7. ***Serving as a Health Information and Education Source for the Public:*** Hospital pharmacists in ambulatory care settings have a good opportunity to provide health information and educational materials to the public. Programs to increase the public awareness and understanding of venereal disease, hypertension and diabetes have been successfully conducted through out-patient pharmacies. Pharmacy directed educational programs for immunization, poison prevention, and drug abuse prevention have also been successful.

8. ***Participation in Drug Use Review and Patient Care Audits:*** Hospital pharmacists are required to participate in those aspects of the overall hospital quality assurance program that relate to drug utilization and effectiveness. This participation may include the determination of usage patterns for a drug according to clinical services or individual prescribers, and assisting in the establishment of drug utilization review studies resulting from such program. As a consequence, prescribing practices have been modified, and for these institutions, an improvement in drug therapy has been realized.

9. ***Providing Education for Physicians, Nurses, and other Health Professionals:*** Many hospital pharmacists conduct drug education programs for nurses, prepare pharmacy news letters for the medical and nursing staff, participate in medical staff conferences as invited speakers and provide education informally on rounds and by participating in conferences.

(ii) Specialized Functions and Services

In addition to these general pharmacy services, the following specialized types of clinical pharmacy services are now being provided in some settings.

- nutritional support services,
- formal (written) drug therapy consultations,
- clinical pharmacokinetics services,
- clinical toxicology services and
- clinical drug investigations.

1.7 Pharmaceutical Care

Pharmaceutical care is defined as the functions performed by a pharmacist in ensuring the optimal use of medications to achieve specific outcomes that improve a patient's quality of life. Further, the pharmacist accepts responsibility for outcomes that ensue from his or her actions, which occur in collaboration with patients and other health care colleagues.

Elements of Pharmaceutical Care

There are six general principles or elements of pharmaceutical care:

1. ***Responsible provision of care:*** The pharmacist should accept responsibility for the patient. The pharmacist should say 'my patient' rather than 'the patient'.
2. ***Direct provision of care:*** Pharmaceutical care is directly provided to patients. This means pharmacists must be in direct contact with patients. They must see and talk to the patients. The patient-pharmacist interface is critical to helping patients and to helping make pharmacy a true clinical profession.
3. ***Caring:*** The virtue of caring, a key characteristic among nurses and physicians, has been the most understated aspect of pharmacy. It is the center piece of pharmaceutical care.
4. ***Achieving positive outcomes:*** Several positive outcomes can occur as a result of taking medication: (a) cure of disease (b) elimination or decline of a patient's symptoms, (c) arresting or slowing of a disease process or (d) preventing a disease or a symptom.

   There are also negative outcomes from taking medication: (a) the medication fails to work as expected, (b) there are undesirable side effects, or (c) there are adverse drug reactions that cause moderate patient morbidity, a life threatening or permanent disability or death.
5. ***Improving the patient's quality of life:*** Many factors determine a person's quality of life, including socio–economic status, educational background, social and business contacts and health. Of these, health status is a major factor of a person's overall quality of life.
6. ***Resolution of medication related problems:*** The task of pharmaceutical care is to resolve medication related problems (MRPs). MRPs are undesirable events a patient experiences that involve (or are suspected of involving) drug therapy that actually (or potentially) interferes with a desired patient outcome. There are eight kinds of MRPs
   - ***Needed drug therapy:*** The patient has a medical condition that requires the initiation of new or additional drug therapy
   - ***Unnecessary drug therapy:*** The patient is taking drug therapy that is unnecessary, given his or her present condition.
   - ***Use of wrong drug:*** The patient has a medical condition for which the wrong drug is being taken.

- ***Dosage is too low:*** The patient has a medical condition for which too little of the correct drug is being taken.
- ***Dosage is too high:*** The patient has a medical condition for which too much of the correct drug is being taken.
- ***Adverse drug reaction:*** The patient has a medical condition because of an adverse drug reaction or event.
- ***Not receiving the drug:*** The patient has a medical condition for which the patient is not receiving the drug.
- ***Drug interaction:*** The patient has a medical condition and there is a drug-drug, drug-food or drug-lab test interaction.

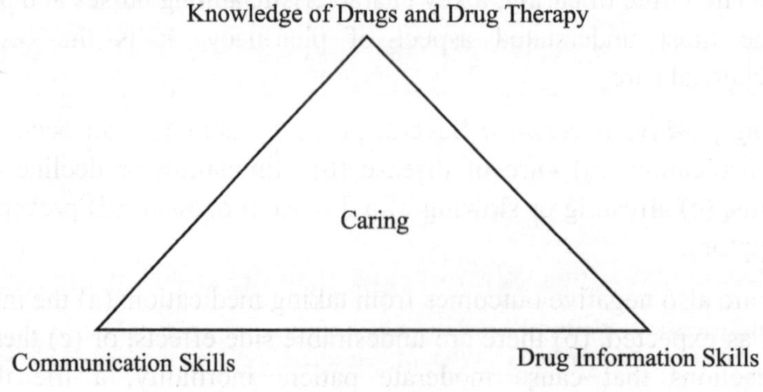

Fig. 1.1 Important factors in being a good pharmacist.

Pharmaceutical Care versus *Clinical Pharmacy*

Pharmaceutical care is not the same as clinical pharmacy, although it evolved from clinical pharmacy. The major difference between the two practice models is the primary recipient of the pharmacist's service. Under clinical pharmacy, the physician was the primary focus of the pharmacist's attention. The pharmacist provided the physician with drug information and performed drug and pharmacokinetic monitoring for the physician. The patient rarely, if ever, knew that pharmacist was involved with their care.

Providing services for the physician was a necessary step for the pharmacist to evolve clinically. It was necessary to establish credibility with physicians before pharmacists could begin to interact directly with patients. Many physicians believed that no one else should have similar relationship, particularly if that new relationship eroded the existing physician-patient relationship. Thus, it is important that pharmaceutical care be done cooperatively with the other health professionals providing care for the patient.

Other major differences between pharmaceutical care and clinical pharmacy are, pharmaceutical care focuses on various patient outcomes, shows caring and can be provided by all pharmacists regardless of educational background or training.

Table 1.1 Comparison of Pharmaceutical Care and Clinical Pharmacy

Pharmaceutical Care	Clinical Pharmacy
More of a primary care model	More of a specialty, consultant model
Patient focused	Physician focused
Provided directly to patients	Usually provided indirectly to patients
Outcome directed	Process directed
Focuses on a variety of outcomes	Mostly focuses on clinical outcomes
Based primarily on caring	Based primarily on competency
Pharmacist responsible for patient outcome	Physician responsible for patient outcome
Quality-of-life role	Quality-of-life role
Practiced in all settings	Practiced mostly in acute care settings
All Pharmacists can provide	Some Pharmacists can provide

Like Medicine, pharmacy needs a standardized approach to the patient, and one that patient recognize. The following approach to pharmaceutical care is suggested:

- Establish the patient-pharmacist relationship.
- Collect and organize information about the patient.
- List and rank the patient's medication related problems.
- Establish the desired outcome for each medication related problem.
- Determine feasible solutions for each medication related problem.
- Choose the best solution for each medication related problem.
- Discuss and negotiate the plan with the physician as needed.
- Educate the patient about the plan and counsel the patient about the medication.
- Design and implement an effective monitoring plan.
- Follow up, measure and document progress.
- Bill for services as appropriate.

1.8 Status of Clinical Pharmacy Practice

International

Initially, the discipline of clinical pharmacy borrowed heavily from other disciplines (e.g., clinical medicine, pharmacology, pharmaceutics, clinical pharmacology, medical subspecialties etc.) to synthesize a body of knowledge which provided the basis for clinical pharmacy practice. Today however, clinical pharmacy is generating a body of literature of its own. Increasing numbers of scientific papers concerning rational pharmacotherapeutic, pharmacokinetics, drug compliance and the identification and solution of other drug-related problems are being published either by clinical pharmacists alone or in collaboration with physicians and biomedical scientists. Clinical pharmacy has by now become firmly established and is recognized as having teaching, practice, and clinical research components, each of which is aimed at promoting rational drug therapy.

A *clinical pharmacist* is usually thought of as one who devotes the majority of his/her professional efforts to the provision of clinical services as opposed to distribution, technological or administrative services. Clinical pharmacists often have advanced education in the pharmaceutical and biomedical sciences and substantial clinical training and experience that enables them to provide a level of service not commonly expected of a general practice pharmacist.

In most hospital pharmacies however, clinical services are integrated into the total pharmaceutical services program rather than being offered as free-standing services. Clinical services are often provided from a satellite pharmacy through the use of a pharmacy liaison service, or through the establishment of a decentralized pharmacist service. Many prominent pharmacy educators and practitioners claim that pharmacy is an inherently clinical profession, a view which is reinforced in those hospitals where clinical services are provided by physicians, rather than by clinical specialists.

Pharmacists can influence drug use control within an institution through the provision of clinical pharmacy as well as other pharmacy services. Although there is great diversity in practice, hospital pharmacy's future depends on its overall contribution to patient care and on the recognition by other health providers of pharmacists as essential and important health care team members.

India

Pharmacy is a science-based health profession concerned with medicines and their use in the treatment and prevention of disease.

The words "Pharmacy" and "Pharmaceutical Sciences" were used as synonyms which in fact are quite different.

Pharmaceutical sciences combine a broad range of scientific disciplines that are critical to the discovery and development of new drugs and therapies. This includes drug discovery and design, drug delivery, clinical sciences, drug analysis, cost effectiveness of medicines and regulatory affairs.

Pharmacy is concerned with medicines and their use in the treatment and prevention of disease. The practice of pharmacy is mainly in the community pharmacies, hospital pharmacies where there is an interaction between the pharmacist and patient and pharmacist and various other health care professionals like doctors and nurses.

Pharmacy has two facets: Technical and Professional. The concept of Pharmaceutical Sciences or the Technical facet is well developed in India, where as, Pharmacy or Clinical Pharmacy or the Professional facet as a discipline as explained above is not well recognized in India.

For the last 40-50 years the Pharmacy education was totally oriented towards the Industrial Pharmacy. Pharmacists were educated to be a technical person who is trained and is capable of handling manufacturing, quality control, quality assurance, regulatory affairs, marketing, research and development etc. The professional angle of the pharmacy profession is not well recognized in our country. The areas of community pharmacy practice, hospital pharmacy and clinical pharmacy are still in a very nascent stage. Little effort was put in this direction. The curriculum is also designed to suit the needs of the industry. The apex bodies controlling the pharmacy education realized this draw back on the part of the pharmacy education and are taking certain measures in this direction to uplift the profession of clinical pharmacy.

Need for Clinical Pharmacy in India

Clinical Pharmacy is very essential in a country like India. India is having a large pharmaceutical industry base with more than 80,000 formulations in the market with a large patient population. The formulations prepared by many of the pharmaceutical companies are irrational combinations and non essential medications such as vitamins and tonics.

The number of prescribers (physicians) is very low when compared to the high patient population. The load on an average prescriber is very high. The physician due to high patient load is not in a position to give proper attention to the patient and is not able to diagnose the disease accurately in the short span of time available. In the process he is prescribing more medications. With the large number of drugs prescribed, the chances of drug-drug interactions and adverse drug reactions are high. Added to this the physician generally relies upon the medical representative for information on the vast number of formulations available. The information provided by the companies through their medical representatives is going to be biased and does not provide the physician with independent and unbiased information on the medication safety and treatment.

The pharmacists who are working in the retail or hospital pharmacies are not properly trained and many of the medical stores or pharmacies do not offer any specialized services to patients such as patient counseling, labeling of medications etc. Pharmacies are mainly managed by non pharmacists and there are no true community pharmacies in India. Even the large corporate hospitals do not have qualified pharmacists who can advise the physicians and patients on matters relating to drug prescribing, drug interactions, adverse drug reactions, medication compliance, medication errors etc. There is no clear policy on this aspect of health care even for the policy makers. The policies of the government are mainly aimed at the industry and not towards the patient.

The majority of the Indian patients are illiterate who cannot read and understand English, the language which is mainly used in labeling the medications containers and closures and in package inserts.

The Clinical Pharmacist can provide help in all the above situations to physicians, nurses and patients. The Clinical Pharmacist can give accurate, unbiased drug information to the physicians, advice the physician on the medication prescribing and various drug-drug interactions, adverse drug reactions; advise the patient on medication compliance through proper patient counseling help in avoiding medication errors. Clinical pharmacists can also advise patients and the physicians on cost effective medications.

Conclusion

The discipline of clinical pharmacy borrowed heavily from other disciplines (e.g., clinical medicine, pharmacology, pharmaceutics, clinical pharmacology, medical subspecialties, etc...) to synthesize a body of knowledge which provided the basis for clinical pharmacy practice. Today however, clinical pharmacy is generating a body of literature of its own. Increasing numbers of scientific papers concerning rational pharmacotherapeutics, pharmacokinetics, drug compliance and the identification and solution of other drug-related problems are being published, either by clinical pharmacists alone or in collaboration with physicians and biomedical scientists. Clinical pharmacy has by now become firmly established and is recognized as having teaching, practice, and clinical research components, each of which is aimed at promoting rational drug therapy.

A *clinical pharmacist* is usually thought of as one who devotes the majority of his/her professional efforts to the provision of clinical services, as opposed to distribution, technological or administrative services. Clinical pharmacists often have advanced education in the pharmaceutical and biomedical sciences and substantial clinical training and experience that enables them to provide a level of service not commonly expected of a general practice pharmacist.

In most hospital pharmacies however, clinical services are integrated into the total pharmaceutical services program rather than being offered as free-standing services. Clinical services are often provided from a satellite pharmacy through the use of a pharmacy liaison service, or through the establishment of a decentralized pharmacist service. Many prominent pharmacy educators and practitioners claim that pharmacy is an inherently clinical profession, a view which is reinforced in those hospitals where clinical services are provided by physicians, rather than by clinical specialists.

Pharmacists can influence drug use control within an institution through the provision of clinical pharmacy as well as other pharmacy services. Although there is great diversity in practice, hospital pharmacy's future depends on its overall contribution to patient care, and on the recognition by other health providers of pharmacists as essential and important health care team members.

Study Outline

Clinical Pharmacy can be defined as an area which deals with procuring and preparation of medications and their distribution to the public.

Clinical Pharmacists are a primary source of scientifically valid information and advice regarding the safe, appropriate and cost effective use of medications.

The three basic components of Clinical Pharmacy Practice are

- Communication
- Counseling
- Consulting

Scope of Clinical Pharmacy Encompasses

- Drug distribution systems
- Drug information
- Drug utilization
- Drug evaluation and selection
- Medication therapy management
- Formal education and training program
- Miscellaneous

Clinical Pharmacy Functions and Services

General

- providing drug information to other health professionals
- obtaining patient medication histories and using patient medication profiles to assure proper drug utilization
- monitoring drug therapy
- Providing patient education and medication counseling
- providing disease screening, monitoring and maintenance care for patients with chronic diseases.
- Participation in the management of emergency medical care
- serving as a health information and education source for the public
- Participation in drug use review and patient care audits
- providing education for physicians, nurses and other health care professionals.

Specialized

- Nutrition support services
- Formal (written) drug therapy consultations
- Clinical Pharmacokinetics services
- Clinical toxicology services
- Clinical drug investigations

Pharmaceutical Care: is defined as those functions performed by a pharmacist in ensuring optimal use of medications to achieve specific outcomes that improve a patient's quality of life. It consists of the following six elements

- Responsible provision of care
- Direct provision of care
- Caring
- Achieving positive outcomes
- Improving patients quality of life
- Resolution of medication related problems

Status of Clinical Pharmacy Practice

International

Clinical Pharmacists have advanced education in pharmaceutical and biomedical sciences, substantial clinical training and experience that enables them to provide a level of service not expected of a general practice pharmacist.

National

The role of pharmacists is more towards technical side dealing with manufacturing, Quality control, Quality assurance, Regulatory affairs, Marketing, Research and Development etc.,

The areas of Community, Hospital and Clinical Pharmacy are still in a very nascent stage.

CHAPTER 2

Ambulatory Pharmacy

Objectives

After reading this chapter the student should be able to:

- Identify, explain and compare the types of community pharmacies
- Discuss the extent of pharmaceutical care being provided in community pharmacies
- Discuss the types of dispensing errors
- Discuss some of the real challenges in providing pharmaceutical care in this environment

2.1 Introduction

The practice of ambulatory (serving those who can walk or move about freely) pharmacy in the community is the oldest type of pharmacy practice. Of the different types of ambulatory practice settings, the most common is the community pharmacy. Community pharmacists serve patients by providing information and advice about health and drugs, provide medication, and refer patients to other sources of help and care such as physicians, clinics, hospitals etc.

There are four types of community pharmacies

- Independent
- Chain store
- Mass merchandise and
- Supermarket

For each type of community pharmacy practice setting, certain things are same whereas other things are unique. Some things that differ among community pharmacies are prescription volume and the changing market share for prescriptions.

Independent Pharmacies: The independent pharmacy is where the profession began, and in many ways it remains the heart and soul of pharmacy. Many independent pharmacies started as family owned corner drug stores in towns both big and small. The uniqueness of the independent community pharmacy lies in the word independent. Independent community pharmacies are owned by pharmacists or where a pharmacist is employed full time or where the pharmacist is a partner in the business. They practice the pharmacy profession the way they choose as long as it is within the law.

Chain Store Pharmacies: The dominant corporations in chain store pharmacies are Medplus, Apollo, Guardian, Medicine Shoppe, Hetero Drugs etc. The practice of pharmacy in chain stores is similar, yet different from the practice of pharmacy in independent community pharmacies. What is similar is dispensing. After that everything is different. First, working in a chain drug store means one is working for a large corporation rather than a small family business. Therefore, the pharmacist needs to be sensitive to the corporate culture and policies.

The positions for pharmacists especially diploma holders in Pharmacy is plentiful in our country. Bachelor in Pharmacy graduates is also having ample opportunities as Pharmacy Managers manning several pharmacies. The growth of chain store pharmacies is rapid and employment in this sector is vast. Salaries are generally higher than in independent and hospital pharmacies. There is also job security and opportunity for moving up to management. Chain store pharmacy practice is fast paced, usually more so than the practice in independent pharmacies, and it needs intense focus, organization, and efficiency. There is usually less opportunity to interact with patients because of the volume of prescriptions to be dispensed.

Supermarket Pharmacies: The emergence of pharmacies within supermarkets, such as Subhiksha, Reliance, Mor, etc. has occurred within the last 5 years. The concept supermarkets use to attract customers is convenience and one-stop shopping. Patients can drop their prescriptions at the pharmacy and do their shopping rather than idly waiting for their prescriptions. This concept is still in its infancy and the takers are not many for this. This kind of set up is well taken in the western countries but in our country the patient would like to go to a pharmacy which is exclusive. The reason may be the availability of all the drugs and also personalized relationships, rapport with the pharmacist or the owner etc. Supermarket pharmacies do not stock all the drugs and brands. They generally stock fast moving products and some kind of OTC medicines.

Supermarkets are trying to create an atmosphere that provides a sense of community and a shopping experience the new wellness consumer is seeking. Consumers are looking for stores, people, brands and products they can trust.

Mass Merchandise Pharmacies: An even more recent development than supermarket pharmacies is the placing of pharmacies inside the stores of mass merchandisers such as the Big bazaar, Hyper market and Shoppers stop etc. These stores are capitalizing on a major shift in the buying practices of the public. Today, the consumers are consolidating their shopping trips and are spending more money for basics – such as prescriptions at discount stores.

2.2 Pharmaceutical Care

Definition:

Pharmaceutical care is defined as the functions performed by a pharmacist in ensuring optimal use of medications to achieve specific outcomes that improve a patient's quality of life; further, the pharmacist accepts responsibility for outcomes that ensure from his or her actions, which occur in collaboration with patients and other health care colleagues.

One of the principles of pharmaceutical care is that it can be practiced in any practice site including the community pharmacy, not just in organized health care settings like the hospitals. Many community pharmacists believe pharmaceutical care is the right direction for pharmacy but some feel they are just too busy to practice it.

The growth of pharmaceutical care in community pharmacy may be inhibited by several factors. First, there is a misconception that it is expensive to practice pharmaceutical care; that is, you need to remodel, buy new computer software and add personnel. The truth is that little money needs to be spent to start practicing pharmaceutical care. If it goes well, money can be spent over time to make improvements in performing, documenting, and billing for pharmaceutical care.

Another challenge to implementing pharmaceutical care in the community pharmacy environment is providing practicing pharmacists with the knowledge and skills to provide pharmaceutical care. Most pharmacists have some understanding of pharmaceutical care and support it, but they lack the necessary tools to practice it effectively. Continuing education programs, certification programs are needed to develop the skills of community pharmacists to practice pharmaceutical care.

Another challenge is generating revenue for pharmaceutical care. Charging for pharmaceutical care seems like the obvious answer to this challenge.

The last challenge and perhaps the most difficult one, is increasing workload and the need for more pharmacists or technicians.

It is becoming clear that pharmaceutical care will not happen in community pharmacies without catalysts such as

- improving the pharmacists clinical skills and knowledge about evidence based pharmaceutical care techniques that work
- freeing the pharmacist for pharmaceutical care by using more pharmacy technicians and automation
- reimbursement for pharmaceutical care
- more privacy for pharmacist-patient interaction
- access to the patient's medical records and
- a closer relationship with patient's doctors

Dispensing Procedures to Improve Pharmaceutical Care

- ***Accept the Prescription and Establish the Pharmacist-Patient Relationship:*** The pharmacist should be the person greeting the patient and accepting the patient's prescription, not a salesman. After establishing the pharmacist-patient relationship, the pharmacist should note the date of the prescription, verify the full and correct name of the patient, and get the patient's address and telephone numbers. During the first visit to the pharmacy the patient should also complete a form that gathers information like demographics, clinical information such as drug allergies and other pertinent information that will be useful to the pharmacy in dispensing right medicines.

- ***Review the Prescription and Patient Information:*** The pharmacist should review the prescription and patient information from a safety standpoint.

- ***Data Entry and Review of the Patient's Medication Profile:*** Each patient should have a patient record or profile in the pharmacy's computer system. The basic information for this profile is gathered on each new patient using a form, and this information should be updated at least once a year on active patients.

  Before a prescription is filled, the pharmacist should check the patient's profile for drug duplication, allergies, and potential drug interactions (software are available which do this job automatically). In order to do this properly, the patients must be asked what medications they are presently taking from any source. Each time a prescription is filled, it is added to the patient's profile by entering the information into the pharmacy computer system, which is the function of a pharmacy technician.

- ***Retrieve the Drug or Ingredients from Storage:*** Once the pharmacist is confident that a prescription is in the best interest of the patient, the prescription needs to be filled. The first step in this process is for the pharmacy technician to retrieve the correct medication or the ingredients to prepare (mix) or compound (make) the medication. The location of the drugs and ingredients for prescriptions are carefully planned for safety, efficiency and inventory control.

To be safe, drugs that can be easily confused should be stored at a distance from each other. Another safe practice is to store potent, potentially dangerous drugs and drugs known to be associated with errors in a separate, special location preferably under lock and key.

Medications can be stored product wise, such as oral medication, ointments and creams, ophthalmic (for the eye) and otics (for the ear). The drugs in each category are placed alphabetically. Some pharmacies store their medications company wise, especially if they are ordering those drugs directly from the pharmaceutical manufacturer.

Irrespective of how drugs are stored in the pharmacy, all must be kept under ideal storage conditions in which they are protected from extreme temperatures and excessive sunlight. Others must be refrigerated. Some drug wholesalers and pharmaceutical manufacturers will take back and credit outdated stock, but they do not like to see this happen often. Thus, the stock needs to be checked on a routine basis for outdated drugs.

- ***Preparation and Compounding:*** Some medications need to be counted (tablets and capsules) or poured out (liquids such as tinctures, syrups and suspensions). Other medications need to be prepared. An example is reconstituting antibiotic suspensions for paediatric patients. The drug comes in a powder or is freeze dried and needs to be made into a liquid for the patient to use.

  Compounding a prescription is more complex than preparation and involves physical chemistry and *secudum artem* – the art of pharmacy. *Secudum artem* involves the careful measurement of ingredients and knowing in what order to make the preparation and what technique to use to make an elegant final product.

- ***Label the Prescription:*** Once the product is counted, prepared or compounded and checked it needs to be labeled. Ideally the label should contain the following - a prescription number unique to that patient, product and pharmacy; date of dispensing, the patient's name, the physician's name, name and amount of the drug, initials of the pharmacist who filled the prescription etc. It may also have the lot number information and expiration date.

- ***Check for Proper Dispensing:*** Once a medicine is prepared and labeled, it needs to have a terminal check before it can be dispensed to the patient. Preferably the pharmacist should do this job. After checking the pharmacists initials are added to the label and the patients record.

- ***Drug use Review and Dispensing:*** The pharmacist must check the medication for the eight medication-related problems (Table 1) sometimes before it is dispensed.
- ***Medication Delivery and Patient Counseling:*** The pharmacist should deliver the medication to the patient, and not the pharmacy technician or sales person. The pharmacist should also counsel the patient about the medication and other related issues. Some pharmacies have even added a separate counseling area for patients. This concept is well developed in the western countries like USA, UK etc., whereas in India this is still not seen even in metro cities.

The three Cs of effective patient counseling are communication, comprehension and compliance.

Communication - To communicate effectively with patients, pharmacists need to remove any barriers to good communication, be good listeners and use open-ended questions.

Comprehension - To counsel patients properly, pharmacists should select only a few key counseling points and verify that patients understand what they need to know.

Compliance - Most patients will not take their medication exactly as prescribed. It is important to stress how often to take the medication and what may happen if the patient does not take it as prescribed.

2.3 Avoiding Errors in Dispensing Process

The primary principle of pharmacy practice is *primum non nocere*, or "first do harm". Pharmacists should not do any mistakes and do all that is necessary to avoid errors.

Types of Medication Errors: There are many types of medication errors, and some are more dangerous than others. The most dangerous medication errors are those involving the wrong dose, when a patient receives the wrong drug, when the frequency of taking the medication is incorrect and some drug interactions. All of these can result in significant harm to the patient. Other errors, such as dispensing the wrong form of the drug (a tablet instead of liquid), misspelling the patients name, and not labeling the container with the drug name will not cause much patient harm to the patient.

Reasons for Medication Errors: Errors happen because of human failing, but they most often occur because of flaws in the medication use process: the prescribing, dispensing, administration, and monitoring of medication. Medication errors are based on a knowledge deficit or a performance deficit. Knowledge deficit errors are also called mistakes. In the case of a mistake, the person committing the error does not possess the knowledge to avoid error. For example, if a pharmacist dispensed an overdose of a medication and did not know that amount of medication was an overdose; this can be called as error due to knowledge deficit or a mistake. Performance deficit errors are also called slips, as the person committing the error knew better but did not perform as expected. Slips are often caused by inattentiveness or distraction.

Some of the major contributors to errors are

- Not reading labels
- Being too busy
- The oral prescribing of medication
- Sloppy handwriting

Community Pharmacy Services

Community pharmacies provide various services for patients.

1. ***Traditional Services:*** Community pharmacies offer the following traditional services like dispensing prescriptions, over-the-counter (OTC) drugs, home delivery, delivering medicines to nursing homes etc. Some pharmacies even may offer to sell general items like greeting cards, telephone cards, cosmetics, magazines, and other sundry items required.

   Prescription services: Dispensing prescriptions is one of the most important jobs of a community pharmacy. It is very difficult for any community pharmacy to store all the medicines or brands available especially in our country. There are more than 80000 formulations. No pharmacy can store all of these brands. Most pharmacies choose to stock the most popular drugs depending upon the prescription habits of the local physicians. The pharmacies can get some medicines which are not available with them, within a day or two from the wholesaler if asked for by the patient.

   Over-the-Counter Drugs: The pharmacist is qualified to advise patients about OTC medications. OTC medicines are an important source of income for the pharmacy. Many patients come to the pharmacist for advice on routine problems before going to a doctor. If the pharmacist is knowledgeable and trust worthy the pharmacy gets good business from these services.

   The pharmacist should counsel the OTC patients which includes several steps:

   - Assess the patient's physical complaint, symptoms, and medical condition
   - Determine if the condition is self-limiting or needs medical intervention
   - Advise the patient on the proper course of action, that is, no treatment with drug therapy, self-treatment with nonprescription products, or referral to a physician or other health care provider.

If self-treatment with one or more nonprescription drugs is appropriate, the pharmacist should assist the patient in product selection, assess patient risk factors, counsel the patient regarding the proper use of the OTC, note the use of the drug in the patient's profile, provide follow up, prevent delays in seeking appropriate medical attention and assess if the nonprescription drug is masking the symptoms of a more serious condition

2. ***Newer Services:*** Community pharmacies can provide new services for the patient care. Some of the newer services that can be offered are
   - Providing immunizations
   - Checking blood pressure, glucose and cholesterol levels
   - Providing for the checkup of height, weight and analysis of weight and fat

Conclusion

Community Pharmacy is the heart and soul of Pharmacy Practice. In our country not many qualified graduate pharmacists work in these pharmacies. The large chain pharmacies are employing Diploma in Pharmacy qualified personnel as Pharmacists and Graduate Pharmacists as Pharmacy Managers supervising few pharmacies in an area. With the advent of large chain pharmacies and some Multi National Companies expected to enter the community pharmacy market, the scenario is going to change in the next few years. There is an ample scope for a large number of graduate pharmacists in these community pharmacies. Community pharmacies and the out patient pharmacies in large hospitals will create good employment opportunities for the future pharmacists.

Study Outline

Ambulatory Pharmacy refers to pharmacy service to those patients who can walk or move about freely, of which community pharmacy is the most common.

Types of Community Pharmacies

- Independent
- chain store
- Mass merchandise
- supermarket

Pharmaceutical Care is the right direction for community pharmacy's growth. Implementing Pharmaceutical Care in community pharmacy involves certain challenges.

- Misconception that Pharmaceutical Care is expensive
- Lack of skilled personnel for effective implementation
- more work load and the need for more pharmacist / technicians
- Need to generate more revenue to employ more pharmacists / technicians

Dispensing Procedures to improve pharmaceutical care

- accept the prescription and establish the Pharmacist-Patient relationship
- review the prescription and patient information
- Data entry and review of the patient's medication profile
- retrieve the drug or ingredients from storage
- Preparation and compounding
- label the prescriptions
- Check for proper dispensing
- Drug use review and dispensing
- Medication deliver and patient counseling

Avoiding Errors in Dispensing Process

The primary principle of pharmacy practice is primum non nocere, or first does no harm. Pharmacists should not do any mistakes and do all that is necessary to avoid errors. Some of the major contributors to errors are

- not reading labels
- the oral prescribing of medication
- being too busy
- sloppy handwriting

Community Pharmacy provides various services to patients

- traditional services
- prescription services
- advising about OTC drugs
- services like diagnostic services, providing immunization

CHAPTER 3

Patient Counseling

Objectives

After reading this chapter, the student should be able to:

- Define and understand patient counseling
- Identify the role of various health care professionals in patient counseling, especially the role of pharmacist
- Decide whom to counsel, what to counsel, where to counsel
- Recognize communication skills that are useful in patient counseling
- Identify the sources of patient-education materials and design strategies for drug-education for a specific institution

3.1 Introduction

Patient counseling is a very important component of Pharmaceutical Care process. With the availability of medical information through advertising in media and easy access to information on the Web, it is important for pharmacists to provide appropriate, understandable and relevant information to patients about their medication. The pharmacist is in a highly visible and readily available position to answer patient concerns and enquiries about their medications and alternate treatments they may read about or hear from others.

Definition: *Counseling may be defined as a one-to-one interaction between a pharmacist and a patient and / or caregiver. It is interactive in nature. It should include an assessment of whether or not the information was received as intended and that the patient understands how to use the information to improve the probability of positive therapeutic outcomes.*

Pharmacists practicing in institutional settings should develop or become involved in the process of educating patients about drugs. The extent of pharmacy or pharmacist involvement in patient counseling as well as the types of services offered is varied depending on the hospital.

Drug-education services may be uniformly provided to all in-patients and/or out-patients, or they may be targeted to specific subsets of these populations. The desired endpoint of patient drug education by pharmacists is a well informed patient who exhibits greater drug compliance, more careful drug use and storage, greater understanding of the purpose of the prescribed drug, and ultimately, better treatment response.

The quality of drug education services that the institutional pharmacy may offer is limited only by financial constraints of the department and the willingness of pharmacists to participate in this activity. An understanding of the need for and process of patient drug education is basic for designing quality programs that can be implemented, maintained, and evaluated successfully.

3.2 Role of Various Health Care Professionals in Patient Counseling

Patient education must be separated from patient information, since the former is associated with a degree of behavioral modification and the later with little change in compliance or therapeutic outcome. The effective pharmacist should be able to motivate the patient to learn and to take an active part in his therapeutic regimen. Historically, health professionals have dealt primarily with diagnosis and prescribing but too often has ignored to educate the patient, to ensure adherence to prescribed regimens. It has been reported that non-compliance occurs in 30 - 50% of patients receiving medications. The cause of such defaulting is multifocal and may range from lack of education concerning therapeutic regimens to financial restraints that preclude drug procurement. Additional studies have shown that intervention by the pharmacist, employing oral and /or written counseling upon the initiation of drug therapy, has resulted in a significant improvement in patient compliance. Upon patient's discharge, hospital pharmacists can seek the assistance of community pharmacists in providing the patient with the follow-up and reinforcement necessary to encourage adherence to the prescribed treatment plan.

Physician

The physician is usually the first individual to discuss the therapeutic regimen with the patient. Often, the patient is worried about his diagnosis and the implications of the disease; thus, anxiety associated with the initial visit may preclude the patient's receiving and understanding the details of prescribed therapy. The physician has this initial opportunity to reassure the patient about therapy and to encourage or motivate the individual to take an active interest in the management of his therapy. Because of multiple demands on his time, the physician may not be able to fulfill this important obligation completely. Thus, opportunities frequently arise for the hospital and community pharmacist to teach and motivate the patient to adhere to and complete his therapeutic regimen by initiating or reinforcing instruction concerning prescribed drug therapy.

Nurses

Nurse's responsibility to counsel and educate patients regarding their drug therapy is very important in many of the hospital and clinic settings. The hospital nurse traditionally has been responsible for ensuring proper drug administration. Hospital nurses frequently conduct patient education concerning drugs. It is important that the pharmacist identify these activities prior to beginning his program in order to avoid duplication of effort and possible conflicts between nursing service and professional matters. Nurses will welcome the pharmacist's input into the counseling and provision of educational materials to patients concerning their drug therapy.

The pharmacist should make a concerted effort to provide available educational materials to the nurses in order to assist in their patient-teaching efforts. A nurse administering drugs to the patient daily is in a position to field any number of questions concerning the individual therapeutic regimen. The provision of accurate information will result in continuity and reinforcement of information for the patient.

Pharmacist

The pharmacist is usually the last professional to see the patient during the course of his hospitalization. The pharmacist has an obligation to ensure that the patient understands the purpose of the therapeutic agent and its appropriate use. To accomplish this goal, the pharmacist must develop the skills necessary to communicate this information and to motivate the patient to adhere to his therapeutic regimen. A good initial patient-pharmacist interaction can encourage the patient to seek the guidance of a pharmacist in the community or to return to the institution for follow-up. The hospital pharmacist has an excellent opportunity to provide the knowledge and motivation necessary for a patient to initiate, maintain and complete his therapeutic program successfully.

The pharmacist who fails to discuss certain contraindications and adverse reactions may be held liable if a significant reaction should occur. For example, a pharmacist has a responsibility to warn a patient of the dangers of operating heavy machinery and driving a car when receiving sedative medications.

Before beginning a patient education program, the pharmacist should determine the needs of his institution by distributing a questionnaire to the physicians and nurses at his hospital. Not only can the pharmacist identify the specific needs of other health professionals, but he can obtain data to support the implementation of a new program.

3.3 Counseling Process- What, Whom, When, How, Where

What to Counsel

A pharmacist must develop, implement and fulfill plans to monitor the patient's progress towards desired therapeutic outcomes, routinely and accurately identify the amount and type of education desired by patients to maximize their chances of solving or preventing their drug related problem(s), routinely and accurately identify the degree of monitoring required by a patient according to the health risks posed by the patient's medication, drug related problems, or disease, routinely, effectively and, in consideration of the above two statements, appropriately educate patients on the following when dispensing prescription and non-prescription drugs, when patient counseling on discharge medications or when providing recommendations about management of specific drug related problems:

- Name and class of the drug (e.g. antibiotic, pain reliever)
- Directions for use including education about drug devices
- Special storage requirements
- Common or important drug-drug or drug-food interactions
- The reason for the drug and the intended therapeutic response and associated time frames
- Common or important side effects and associated time frames
- What the patient should do to monitor his/her therapeutic response or development of side effects
- Actions the patient should take if the intended therapeutic response is not obtained or side effects develop
- When appropriate, the actions the pharmacist will undertake to monitor the patient's progress

Whom and When to Counsel

Time and manpower available often will determine whom one can teach and what type of educational programs or materials the pharmacy can provide. By reviewing and compiling the results of an institutional survey, the pharmacist should be able to identify and prioritize those patients or patient types who are in need of drug-education services. Once patient needs, manpower constraints, and services offered by others are identified, the decision concerning which program(s) to implement can be made. The types of services implemented will vary depending on the institution and its patient population.

- Referral Patients

  If the need for pharmacist-based patient education and counseling is recognized by both the medical and administrative staffs, it is often easiest to begin a program based on consultation. This may involve a written order or phone call placed by the physician that requests the pharmacist to see a patient and counsel him concerning the individual's therapeutic regimen. The physician, by requesting consultation, makes the ultimate decision on who will receive pharmacist counseling and who will not.

  An advantage of this particular system should be to limit and possibly target the counseled population through a collaborative pharmacy-medical staff effort. Disadvantages of this type of service include the exclusion of many individuals because of physician disinterest as well as the inability to identify patients who would most likely benefit from consultation. This form of patient-education effort however, is an excellent way to initiate a service with further demand for expansion being proportional to the quality and perceived value of the services provided.

- Patients with Specific Disease States

  Patients who have chronic diseases like cardiovascular disease, renal disease etc. who are placed on long-term therapeutic regimens have a difficult time adhering to them. The hospital setting can be used to great advantage in teaching newly diagnosed cardiac patients about their drugs. This group might include patients with congestive heart failure, angina pectoris, hypertension, or post-myocardial infarction. In these cases, educational strategies are developed that are centered on a disease entity and its therapy. Cardiovascular rehabilitation and education programs have been shown to be very effective in providing cardiac patients with the interest and desire to continue treatment regimens that were initiated in the hospital.

  Advantages of identifying specific populations for patient education include the availability of data in the literature to support such activities (i.e. positive effects on patient outcomes already established by others) and a defined area for the development of specialized educational programs. The pharmacist may narrow his educational efforts to a particular class of drugs based on disease state. Disadvantages include the limited number of patients to be counseled and the possibility to overlap with the activities of other health professionals.

  Group counseling sessions can be conducted utilizing audiovisual aids such as slides or flip-charts, and the pharmacist periodically can teach a group of patients receiving a comparable drug regimen for a single disease entity. This is a very time efficient way to conduct a counseling session but does not assure that the individual patient will retain pertinent information without subsequent follow-up sessions. When conducting group sessions, it is imperative that the pharmacist provide written materials such as pamphlets or brochures that will reinforce important facts concerning drug therapy.

- Patients treated with Specific Classes of Drugs

  Patients who are using specific classes of drugs need to be counseled depending upon their record of use and known liability for incorrect use. Examples include drugs with documented drug-drug, drug-food, drug-alcohol and drug-environmental interactions (e.g., warfarin). Drugs most commonly discontinued by patients and drugs with narrow therapeutic indexes are other examples for which the hospital pharmacist may define a group of non-compliers who may benefit from various educational techniques. This type of service is an excellent initial endeavor since it requires the preparation or acquisition of educational material for only a limited number of therapeutic agents.

- Geriatric Patients

  Drug compliance is very poor in old patients above the age of 70 years. These patients generally have multiple diseases and are on complicated therapeutic regimens and are required to take medications throughout the day. The reasons for drug defaulting within this patient population are many. Frequently, health professionals fail to take the time to ensure the proper understanding of prescribed regimens, and this results in confusing the patient. In the older patients often there is a problem of hearing and sight impairment. Many a times these patients are responsible for taking their own medications. In view of these facts, the elderly patient often benefit from the provision of education aids during counseling sessions.

- Pediatric Patients

  The pediatric population is a unique group of patients who can have significant problems adhering to and completing their treatment. In this situation, the pharmacist must educate the child and/or guardian about the importance of the therapeutic regimen and its completion. Cost of therapy, product palatability, and dosing schedules are all factors that may influence significantly the therapeutic outcome in the pediatric patient. It is important to motivate the young patient to take an active interest in his drug therapy for the present and the future. The most useful approach to ensuring adherence to the therapeutic regimen is to gear counseling efforts to the child. By incorporating additional educational aids such as illustrated written materials and drug calendars, the pharmacist can greatly improve the patient and / or guardian's awareness of the importance of prescribed drug therapy.

- Discharged Patients

  In-patients have the advantage of drugs being administered by the nursing staff. When these patients are discharged they need to be counseled on the medication use process, with organized follow-up from the hospital pharmacist. A program of this type could ensure uniform teaching for all patients, provide the best opportunity to ensure completion of therapeutic regimens, as well as serve to define a role for the pharmacist in the care of the hospitalized patient.

- Patients using OTC Drugs

  Patients who are using OTC drugs will also be using some of the prescription drugs. Such patients need to be counseled, as many a times there is a possibility of severe drug-drug interactions among these drugs.

How to Counsel

The Pharmacist must emphasize on patient education, and not patient information. There are two phases in the pharmacist-patient interaction process.

- Assessment Phase
- Planning and Implementation Phase

  Assessment Phase: The Pharmacist assesses the individual patient's knowledge and understanding of his disease process and what drug therapy he is taking and its relation with the disease. He will use certain questioning techniques such as open ended questions, close ended questions, reflective questions and suggestive questions.

  - *Open ended questions* require maximum participation on the part of the patient. This is a very good technique.
  - *Close ended questions* are simple questions which require only a Yes or No response.
  - *Reflective questions* provide the patient with the opportunity to explain his previous statements in more detail and provides with more information concerning the patient's anxiety and fear.
  - *Suggestive questions* should be avoided since the pharmacist's opinion is imposed on the patient automatically.

  Planning and Implementation Phase: This phase encourages behavioral modification on the part of the patient to ensure adherence to the therapeutic regimen. Proper *verbal communication, Non verbal communication, listening and evaluation techniques* are to be used in this phase. The language (verbal) used by the pharmacist should be appropriate that is understandable to the patient without using medical jargon. Body language and gestures (non verbal) are also very important. Apart from the above the pharmacist must also be a good listener. The pharmacist should evaluate by asking follow up questions.

Where to Counsel (Counseling Area)

The patient should be counseled in a semi-private, or private area away from other people and distractions, depending on the medication(s). The patient should perceive the counseling area as confidential, secure and conducive to learning. This helps ensure both parties are focused on the discussion, and minimizes interruptions and distractions. It provides an opportunity for patients to ask questions they may be hesitant to ask in public.

In-patient: The pharmacist is having an excellent opportunity to present information to the patient and there will be a good patient-pharmacist interaction in an inpatient setting. Inpatients have time to learn and are readily available to discuss their therapy. One of the most useful and practical way to counsel patients while they are in the hospital is by instituting a self medication program. Most commonly counseling takes place while the patient is being discharged.

Out-patient: The pharmacist has an opportunity to monitor compliance and to reinforce understanding of educational facts in an outpatient setting. The counseling principles like communication and teaching that apply in inpatient setting will hold good for outpatients also.

3.4 Counseling on Non-Prescription Drugs

Effective non-prescription drug counseling requires a thorough description of patient's symptoms. Before advice can be given, the pharmacist will need knowledge on the nature, severity and circumstances surrounding those symptoms, as well as, other aspects of the patient's health e.g. other diseases, drugs, contraindications, allergies, must be examined. This information gathering stage is most important. When non-prescription drugs are indicated, the pharmacist must be able to give information to the patient, so products are used both safely and effectively. When providing care to patients involving over-the- counter (OTC) medications, it is necessary to perform an adequate assessment of the client's problem, in the following way:

- properly identifying the person who will be using the product and determining their approximate age;
- inquiring about any current medical conditions;
- asking about current prescription drug use;
- inquiring about the symptoms and duration of the complaint;
- asking about whether the patient has any medication allergies; and
- asking whether the patient has consulted a health care professional about the problem.

The pharmacist should refer the patient for medical attention if:

- his condition is potentially severe, and is uncertain about their symptoms
- his self-diagnosis is likely to be incorrect
- his condition has not responded to previous appropriate therapy, or
- he has other risk factors that should be assessed.

When the pharmacist has assessed the patient and the problem, and feel that a referral is not necessary, he may recommend an appropriate product or course of action, including non-drug measures. If a non-prescription drug product is recommended then the pharmacist should discuss:

- Directions for use
- Expected outcomes of therapy, including a time-frame for a response
- Common adverse effects and precautions
- Correct storage and
- When to seek medical attention.

Ideally, the pharmacist should document nonprescription drug use on the client's medication profile. This is especially important for patients who have a medical condition and/or are taking prescription medication.

3.5 Material (Aids) for Counseling

The pharmacist can make use of a variety of teaching aids to conduct the counseling process. The use of teaching aids is helpful in reinforcing the information communicated by the pharmacist. Printed materials like patient information leaflets, illustrated information, audio visual aids like video tapes, audio tapes; dosage compliance aids like drug calendars and educational displays are used.

3.6 Patient Counseling – Check List

Effective patient counseling is not simply the provision of information. Information is prerequisite to compliance, but the timing and organization of the message and involvement of the patient are also critical in determining what the patient understands and remembers. The counseling encounter should be thought of as an opportunity for information exchange. The pharmacist is the expert on drug therapy, but patients are experts on their daily routines, how they understand their illness and its treatment, whether they anticipate any problems taking the medicine as prescribed, and so forth. Each of these points needs to be assessed if counseling is to be effective. The counseling checklist provided here is developed to increase the probability that the patient will comply with the treatment regimen. It is assumed that before the pharmacist counsels the patient, he or she will first assess the appropriateness of the drug therapy.

- ***Introduce yourself:*** It is important for patients to know they are speaking with the pharmacist. They may be reluctant to ask questions or express concerns if they believe they are speaking to a technician or clerk.
- ***Identify to whom you are speaking:*** If you are talking to the patient directly, information is less likely to be confused or distorted than if you are talking to the patient's agent, who must pass the information on to the patient. In third party communication, written information becomes even more important than when directly communicating with the patient. Pharmacists may need to call patients if they believe that the information truly needs to be communicated directly to them.
- ***Ask if the patient has time to discuss the medicine:*** If patients do not have time to listen, the information will be ineffective. The information should be written and/or the patient should be contacted at a more convenient time. For a new patient, a database should be established so that appropriate decisions may be made in the future.
- ***Explain the purpose/importance of the counseling session:*** People listen and learn more effectively when they are given reasons for what is being asked of them. For example, patients are less likely to take tetracycline with food or dairy products if they are told that decreased absorption and effectiveness of the drug may result. For new patients, it will be necessary to explain why the information being gathered is needed.
- ***Ask the patient what the physician told him/her about the drug and what condition it is treating:*** Find out what the patient knows or understands about his or her disease. There is no reason for the pharmacist to present information that the patient already has mastered. Generally speaking, in any effective counseling session, the patient should speak more than the healthcare provider. The purpose of the session is to ensure that patients leave the pharmacy with knowledge about the proper use of the medication. Accurate information that the patient supplies should be supported and praised. Inaccurate information should be corrected, and information that is omitted should be added. Use any available patient profile information.
- ***Prior to providing information, ask the patient if he/she has any concerns:*** Often, patients will not vocalize concerns about the drug(s) they are about to take or the condition the doctor is treating unless they are asked. It is important to address these concerns immediately, with as much understanding as possible. Until the concern is addressed, the patient will not register or internalize any other

information that is provided. The pharmacist should make every effort to understand the concerns of the patient and treat the concerns with the attention they deserve.

- ***Listen carefully and respond with appropriate empathy:*** These skills are absolutely essential to an effective counseling session. The relationship between the patient and practitioner is a key variable in predicting compliance with treatment regimens. Patients need to view healthcare providers as competent, trustworthy professionals who care about what happens to them. Listening and empathic responding are effective tools for communicating caring.
- ***Tell the patient the name, indication, and route of administration of the medication:*** This and the steps that follow will, are generally performed after determining the appropriateness of the medication and filling the prescription. Telling patients the name of the medication, helps them get used to identifying it. This is especially important in case of an emergency (e.g., a child ingesting it, overdose). Stating the indication reinforces the diagnosis and creates confidence in the appropriateness of the therapy. While the route of administration often seems obvious, pharmacists often encounter cases of patients taking a medication by the wrong route. It should not be assumed that printing this information on the label will cover these points. Many patients cannot read, and those who can read often don't.
- ***Inform the patient of the dosage regimen:*** Patients should be told the dosage regimen in order to either reinforce what the doctor instructed or informed them for the first time. While a particular dosage regimen may seem straightforward or obvious, it may be interpreted incorrectly. For example, not everyone eats three meals a day. Patients with diabetes may eat six or seven mini-meals each day. Therefore, directions that state, "Take one tablet after meals and at bedtime" may prompt some patients to take their medications more than the intended four times per day.
- ***Ask the patient if he/she will have a problem taking the medication as prescribed:*** This is an important question that is seldom asked by any healthcare provider. Yet, research shows that the complexity of the dosage regimen can greatly affect compliance. This has significant implications for the pharmacist. The total cost of care needs to be considered, not just the cost of the drug. Noncompliance as a consequence of complex dosage regimens may result in hospitalization of the patient. Pharmacists should attempt to resolve problems related to the dosage regimen, either through tailoring the regimen or working with the physician to change the medication to a less complicated dosing schedule.
- ***Tailor the medication regimen to the patient's daily routine:*** Making a connection between taking a dose of medication and a regular daily task will enhance compliance. This could include identifying when the patient wakes up and goes to

bed or which meals the patient eats. Pharmacists should not assume that patients follow a common routine (e.g., eating three meals a day). They should ask patients about their routines before suggesting a plan.

- ***Tell the patient how long it will take for the drug to show an effect:*** If patients are not told when to expect onset of action, they may believe the medication is not working. Patients may cease taking a medication, or they may take too much because they believe one dose did not work.
- ***Tell the patient how long he/she might be taking the medication:*** Patients need to have a reasonable expectation of how long they will need to take the medication. This helps them get into a "mind set" of compliance. It also helps to eliminate unrealistic expectations. Moreover, it gives patients a chance to express concerns about the length of treatment.
- ***Tell the patient when he/she is due back for a refill (and the number of refills needed):*** Patients need to plan in order to be compliant, and this information assists them in doing so. The information may be given in the form of a verbal contract.
- ***Emphasize the benefits of the medication:*** Pharmacists should make every effort to support the chosen therapy and tell patients about the benefits of the treatment before they discuss potential side effects. This not only helps to put side effects in perspective, but it also promotes patient confidence in the therapy. If the pharmacist and the physician cannot instill confidence in the patient regarding the therapy it may result in noncompliance.
- ***Discuss major side effects of the drug:*** The pharmacist should discuss very clearly about the major side effects of the drug(s). The pharmacist should be very specific about the side effects. He should tell the patient about the severity, will the side effects go away on its own and if so how much it may take etc. What should they do if side effects don't go away or become intolerable? Effective counseling helps patients understand the extent of the risk they are taking by using a medication. It is possible that some patients will not want to know about any side effects, and some will want to know all possible side effects. Pharmacists must develop a flexible approach to the dissemination of information. Leaflets are an excellent way to provide patients with additional information.
- ***Point out that additional, rare side effects are listed in the information sheet:*** An information sheet summarizing facts about the medication should be given to the patient at the end of the counseling session. Emphasize the rarity of some of the side effects listed, and encourage the patient to call if he/she has any concerns about these.
- ***Use written information to support counseling when appropriate:*** For literate patients, written information has been shown to reinforce verbal instructions. It gives the patient tangible information to refer to in case he/she forgets what the

pharmacist has said. In addition, it can be used to promote more effective counseling. Written information may be given to patients to look over while their prescription is being filled. This can prepare patients to ask better questions and the pharmacist will do less talking.

- ***Discuss precautions (e.g., activities to avoid) and beneficial activities (e.g., exercise, decreased salt intake, diet, self-monitoring):*** It should not be assumed that the physician has discussed these things with the patient. Ask patients what they have been told, and discuss if necessary.
- ***Discuss drug-drug, drug-food, and drug-disease interactions:*** Patients generally are not aware that other medications, foods, or diseases may interfere with the drug they are taking or affect the condition for which they are being treated. For example, a patient with high blood pressure should be told to ask the pharmacist before taking any medicines for coughs or colds. The patient should also be told why these precautions are necessary.
- ***Discuss storage recommendations, ancillary instructions (e.g., shake well, refrigerate):*** Many patients still store their medications in medicine cabinets in the bathroom, probably the worst place in the house to keep medicines because of heat and humidity. Give general storage recommendations for all medicines, and specific storage recommendations (e.g., refrigeration) and ancillary instructions to the patient.
- ***Explain to the patient in precise terms what to do if he/she misses a dose:*** Actual times of day and specific examples should be used to make this clear. The patient should then be asked, for example, "What will you do if it is 3:00 in the afternoon and you realize you have missed your noon dose?" The only way you can assess whether patients understand is by asking them to repeat back the information. If you ask them if they understand, patients may say yes even if they do not.
- ***Cheek for further understanding by asking the patient to repeat back additional key information:*** To fully assess whether the patient understands the dosage regimen, you could say, "Mrs. Ravi, sometimes information can be a little confusing. Just to be sure I was clear, could you tell me how you are going to take your medication?" The same would be done with side effects, storage conditions, etc. Correct answers should be praised and incorrect information should be corrected. Praising has been shown to reinforce compliance.
- ***Check for any additional concerns or questions:*** The counseling session may have raised additional questions or concerns. The pharmacist should ask if this is so and listen respectfully and carefully to what the patient has to say.

- ***Advice patients to always check their medicine before they leave the pharmacy:*** This helps to familiarize patients with their medicine and makes them a partner in ensuring an error has not been made. The pharmacist should say, "Please always check your medicine before you leave the pharmacy. If you have any questions or problems about the way it looks, please notify me. I don't intend to make any mistakes, but it's good to be cautious. You are the final check." By doing this you are emphasizing that this is a partnership in which the patient also has responsibilities.
- ***Use appropriate language throughout the counseling session:*** On occasion, pharmacists use language that is unnecessarily confusing (e.g., hypertension rather than high blood pressure; GI instead of gastrointestinal or stomach). Many patients will not say they are confused because they do not want to appear stupid. Language that is simple and understandable promotes compliance.
- ***Maintain control of the counseling session:*** A great deal of information needs to be covered in order to counsel the patient effectively. Concerns take time to address. Therefore, keep superfluous conversation to a minimum. Small talk is helpful to start the counseling session, but it needs to be brief and simply serve to break the ice.
- ***Organize the information in an appropriate manner:*** Generally speaking, the most important information should be provided at the beginning of the counseling session and repeated at the end. In addition, support of the drug should precede side effects. This checklist has been formulated to reflect the recommended organization of the counseling session.
- ***Follow up to determine how the patient is doing:*** Follow-up care is a good way to
  - Differentiate your services
  - Let patients know you are concerned and
  - Increase your refill prescription business.

  Very few healthcare providers offer follow-up care. Yet abundant evidence indicates that patients tend not to get their refills on time and some never return at all. Advise patients that not refilling chronic medications on time places them at risk for further problems, and offer reminders about refills. Follow-up care should be done voluntarily and should be as flexible as possible. Keep in mind that some patients may not want it. Patients should be enrolled in a follow-up care program and given options as to how they receive it. For example, some may prefer a telephone call, while others may prefer a postcard, a letter, or a fax. The more flexible you can be in providing this service, the more likely it will work.

The above checklist is provided as a general guide to effective counseling. Many a times the Pharmacist is very busy in his practice and may not have the time to thoroughly cover every item. Time, severity of the illness, and type of medication will be major factors in determining how much or how little of the checklist the pharmacist uses.

It is important to be as thorough as possible to make sure that your patients leave the pharmacy knowing how to take their medications.

Documentation

The counseling session should be documented. This may be as simple as a check list or as detailed as recorded notes in the patients' medication profile. Any follow-up required should be noted. It should also be recorded if the patient does not wish to be counseled.

3.7 Patient Counseling Tips

The pharmacist should caution the patient with the following instructions depending on the medication being taken and the interacting drug, food etc.

Medications

- Alcohol is known to alter the activity of most anti-diabetic drugs, potentiate the activity of antihistamines, depressants etc. and is dangerous when taken with barbiturates since the depressant effects of both the alcohol and the barbiturates can be fatal.

  Caution/Advice

  - May cause drowsiness. Avoid taking with other depressants or when operating a motor vehicle.
  - Avoid taking alcohol with medication.

- Some drugs that are not irritating to the gastrointestinal tract are absorbed best when taken on an empty stomach, whereas drugs that are irritating but absorbed well in the presence of food are best taken on a full stomach. Food is often used to mask medications with disagreeable tastes, but this is a questionable practice for children as it may destroy their taste for the food. Infants should not receive a drug in milk if the drug alters the taste or odor of the milk. Drugs may sometimes be administered in foods that have dietary usefulness.

  The time of administration generally modifies the action of most drugs. A full stomach delays general and lessens local action. Consideration must also be given to food-drug interactions that might occur when certain substances are taken concurrently (i.e., antibacterial agents/milk and dairy products; anticoagulants/leafy green vegetables; antihypertensives or monoamine oxidase inhibitors/aged cheeses, chocolate, chicken liver, licorice; cardiac glycosides/dairy products and licorice; and oral diuretics/licorice).

Caution/Advice

- Do not take aspirin with medication.
- Avoid taking mineral oil with medication; take with water.
- Do not drink milk while taking this medication,
- Avoid aged cheese, wine, beer, other alcoholic beverages, or antihistamines when taking this medication.
- Take a potassium source with medication.
- Take medication with plenty of water. Fluids administered with medicaments normally hasten their absorption
- Take medications with meals or at a certain interval before or after meals.
- Take medication on an empty stomach.
- Take medication with milk.

  Iodine preparations are given well diluted in milk if possible, or in water or fruit juice.
- Chill medication before taking.

  Because cooling decreases taste sensation, chilling also may be used to help solve the problems of administering disagreeable remedies. Unpalatable drugs may be given ice cold if condition permits.
- Do not dilute this medication.

  Cough syrups should be given undiluted and should be the last medication given if taken with other medication.
- Use medication carefully because of possible staining on contact with skin or clothing. If tablets, do not chew; if liquid, avoid contact with skin and clothing. Giving acids through a straw will prevent discoloration of teeth.
- Avoid undue exposure to sunlight or sunlamps.

  This caution is warranted with all drugs that produce photoallergic or photosensitive reactions.

- Darkening or change in stools may occur while taking this medication.
- Medication may color urine.

  Examples: Pyridium—red, Methylene blue—bluish green, Sulfonamides—rust yellow or brownish
- Shake well before use.

  This instruction should accompany any suspension that separates or deposits at the bottom of preparations.

Dosage Forms

Each dosage form requires separate consideration in its use. Examples of information that should be relayed to the patient by the pharmacist are given below for commonly prescribed items

- eye drops:
  - Position of head
  - Method of inserting without touching lid
  - Importance of keeping dropper sterile
  - Use may cause discomfort.
- Ophthalmic ointments:
  - Need to cleanse eyelids before application
  - Where to place ointment
  - How much to use
  - Importance of not touching tube to lid
  - Information that impaired vision may occur briefly.
- Capsules:
  - Type determines need to be swallowed whole or whether contents may be removed
  - Hot liquid could affect time-drug levels of some time-release capsules.
- Oral liquids:
  - Shake well before using liquids that separate on standing
  - Use standard measuring device for accurate and uniform dosage
  - Instructions on storage area and expiration dates, if warranted.

Table 3.1 Instructions for Administering Specific Dosage Forms

S.No.	Dosage form	Instructions
01	Oral liquids	• Shake well before use for liquids that separate on standing • Use standard measuring device for accurate and uniform dosage • Store in cool and dark place • Replace the cap tightly immediately after use • Check expiry date
02	Capsules	• To be swallowed whole without breaking the shell • To be swallowed with full glass of water • Hot drinks could affect timed release capsules
03	Tablets	• Store in cool and dry place • Sublingual tablets to be placed below the tongue • Chewable tablets to be chewed, not to be crushed and swallowed • Oral controlled release and coated tablets to be administered with caution as directed by the physician
04	Eye and ear drops	• Method of insertion without touching head • Explain position of head while administration of the eye drops • Importance of keeping dropper clean and sterile • Use may cause temporary discomfort
05	Ophthalmic Ointments	• Clean the eyelids before application • Place the ointment in the cup of lower eye lid • Quantity to be used at a time • Do let the tube touch the lid • May cause temporary blurring
06	Injections	• Rotate the injection site • Watch for infiltration or oozing of medication from injection site • If there is localized swelling, pain or inflammation at injection site, inform the physician
07	Inhalation Aerosols	• Check the mouth piece and actuator for cleanliness • Shake the inhaler, vigorously before actuation • Breath out gently and then trigger the spray in the mouth, breath deeply to inhale • Hold your breath for a few seconds, before breathing out slowly

Table 3.2 Instructions while dispensing certain medications

S.No	Instruction	Examples of drugs
01	May cause drowsiness, avoid taking with other depressants or when operating a motor vehicle	Chlorpromazine, Chlordiazepoxide, Diazepam
02	Avoid taking alcohol with medication	Chlorpheniramine, Chlorpropamide
03	Do not take aspirin with this medication	Phenylbutazone, Warfarin
04	Avoid taking mineral oil with medication	Griseofulvin
05	Take a potassium source with medication. Ex. Carrot, Cabbage	Prednisolone, Hydrocortisone
06	Take medication with plenty of water	All sulpha drugs
07	Don't drink milk while taking this medication	Tetracycline
08	Take medication with milk	Iodine preparations
09	Chill medication before taking	Magnesium citrate solution
10	Do not dilute this medication	Cough syrup
11	Do not chew the tablets	Pyrovinium pamoate, Dulcolax tablets
12	Avoid contact with skin and clothing	Non staining iodine ointment
13	Avoid contact with teeth, use straw to drink	Syrup of ferrous iodine
14	Avoid undue exposure to sunlight	Sulphasalazine
15	Shake well before use	All emulsions and suspensions
16	Take medication on empty stomach	Penicillin, Cloxacillin
17	Take medication half an hour before meals	Propenthallin, Ampicillin, Erythromycin
18	Take with meals	Reserpine, Tolbutamide
19	Take after meals	Aminophylline, Isoniazide, Hydrocortisone
20	Medication may colour the urine	Rifampicin (orange), Pyridium (red)
21	Complete the course of treatment unless otherwise directed	Antibiotics

Conclusion

The need for counseling the patients regarding their drug therapy is evidenced by documented deficiencies in patient education and a growing patient demand. The practicing pharmacist has an excellent opportunity to provide a clinical service that is directly involved with and accepted by the patient. The pharmacist is in a unique position to provide this information and reinforce the importance of compliance by the patient with the therapeutic regimen. Pharmacists must realize their ethical responsibility to provide this very important service to patient education.

Study Outline

Patient counseling is one to one interaction between a pharmacist and a patient or his care taker. The pharmacist should provide appropriate, understandable and relevant information to patients about their medication.

Various health care professionals involved in the patient counseling process are:

Physician has initial opportunity to reassure patient and to encourage patient to take active interest in management of his therapy. The physicians are too busy and cannot spend much time with the patient.

Nurses ensure proper drug administration in hospital and clinical setting

Pharmacist is the last professional to see the patient during the course of his hospitalization. He has an excellent opportunity to provide knowledge and motivation necessary for a patient to initiate, maintain and complete his therapeutic program successfully.

What to Counsel

- name and class of the drug (e.g. antibiotic, pain reliever)
- Directions for use
- Special storage requirements
- Common or important drug-drug or drug -food interactions
- Intended therapeutic response and associated time frames.
- Common or important side effects and associated time frames
- What the patient should do to monitor his/her therapeutic response or development of side effects
- Actions the patient should take if the intended therapeutic response is not obtained or side effects develop
- When appropriate, the actions the pharmacist will undertake to monitor the patient's progress.

Whom and When to Counsel

- Referral patients
- Patients with specific disease state
- Patients treated with specific classes of drugs (egg. anticoagulants)
- Patients receiving more than a specified number of medications
- Patients known to have visual, hearing or literacy problems
- Pediatric patients
- Pharmacists should counsel on all new prescriptions, including transferred prescriptions
- Patients being discharged from the hospital
- Medicines picked up by third party
- Patients who come for refills
- Patients using OTC medications

Counseling on Non Prescription Drugs

When non prescription / OTC drugs are indicated, the pharmacist must be able to give information to the patient so that they are used safely and effectively after adequate assessment of the patient's problem.

How to Counsel

Assessment phase – Pharmacist with the help of questions must assess the patients knowledge and understanding of his disease process, drug therapy he is taking and its relation with the disease.

Planning and implementation phase – Pharmacist must motivate the patient to ensure adherence to therapeutic regimen.

Format of Counseling

Counseling should be verbal and accompanied by written material for the patient to refer at home.

Where to Counsel

Semi-private or private area which the patient perceives as confidential, secure and conducive to learning.

Material (Aids) for Counseling

Patient information leaflets, illustrated information, audio visual aids, dosage compliance aids like drug calendars and educational displays.

Medication Counseling Tips

- ✓ Establish relationship — show interest in patient (verbal & nonverbal)
- ✓ Verify Patient's name and prescriber's name
- ✓ Why the patient is being prescribed the medication (if known) or the medication's use, expected benefits and action.
- ✓ Open the medication containers and show patient what the medication looks like, or demonstrate use
- ✓ How to take the medication
- ✓ When to take and how long to take the medication
- ✓ What to do if a dose is missed
- ✓ Any special precautions to follow
- ✓ Foods, alcoholic beverages or OTC drugs to be avoided
- ✓ How the patient will know the medication is working
- ✓ How to store the medication
- ✓ If the prescription can be refilled, and if so, when
- ✓ Verify the patient's knowledge and understanding
- ✓ Ask the patient if they have any questions
- ✓ Document the interaction.

CHAPTER 4

Medication History Review

Objectives

After reading this chapter, the student should be able to:

- Understand the importance of Medication History Review
- Select patients who are in need of a Medication History Review
- Recognize specific objectives and identify questions that are appropriate for accomplishing the objectives of a Medication History Interview.
- Plan and conduct a Medication Review by selecting appropriate interview techniques
- Communicate the findings of the interview to the physicians, nurses and patients.

4.1 Introduction

The tradition of the physician taking a drug history along with the patient's admission medical history dates back to the time when there was little drug therapy that could alter the course of most diseases, and little importance was attached to the previous drug therapy. With the vast number of today's potent drugs that are capable not only of profoundly influencing the outcome of a disease, but also of producing clinical features simulating various disorders, thereby obscuring a correct diagnosis, a re-evaluation of the role of drug therapy is essential.

There is a need for information regarding past medications of patients, along with the implications of the information. However, since it is nearly impossible for physicians to keep abreast of current drug literature, qualified personnel are needed to assume the functions of obtaining and interpreting this data and making it available to the physician. These tasks are becoming more and more a part of the pharmacist's clinical role.

With the increasing role of Pharmacists in the health care system the Clinical Pharmacist has the opportunity for direct patient contact in various areas. In addition to the traditional dispensing and counseling encounter that occurs at the time medication is given to the patient, pharmacists also participate in programs for monitoring drug utilization or adverse drug reactions and obtain medication histories, particularly in the institutional setting. The success of these confrontations with the patient will depend to a great extent on the pharmacist's skill as an interviewer in eliciting pertinent information.

4.2 Need for Medication History Interview

The number of potent drugs available to the patients along with the ever increasing frequency of adverse drug reactions and drug misuse increases the importance of a well documented drug history and medication history review. Pharmacists have contributed significantly to patient care by taking thorough medication histories.

Successful performance of many clinical services by pharmacists depends upon the possession of effective communication and interviewing skills. Clinical activities such as drug therapy counseling and consulting usually require a data base that includes information obtained from a medication history interview. Direct patient-pharmacist communication in an interview format frequently provides significant data upon which other clinical activities are dependent.

Pharmacists can contribute significantly to the care of patients by

- obtaining information regarding past and present medications,
- history of allergies and side-effects, and
- attitudes toward drugs as well as determining compliance behavior and therapeutic response to drugs.

These activities are dependent on the pharmacist's understanding of interpersonal relations and use of appropriate interviewing techniques and communication skills.

4.3 Preliminaries to the Interview – Understanding the Patient

The Patient's Feelings

The patient is undergoing an unfamiliar experience in a strange environment that is governed by a strange set of customs. He is expected to be dependent, cooperative, uncomplaining and to have limited contact with the outside world, including his family.

Meaning of Illness

The meaning of illness to a patient depends upon his unique experience and life position. He may welcome the opportunity to escape his responsibilities; he may fight the idea of being ill out of fear and frustration that arise from being unable to continue his life style; or he may regress to a childlike passive dependency, taking no responsibility for his own illness or needs, expecting everyone else to meet his needs. On occasion a patient may simply give up and turn toward suicide as his preferred alternative.

Role Characteristics of the Patient and the Interviewer

Having established these preliminaries and a broad definitional base for the microcosm and its inhabitants, we now turn to pre-interview planning. The patient interview (utilized to obtain a medical or drug history) is simply a specialized interaction. To understand this interaction, it is helpful to review a description of the ideal patient's social role and the ideal interviewer's role.

The interviewer's role might also be defined as follows:

- try to understand the patient
- be honest with the patient
- show concern for the patient
- show respect for the patient
- show interest in the patient
- refrain from making judgments about the patient; do not criticize the patient
- help the patient gain control of his life and health.

Nonverbal Communication

Patient's Room: Upon entering a patient's hospital room, one learns a great deal about the patient before any words are exchanged. A quick glance around the room will yield to the perceptive interviewer invaluable preliminary information.

Appearance of the Patient: Next the interviewer turns his focus to the bed and the patient. This tacit inquiry will also yield useful information. The interviewer should attempt to equate the patient's attire, appearance, etc., with what is known about the actual state of the patient's illness.

Another focus of nonverbal communication is the patient's head. One can note the state of the hair, whether a male patient has shaved, or whether a female patient is wearing make-up, etc. Is the patient's face tense, relaxed, sad, comfortable, angry, or fighting for breath? Some faces demonstrate signs of chronic tension with deep furrows in the forehead or around the eyes.

Finally, note the body posture. Many people can control their facial expressions and are said to wear a mask. Very few people are able to control the feelings that their body expresses. Their posture, movements, or gestures belie their inner feelings of anger, tension, sadness, depression, pain or hurt. Thus, upon entering the room, the observant person can learn a great deal about a patient before a word is spoken.

Patient- Interviewer Introduction

How one should approach or introduce himself to a patient? What should take place in the introduction? Optimally, the introduction should; (1) make positive identification of the patient; (2) introduce the interviewer by name; (3) demonstrate that the interviewer is sensitive and considerate; (4) show respect to the patient; and (5) demonstrate confidence and strength of the interviewer.

The initial contact may be handed through any means within the boundaries of propriety and decorum. However, the interviewer should be certain that positive identification has been established between both parties. The tenor of the interviewer's voice will convey his confidence and strength. The interviewer must demonstrate, without asserting, that he knows what he is doing and that he is in control. A sick patient doesn't want to actively or emotionally support a visitor – he has all he can do to maintain his own composure.

Throughout the discourse the interviewer should show respect and consideration for the patient. Be as empathic as possible, realizing that such intrusions may be received somewhat less than enthusiastically by the patient. Be clear and precise. The interview technique is a skill acquired only through experience, feedback, modifying behavior and repetition. However, the process may be expedited somewhat by role-playing and tape recording a practice interview with a classmate, and listening to it with your peer to see how you can improve your style.

Patient Attitudes toward Medication

Patients attitude toward drugs vary greatly depending upon the individual patient, ethnic-cultural background, illness, age, socio-economic level, and his own attitude toward self-reliance.

Almost everyone takes drugs of one kind or another every day: aspirin for pain, coffee to get started, alcohol to avoid anxiety, tobacco for reassurance, sedatives for sleep, tranquilizers for comfort, vitamins for health, and laxatives to join the regulars. However, there are those individuals who view the use of medicine as an indication of illness, frailty or retribution. Some people have a fear of becoming dependent upon any drug, even aspirin. Others believe drugs have powerful magical qualities, and feel they really only need one half or one fourth of what their doctor prescribed. Moreover, if such a patient progresses satisfactorily with a reduced dosage, then from his perspective he is not as sick as was perhaps originally suspected. In addition, there are those individuals who err in the opposite extreme, i.e., they want to take large amounts of medication so they will recover faster. For example, such an individual might decide that if one tablet will get him well in five days, then taking five tablets at once should get him well in one day. Finally, there are those individuals for whom medication symbolizes their doctor's concern, interest, devotion, or love. For such individuals, medication means that part of the doctor is always with them.

The patient's expectations of a medication and the circumstances under which it is taken frequently have as much influence on the overall result as does the medication's chemical composition. The truth of this statement becomes apparent when one considers that experimental figures usually show that approximately 30 per cent of all patients are placebo reactors. This means that when an inert chemical is given to a patient who is led to believe that it is a specific medicine, he will respond as though he had taken the actual medication.

The doctor-patient relationship may sometimes govern whether or not a patient takes his medication. Obviously, whether or not the patient takes a medication also depends upon the extent to which he has access to the medicine.

Recognition of Suicidal Patients

The pharmacist should learn to recognize subtle statements, behaviors, and actions that might cause one to suspect suicidal intentions. Some situations and symptoms especially associated with suicidal predispositions are: (1) recent death, separation, divorce or loss of a job; (2) withdrawal from activities; (3) sudden giving away of one's possessions; (4) alcoholism; (5) recent behavioral changes; and (6) attempts to bring one's affairs to a final state of orderliness.

Once you become suspicious that you might be dealing with a suicidal individual, seek immediate professional assistance and notify that person's relatives.

4.4 Planning Medication History Interview

Before beginning the medication history interview, the pharmacist will need to organize his activities. The pharmacist first should select those patients who need to be preferentially interviewed. A brief review of patient's charts will give the pharmacist information on which to base this selection and will help establish specific objectives for the interview.

Patient Selection

Pharmacists generally will not have time or opportunity to interview every patient admitted to a particular hospital service. A selective process can be initiated by a brief review of patient's chart.

Some of the criteria by which a Pharmacist can prefer to select the patient over other patients for an interview are as follows:

- Patients with symptoms or signs suggestive of possible drug-related problems should be interviewed initially. e.g., a patient with an acute, severe illness may be selected over a chronic care patient with a stable drug regimen.
- Patients with a documented history of poor compliance, inadequate therapeutic response, or adverse drug reactions are prime candidates for a medication history interview.
- Patients receiving a drug with low therapeutic index that requires serum drug concentration monitoring should be interviewed.
- Patients on multiple drug regimens or with multiple disease states should receive pharmacist's attention.
- Psychiatric patients and elderly patients require medication histories because of the frequency of multiple drug use and drug-related problems in these patients.

Objectives of the Interview

The goal of taking a medication history is to obtain information on drug use that may assist in diagnosis and / or treatment of the patient. The major objectives of the medication history interview can be to:

- document allergies and drug reactions that might be omitted from or erroneously added to the patient's records;
- provide admission screening for drug interactions;
- determine patient medication compliance; and
- determine the patient's therapeutic to medication.

The medication history interview also should obtain information concerning the patient's general attitude toward drugs;

- tendency for drug abuse;
- diet restrictions;
- caffeine, alcohol, and nicotine use; and
- past history of adverse drug reactions.

Questions can be also directed to obtain information concerning the appropriateness of drug administration techniques and the adequacy of storage precautions for drugs. In addition, information on possible difficulties in obtaining prescribed drugs (e.g., financial problems, transportation problems) should be identified.

There will be no standard questionnaire and the interview process should be tailored to the individual patient. The thoroughness of the questioning in each category will depend on specific clinical data and patient characteristics. For example, a patient with a history of noncompliance with prescribed regimens should receive more intensive questioning in this area of medication use as an objective of the interview. On the other hand, questioning on alcohol and nicotine use in a five-year-old child would be inappropriate as an objective of the interview.

All information should be obtained with the purpose of examining the patient's drug use history for appropriateness and safety.

Preparation for the Interview

Prior to meeting with the patient to obtain the medication history, the patient's chart should be reviewed. The letters of referral, physician's admitting medical history and physical examination, laboratory data, progress notes, and other reports can provide information to assist the pharmacist in preparing for the interview. Other health professionals who have seen the patient can be consulted to obtain information prior to the interview. The pharmacist should make special note of any data that indicate a history of noncompliance, reported allergies, past adverse drug effects, responses to past therapy, or abnormal laboratory values or physical findings. These data can be used to direct the emphasis of questions in the interview.

Reference textbooks can also be reviewed to update the pharmacist's knowledge of the patient's disease state and drug therapy. This information may help the pharmacist ask more specific questions in order to assess the patient's therapeutic response to medications.

The pharmacist should use a form *(Medication Review Form)*[*] that covers the important areas in every interview:

- prescription and nonprescription medications
- allergies and manifestations
- adverse drug reactions other than allergies
- home remedies
- diet
- fluid intake and
- social drug use

[*] Sample form provided at the end of chapter.

The form may also contain statements reminding the pharmacist to ask questions to ascertain the patient's understanding of the use of medications, compliance behavior, and opinion of drug effectiveness.

The pharmacist should discuss each of the patient's prescription medications in detail. Questions like 'what drug', 'for what purpose', 'how much,' 'how often,' 'how long', 'how effective,' and 'any problems' should be asked for each prescription and nonprescription drug. If the patient has brought prescription vials into the hospital or clinic, data such as the prescription number, name and telephone number of the pharmacy filling the prescription, and the name of the physician who wrote the prescription should be recorded. An estimate should be obtained as to the approximate number of doses administered over the course of a week or month. Also, if the patient has discontinued the use of medication, an estimate of the approximate time of cessation of therapy should be obtained.

After the patient has related all of the prescription and nonprescription medications that can be remembered, the interviewer should use a checklist to stimulate the patient's recall of additional medications. The use of this checklist should prove highly effective and frequently, will induce the recall of additional medications. As each category of medication or symptom is reviewed, examples of preparations should also be mentioned.

The patient should be asked whether any homemade medications are used. As in the receding discussion, it is best to cite examples of common homemade medications, such as honey and lemon juice or castor oil and lemon juice. If the patient is taking an unusual concoction, the reasons for its use and contents of the formulation should be described.

The form used by the pharmacist in an interview should serve only as a reminder. It should not be followed so strictly that the pharmacist does not allow time to explore comments made by the patient concerning different aspects of the medication regimen. The taking of a medication history is a dialogue between patient and pharmacist. If it were simply a routine interrogation, a standardized questionnaire would suffice for literate, intelligent patients.

The essential difference between taking a history and performing an interrogation with a standardized questionnaire centers upon analysis. The expert interviewer weighs and analyzes each response of the patient. Subsequent questions depend greatly upon the patient's response to previous questions. The pharmacist should be prepared to analyze data while acquiring it and then to direct questions to the patient in order to accomplish the objective of the medication history interview process.

4.5 Conducting the Medication History Interview

The medication history, must elicit all pertinent data relating to the patient's drug history. However, certain basic questions which can serve as a guide in the interview are discussed.

Medication History Data

- What prescription drugs were being used prior to hospital admission (name, dose, duration)?
- What other drugs have been taken in the last six months?
    - OTC products:
      analgesics (pain, headaches)
      laxatives
      sedatives (nerves)
      hypnotics (sleep)
      antihistamines (hay fever, colds)
      antidiarrheals
      cough syrups
      antacids (stomach)
      vitamins
      diuretics
    - 'heart'medications,
    - 'shots' in a physician's office,
    - external preparations (lotions, ointments),
    - sprays or drops
    - another person's prescription medications.
- Were there any known allergies or reactions to any drugs?
    - What happens when this drug is received?
    - Was any medication given to counteract the reaction?
- Were there any chemical poisonings or exposure to noxious or environmental factors (household products, industrial or agricultural chemicals)?
- Is there any dependence on drugs?
    - Does the physician know of this?
- Did the patient take prescription drugs regularly or as directed by the physician?
    - If not, why?
- Were large amounts of any of the following consumed?
    - alcoholic beverages (amount),
    - soft drinks (amount),
    - coffee, tea (amount).

- Have there been any particular problems with drugs (difficulty swallowing, bad taste, etc)?

During any patient interview the pharmacist must always think how the interview will help the patient and how as a pharmacist I can help this person. The medication history interview is usually the pharmacist's introduction to the patient. This should help the pharmacist to develop a good rapport with the patient. It is essential that this relationship get off to a good start. A style of communication should develop that will support the patient's efforts to express himself fully and, therefore, will support the pharmacist's ability to respond sensitively and appropriately to the patient's needs.

The pharmacist should be aware of the patient's perceptions and feelings in coping with illness and hospitalization. Illness disrupts the social and psychological balance within an individual. Fear and anxiety may be enhanced by several factors, such as loss of mobility and control over environment and finances. Patient's feelings of anger, distrust, and dependency may be displaced onto health care professionals.

The patient usually views a health care professional as a person who can help relieve the fear, anxiety, pain, and discomfort associated with illness. The helping relationship will be most effective if the pharmacist is sensitive and empathetic and expresses warmth and a genuine desire to help the patient. These attributes of the pharmacist of warmth, empathy, and openness will give permission to the patient to interact more openly with the pharmacist.

During the interview, the pharmacist should encourage a sense of mutual trust between the patient and himself. This can be achieved by including the patient in the treatment process. The pharmacist can discuss matters like reasons for the drug therapy and the need for a complete, accurate history which can motivate the patient to greater participation in the interview. The process of allowing the patient to involve in the treatment schedule may help alleviate any feelings of distrust or anxiety and stimulate the patient to provide more information.

The pharmacist must give adequate time to the interview process and should not have distracting concerns or commitments, so that the patient can tell the whole story and can feel comfortable talking to the pharmacist. The patient should feel that the pharmacist is an understanding listener. The pharmacist genuinely should appear interested, unhurried, tactful, and considerate. The pharmacist's manner should communicate, without coldness or arrogance, that he knows what to do and that the situation is in control. A sense of confidence and strength should be conveyed in tone of voice.

The pharmacist should be forthright and honest in dealing with patients. Direct questions from the patient regarding the severity and prognosis of the illness or the effectiveness of therapy or procedure should be handled with common sense and usually should be referred to the attending physician. If the condition of the patient is a sensitive issue, the pharmacist should review the situation with the physician and/or nurse prior to the interview. The pharmacist must use discretion and tact and refrain from making professional judgments or clarifications to patients concerning matters outside the realm of the medication history.

Beginning the Interview

The introduction by the pharmacist should include:

- a positive identification of the patient;
- a statement of the interviewer's name, title, and position; and
- a brief statement on the purpose of the interview.

In addition, the pharmacist should inquire whether the patient feels well enough to talk. The question, "Do you feel like talking to me now?" allows the patient to say "no" without guilt. An estimation of the amount of time required for the interview should be expressed to the patient.

The purpose of the interview should be stated in order to motivate the patient to participate actively in the medication history interview. The patient who feels that the information given in the interview will help him recover will be more willing to cooperate. The pharmacist should emphasize that complete information about the patient's drugs can assist the physician in diagnosis and treatment.

A complete introductory statement could be similar to this:

Pharmacist : Hello, Mr. Ravi, I'm Ram, the pharmacist for this hospital floor. I'd like to talk to you for about 20 to 30 minutes about the medications you are taking. Do you feel well enough to talk now?

Patient : Yes.

Pharmacist: A review of your use of and response to medications may assist your physician in the treatment of your condition.

The pharmacist may enhance a state of rapport by opening the initial exchange with comments about matters of mutual interest, such as the weather or a common event. The interviewer should not take too much time in 'small talk', since it may be difficult to move from a conversational attitude to the business at hand also, the patient's anxiety may be heightened by not discussing what the pharmacist came to talk about. Of even more concern is the possibility that the patient may interpret the small talk as reluctance to hear about his problems. An effective way to help a patient feel comfortable and cared for is to help him get directly to what is of concern and begin work rather than attempt to charm or superficially comfort that person. The patient's confidence may be best gained by letting him know quickly and caringly that this time is the patient's and that the pharmacist is ready to deal with the medication history interview. Small talk should be reserved for public areas, such as the hallway. The pharmacist should not ask the patient about his concerns until the patient is in a private area.

Interviewing Techniques

There is no set pattern for interviewing. Techniques must vary with the temperament of the interviewer, and personality and physical condition of patient. Although interviewing can take place anywhere, the more formal, private, face-to-face settings are to be preferred.

- *Provide Privacy:* The pharmacist should ensure that the interview will proceed in privacy and without interruption. The more formal and private the setting the better the communication. If circumstances require the pharmacist to interrupt the visit, however, family and friends can be courteously asked to leave for 20 to 30 minutes. At times, a family member or friend of the patient may need to participate in the interview depending on the patient's condition or ability to communicate. The patient should be made to feel comfortable and at ease during the interview. If the patient is ambulatory and feels inhibited by the lack of privacy in the room, the interview may be performed in an interview room or semi-private lounge area.

- *Be Attentive to Nonverbal Communication:* Communication, by definition, is the process of transmitting information by words, pictures, gestures, or other action; hence, communication may be verbal or nonverbal. From the initial contact to the end of the interview, the pharmacist should be attentive to the nonverbal communication of the patient.

  The pharmacist should maintain eye contact throughout the interview. As much as 50 to 80% of what is communicated in an interview has been estimated to be done nonverbally. Although it is not universally agreed that a majority of the communication takes place nonverbally, it is recognized that for one to be most perceptive of another person, an awareness of nonverbal behavior is extremely important. Eye contact should not be broken frequently.

  The pharmacist should sit in a relaxed position, leaning slightly forward toward the patient. The appropriate distance between persons in an interviewing situation is about 3 to 4 feet from face to face. The relatively close proximity allows for easy hearing and private conversation.

  The interviewer's voice tone and volume, length of the interview, physical distance between patient and interviewer, and questioning strategy will be influenced to some degree by initial perceptions.

- *Encourage the Patient to Talk:* Once the interview has begun, the patient is given the initiative. The pharmacist should prompt the patient to discuss his medications and should avoid dominating the conversation. This does not mean that the patient controls the interview, but only that he should do most of the talking. The pharmacist should provide timely interjections or lead the discussion to new areas by asking questions.

Questions or statements that allow the patient to divulge feelings, thoughts, attitudes, etc., can be very useful in obtaining significant information.

Reflective statements can also be used to keep the patient's concentration on a specific topic. This will prompt the patient and encourage further details on the topic under review.

Questions from patients about their disease states, diagnoses, and treatments should be answered briefly and concisely. Extended explanations to "teach" the patient should be avoided. However, patient education within the interview process is often necessary, and it is an acceptable, technique for expressing the pharmacist's interest and concern for the patient. Extended counseling or advice can be delayed until after the interview.

- *Approach Topics from the General to Specific:* Another technique is to approach topics by asking questions from the general to specific. For example, the topic of prescription drug use may be approached by asking, 'What prescription drugs have you used within the last 30 days?" The Pharmacist then can proceed to ask questions concerning "how much," "how often", and "how long" or each drug mentioned.

  By increasing the proportion of exploratory, open-ended questions, the pharmacist will facilitate narrative discussion on the part of the patient. Contrast the following statements:

  "What kind of health problems have you been having?"

  "Do you have, or have you ever had, diabetes, heart trouble, urinary tract problems, etc., etc.?"

  The first question is a patient-centered one that permits the patient to consider and express his problems, as he sees them. The second is an interviewer-centered question, which in effect may be communicating, "I know what information is important and what I need in order to get on with my work. Your opinion and feelings do not concern me; all I want are the facts".

  Although this method may be more time consuming, the amount of significant information obtained will be greater.

- *Encourage Spontaneity and Listen:* More useful information can be obtained if the patient is encouraged to speak spontaneously. If the patient is allowed to give an account of some event, without frequent interruption, a great deal of relevant information can be obtained.

Furthermore, the pharmacist should be a good listener, in the sense of using minimal verbal activity, so that the initiative given to the person being interviewed produces spontaneity.

An interested, attentive, and relaxed silence is the least-controlling response the pharmacist can make. Even brief silence tends to become uncomfortable, but it usually is best that the patient be given time and opportunity to fill the silence.

Listening must include being attentive to the affective message being presented by the patient in its verbal and nonverbal forms in addition to following the cognitive line being expressed. The responses of the pharmacist often should reflect the feeling tone rather than the storyline of what is being heard. The pharmacist's response should convey a willingness to recognize the patient's feelings, attitudes, and values. To identify and express affective messages while obtaining cognitive (factual) information is one of the most powerful ways of letting the patient know that the pharmacist is not only listening but also hearing and comprehending what is being said.

Avoid judgmental questions or statements that imply social criticism. Similarly, the pharmacist should not react in a strong judgmental manner if the patient says something that seems incredible. In addition, the pharmacist should refrain from making social criticisms of the patient's behavior. If the patient is an alcoholic, the pharmacist should not allow personal feelings of dislike to interfere with the questioning. A judgmental attitude will not facilitate communication; rather, it will inhibit the patient's willingness to provide information.

Exploration of the patient's personal and emotional life should be pursued cautiously and only if it is relevant in obtaining necessary data regarding use of medications. The techniques of getting the patient to express feelings and attitudes are instituted to facilitate communication, establish rapport, and obtain insight into how these feelings and attitudes may affect the patient's response to prescribed drug therapy. The interviewer should never explore areas of the patient's history only because of the interviewer's own interest, need, or curiosity when such material is not relevant to the patient's medication history.

- *Be Specific in Questioning:* The interviewer should be as specific as possible in determining the patient's history. When the patient says that the physician has prescribed a restricted diet, questions should be asked to determine the type of diet, the attitude of the patient towards the diet, the patient's understanding of the reason for the diet, and the patient's method of complying with the diet. The patient should be asked whether any drugs have ever made him sick and, if so, what the symptoms were.

Closed questions have a place in the interview. These questions are essential for documentation of the information. The pharmacist should avoid asking more than one question at a time during the interview. Questions or statements that contain multiple thoughts can heighten the patient's anxiety because he does not know where the interviewer is heading. Patients can become confused when trying to answer complex questions and may not relate important pieces of information in their answers.

Furthermore, the pharmacist should not use leading questions or statements to obtain specific information... Some patients, in fact, will agree to the implied thought in a leading question even though they really do not have an opinion or they disagree.

During the interview, the patient may make statements the pharmacist assumes he understands. For example, the patient may say, "I take three tablets every day". While the pharmacist may assume the patient means that he takes one tablet three times a day, further questioning may reveal that the patient takes two tablets in the morning and one tablet at bedtime. Similarly, if the patient states, "That medicine just doesn't go down right with me," he probably does not have a swallowing problem but is expressing in a colloquial manner that he feels the medication is not helping. There is a need for questions that clarify such as, "What do you mean?"

The pharmacist should attempt to understand the patient's frame of reference and to use words the patient can understand. The pharmacist should be careful not to assume completely the speech mannerisms of the patient. Using too many colloquial terms or including profanities in the conversation because the patient has done so is not appropriate. The pharmacist should maintain a professional role and use colloquial terms only as a means of communicating to the patient a shared frame of reference.

The patient's behavior may contradict what the pharmacist has been told previously. Further probing is justified when this is suspected.

Terminating the Interview

Once the essential topics of the interview have been covered, the pharmacist should summarize significant data for the patient; however, not every detail should be repeated to the patient. This technique helps stimulate the patient's memory so that more information can be obtained, and it provides a means for the patient to correct any information recorded incorrectly.

The pharmacist should ask the patient whether he has any questions concerning the medication history. If the patient does have questions, the pharmacist can use this opportunity to provide further details in advising or counseling the patient about medications.

The patient should be thanked for his cooperation and time devoted to the interview. A closing statement should be made assuring the patient that the information is confidential and will be shared only with those physicians and nurses directly concerned with the patient's care.

4.6 Evaluating the Medication History Interview

Obtaining a complete medication history is not going serve much purpose unless the results of the interview are evaluated and communicated.

Review of the Data

The data should be critically reviewed for present and potential drug-related problems. The pharmacist should review the history for data that could indicate:

- allergies or adverse drug reactions
- lack of therapeutic response
- drug-drug, drug-food, or drug-laboratory interactions
- poor compliance
- unusual self-medication habits
- difficulties in drug administration
- inappropriate dosage
- inappropriate dosage schedule; and / or
- inappropriate dosage formulation

Communication of the Results

A report of the medication history, indicating problems and recommendations should be shared verbally and in written format with the physician directly responsible for the patient's care. The method of incorporating the medication history into the patient's chart will vary from hospital to hospital. A form can be attached to the front of the medical history section of the chart. A write-up of the medication history in the progress notes section of the chart also might be used to communicate the information.

Nurses can be informed of the medication history through the patient's chart and/or by a review at the change of shift during the day. Drug allergies should be posted appropriately on the front of the chart, in the nurse's card file, and on the unit dose profile in the pharmacy dispensing area.

Significant results and clarifications of the medication history should be reviewed with the patient and/or family. Any information on compliance strategies, clarification of allergy manifestations, change in drug dosage or formulation, or explanation of the indication and rationale of the drug therapy can be discussed with the patient before or at the time of discharge from the hospital. It is preferable to discuss these matters in a patient counseling or advisement session at least one day before the patient's discharge in order to ensure that the pharmacist has the patient's full attention.

Significant data from the medication history can also be shared with the patient's local pharmacist. A telephone call or letters to the pharmacist can provide-up-to-date information for the patient's medication profile.

4.7 Case Presentation

Introduction and Objectives

The clinical case study represents an effort to present a comprehensive guide for the assembling of all pertinent information relative to the drug therapy being used in an individual patient. Individual case study is an attempt to bridge the constant gap in therapeutics that exists between the pharmacist and the physician. By actual clinical experience the pharmacist will have first-hand knowledge of clinical pharmacology, medical terminology, the clinical environment and the complex nature of patient care to support his theoretical information. Drug therapy can then be placed in a greater realistic perspective when the actual clinical findings and other types of treatments being used are considered together.

Without this type of experience, the pharmacist is unable to adequately fulfill his role as a medication expert and drug advisor to the patient, physician, and other members of the health care team. These services are being increasingly demanded by the public and the physician. Clearly then, the pharmacist must be prepared to deliver such services.

Data obtained in the medication interview by the practicing pharmacist will be recorded on a card or drug history form and included in the patient's medical record.

The following outline of a case study presentation comprises minimal information necessary for an adequate knowledge and in-depth study of the drug therapy for an individual patient. Cases for study should be selected by the pharmacist in collaboration with another member of the health team-the nurse, resident or attending staff physician. The pharmacist then extracts the hospital record, interviews the patient, and prepares a written case summary for oral presentation.

Case Presentation Outline

I. Identifying Information.

Data that can be prepared for distribution in written form to instructors and other class members includes:

- name – it is better to address and discuss the patient by name rather than by continually referring to 'the patient' or to his clinical diagnosis

- address – gives information as to environment and the possibility of drugs
- age-important relative to dose and routes of administration sex
- race – color, birthplace, nationality, religion, and social status all give clues concerning the interview approach to the patient and his probable response
- occupation – important in considering drug side-effects. Find out exactly what the patient does and how he carries this out date of admission to the hospital
- informant(s) – perhaps information from the spouse or other relatives might be considerably different from that given by the patient. Parents of all pediatric patients must be interviewed
- previous hospital admissions – dates and length of confinement, diagnosis, and drugs continued at time to discharge,
- names of physicians in charge and writing orders
- other members of the therapeutic team – nurses, social workers, etc.

II. Summary of the Medical History and Physical Examination (obtained from the active hospital record).

- chief complaint
- brief summary of the history of the present illness
- brief summary of the past medical and surgical history
- other significant symptoms and complaints
- pertinent family and social information (familial diseases, environmental problems, etc).
- brief summary of pertinent abnormal physical findings
- consultant physician reports and comments
- other pertinent data from the nurse's admission notes or social worker's comments.
- physician's impressions and diagnosis.

III. Treatment Summary.

- pertinent clinical laboratory tests and studies.
- other diagnostic tests and procedures (ECG, x-rays, EEG, isotope studies, skin tests, provocative tests, etc.)
- progress in hospital and later as an out-patient,
- therapies used other than drugs (e.g., diet, physical therapy, psychotherapy) and patient's response,
- if patient expired, a summary of autopsy findings, if available.

IV. The Disease.

A brief general discussion of the natural history of the disease (or diseases, if more than one major diagnosis is made) should be given so as to produce a more complete understanding of the pharmacologic actions of drugs and the rationale of drug therapy.

- definition
- etiology
- incidence
- pathology, physiology and anatomy (include expected abnormal laboratory tests and diagnostic procedures)
- symptoms and signs (clinical manifestations)
- diagnostic criteria
- prognosis.

V. Medication Therapy.

- Information concerning medications taken prior to admission.

  Drugs taken for a protracted period such as peptic ulcer remedies, nasal spray, allergy shots, sedatives, insulin, or common OTC medications may be used so routinely that the patient may forget that these are medications and fail to mention them. An attempt should be made to see these medications and obtain as much identifying information as possible from all available sources. In many instances the family physician must be contacted if the patient has been referred from another institution.

- Information concerning drugs used in previous hospitalizations.

  The previous hospitalization records, those from other locations, and perhaps letters from referring physicians and consultant physicians should be searched. Especially included in this topic should be drugs used as therapy, drugs used in diagnostic tests or trials, special drugs used in x-ray and radioisotope procedures, and drugs used in provocative tests.

- Drug sensitivities or reactions.

  After scanning the hospital records for this type of information, the patient should be allowed to tell his own story, then asked for specific information concerning:

  - drug implicated
  - the onset, age of patient, time of year, environmental situation at that time and other drugs being taken concurrently
  - the first signs and suspected causes
  - symptoms and evolution of the illness
  - treatment given
  - subsequent reactions to the same drug
  - predisposing physiologic factors.

  A check list of the various drug groups might be helpful so that common drugs are not overlooked.

- Drug intoxications.

  Here, the patient should tell his history after the hospital records have been searched. As much specific information as possible concerning the following should be obtained:

  - when
  - circumstances
  - symptoms, whether chronic or acute
  - treatment given (if suicide attempt, did patient receive psychotherapy?)
  - substantiating laboratory data
  - subsequent intoxications involving use of the same drug.

- Drug abuse; habituation and /or addiction.
  - drugs used
  - dosages
  - adverse reactions
  - source
  - Hospitalizations
  - withdrawal reactions
  - psychiatric therapy.

- Drugs the patient is presently taking (discuss this subject in considerable detail).
  - schedule, dosage, route of administration, and last dose. This information will coincide with the 'five rights' of medication administration usually presented in nursing texts:

    the right drug

    to the right patient

    given at the right time

    in the right dose (including dosage parameters)

    by the right route (determined by the drug and patient's condition)
  - discuss thoroughly the drugs of choice for this particular disease or diseases.
  - discuss the pharmacology (including excretion pathways and half life) and more of action (when known).
  - discuss drug-drug interactions.
  - discuss drug-lab test interactions,
  - patient's response.

  Patients' reactions and feelings concerning the medications identified in the medications history can best be obtained throughout the interview as various medications are discussed. Also included here should be a discussion of how the patient feels about his need to take medications, especially if long-term therapy has been used or is anticipated, or if the patient is habituated or addicted for certain drugs.

VI. Forecasting Drug Needs for the Patient.

Knowledge of the present clinical condition, prognosis of the disease state and the patient's response to drug therapy will assist the pharmacist in making pertinent suggestions and recommendations on future drug needs.

Conclusion

Pharmacists can contribute significantly to patient care by obtaining a complete medication history. The pharmacist should develop a style of communication that will support the patient's efforts to express himself fully. The pharmacist should be prepared to analyze data while acquiring it and then direct questions to the patient in order to accomplish the objectives of the medication interview. Pharmacists must possess effective communication skills for successfully performing an interview. The information obtained from the interview should be analyzed for drug related problems and then communicate the same to other health professionals and the patient.

Study Outline

Pharmacists can contribute significantly to patient care by obtaining a complete medication history. A style of communication should develop that will support the patient's efforts to express himself fully and, therefore, will support the pharmacist's ability to respond sensitively and appropriately to the patient's needs. Successful performance of an interview depends upon possession of effective communication skills. These skills include an awareness of the nonverbal communication of the patient and pharmacist and the use of reflected statements, open-ended questions, and probing responses to encourage the patient to talk. The information obtained from the interview should be analyzed for drug-related problems and then communicated to other health professionals and to the patient.

Purposes of patient interview:

- Gather information and monitor progress
- Establish a relationship and develop rapport
- Educate the patient and implement treatment plans

Patient History:

- Standardized format is used
    - Ensures all needed information is obtained
    - Outlines information in a clear, concise manner
- Facilitates communication among other health care professionals

Standardized format for Complete History:

- Identifying information
- Chief complaint
- History of present illness
- Past medical history
- Drug history
- Family history
- Social history
- Review of systems

Patient interview guidelines

Before the Interview:

- Prepare the physical environment
    - Ensure privacy

  - Optimize comfort
  - Minimize distractions
- Prepare yourself
  - Eliminate internal and external distractions
- Review patient information

Beginning the interview:

- Greet the patient, using the patient's name
- Introduce yourself
- Explain purpose of the interaction and expected time
- Smile

During the Interview:

- Invite the patient's story
  - Use open ended questions
  - Give time to think
  - Allow the patient to talk without interrupting
  - Encourage elaboration
  - Elicit and understand patient's perspective
- Clarify information
  - Summarize what you need
  - Request clarification , if needed
  - Ask closed-ended questions
  - Ensure a complete history and review of symptoms
- Negotiate a plan
  - Indicate what you plan to do with the information you have
  - Prioritize problems to be addressed now and at a later date
  - Avoid jargon , keep it simple and succinct

Closing the Interview

- Inquire about any other questions or concerns
- Thank patient for his/her time

Arrange for follow-up

Medication History Taking TIPS

- Balance open-ended questions (what, how, why, when) with yes/no questions
- Ask non-biased questions
- Avoid leading questions
- Explore vague responses (non-compliance)
- Avoid medical jargon – Keep it simple
- Avoid judgmental comments
- Various approaches can be used:
  - 24 hours survey (morning, lunch, supper, bedtime)
  - Review of Systems (head to toe review)
  - Link to prescribers (family physician, specialists)
- Prompt for:
  - Pain medications
  - Stomach medications
  - Medications for bowels
  - Sleeping aids
  - Samples
- Prompt for:
  - Eye or ear drops, nose sprays
  - Patches, creams & ointments
  - Inhalers (puffers)
  - Injections (needles)
- If medication vials available:
  - Review each medication vial with patient
  - Confirm content of bottle
  - Confirm instructions on vials are current and up to date
- If medication list available:
  - Review each medication with patient
  - Confirm that it is current
- If bubble packs available:
  - Review each medication with patient
  - Confirm patient is taking entire contents

Other questions

- Have you recently started any new medications?
- did a doctor change the dose or stop any of your medications recently?
- did you change the dose or stopped any of your medications recently?
- Are any of the medications causing side effects?
- Have you changed the dose or stopped any medications because of unwanted effects?
- Do you sometimes stop taking your medicine whenever you feel better?
- Do you sometimes stop taking your medicine if it makes you feel worse?

Data Collection Form *

(Personal Medication Review)

Instructions for Use

Objectives for the Medication Review:

- To maximize patient adherence to drug therapy
- To help patients better understand their medication therapy
- To ensure medications are being taken as prescribed

By the end of the review, the pharmacist **MUST provide the patient with an up-to-date and accurate medication list**. A sample form is provided (see Form 4: Personal Medication Record).

Note: *The information provided is intended only as a guide to the medication review process. There are many different approaches to conducting medication reviews. These forms can be used or may be adapted for individual practice needs.*

Conduct the in-person interview with the patient in an acoustically private area. This may be done in the pharmacy or at the patient's home, but the interview must be done face-to-face with the patient. While the process of collecting information should be systematic, patients should be given opportunities to raise questions.

Conducting the Medication Review

The following outlines a suggested process for conducting a medication review and preparing a personal medication record.

Identifying Patients

Determination of eligibility:

- Taking three or more chronic prescription medications
- A patient discharged from hospital
- A pharmacist's documented decision
- A physician referral
- A planned hospital admission

Promotion of service by:

- Dialogue with patients on availability of service
- Notification through a prescription insert with dispensed medications
- Advertisement

Scheduling of appointment:

- Indicate to patients that the appointment will last twenty to thirty minutes
- Provide appointment card
- Remind patients to bring all medications to their appointment (including prescriptions from other pharmacies, non-prescription medications, herbal supplements etc.)

Prepare for Medication Review

Step 1: Complete as much information as possible in Patient Background Form (Form 1)

Form 1 may also be filled out by the patient or caregiver prior to the Medication Review.

Step 2: Complete columns A-D in Table 1 (prescription) of the Patient Medication History Form (Form 2)

The **Patient Medication History Form** may be used to verify current patient medication use and assess understanding of medications. It is to be used as a tool to help the pharmacist identify and document discrepancies. Complete this form as much as possible prior to the interview based on your pharmacy records. This form is not intended to be a medication record for the patient. At the end of the review the pharmacist will prepare the patient's **Personal Medication Record (PMR) (Form 4).**

Review Medications with Patient

Step 1: Complete Patient Background Form (Form 1)

Explain the purpose of the interview and complete the **Patient Background Form**; confirm all data, obtain consent, and confirm date of last *MedsCheck* Review.

Q. I would like to review your current medications with you today. I will be taking notes that will be kept confidential. After we review your medications, I will provide you with a complete medication list for your own reference that you may provide to all health professionals (e.g., doctor, home care nurse) that you see, and take with you to the hospital. Do you consent to this process? After our meeting, may I have your permission to contact your doctor with any recommendations that we have discussed? Do you have any questions or concerns at this time?

I would like to ask you some general questions about taking your medications:

Q. Do you administer all the medications yourself? If not, who helps you with your medications?

Q. Do you have any difficulty swallowing?

Step 2: Complete Table 1 (Prescription) of the Patient Medication History Form (Form 2)

Q. I would like to review all of your medications with you today, including any non-prescription and natural products you may be taking. Let's start with the prescription medications you receive from this pharmacy. (Check against pharmacy records).

While completing the medication review, pursue the patient's unclear answers until they are clarified. Vague responses may indicate difficulty adhering to medications. Ask simple questions, and avoid using medical terminology/jargon.

For each medication ask the patient the following questions. Place "✓" to acknowledge discussing each item and to verify understanding. Cross-reference the patients' knowledge of their medications with your records and document any discrepancies in Table 1 under Comments.

Patient Knowledge

Column E (Name): *Do you know the name of your medication?*

Column F (Reason for Use): *Do you know why you use this medication?*

Column G (Dosage/Frequency): *Do you know the strength of your medication? Do you know how often to take or use this medication?*

Column H (Special Instruction): *Are there any special instructions you are aware of with this medication?* This is an opportunity to find out if the patient is aware of special administration issues such as dietary restrictions, technique etc.

Usage

Column I (Labeling & Packaging Appropriate): *Is the labeling and packaging appropriate for you?* This is an opportunity to find out if the patient has any difficulty opening their vials, reading the labels on the vials etc. You may wish to suggest the use of a dossette for those on multiple medications.

Column J (Storage Appropriate): *How do you store this medication?* Assess for proper storage conditions and containers.

Column K (Expiry Date): *Is this an expired medication?* Check if the medication is expired or out-of-date. If so, advise patient of this and offer to dispose of them properly.

Column L (Patient Adherence): *Do you ever skip doses? Do you ever take more, or less, than the prescribed amount of your medication?* If YES to either of these questions, document reason for doing so in Table 1 under Comments.

Do you take or use your medications as prescribed? This may be an opportunity to identify adherence issues not addressed in column G. For example, the patient may not be taking the medication because the tablets are too large or because they dislike the taste. Document any findings in Table 1 under Comments.

Column M: *Do you experience any side effects from this medication? If you do, how bad are they and how often do they occur?* Prompt for commonly reported and serious adverse effects (e.g., nausea, diarrhea/constipation, dizziness, rash, visual disturbances, respiratory effects, etc.)

Determine if the patient is taking any other prescription medications not already discussed.

Q. Are you taking any other prescription medications that you have filled from any other pharmacies other than this one? Repeat above steps (Add to Table 1)

Q. Are there any other medications that you receive by prescription, such as:

- *patches*
- *creams*
- *eye drops*
- *inhalers*
- *samples*
- *injectables*

Repeat above steps (Add to Table 1)

Step 3: Complete Table 2 (OTC/Herbal) of the Patient Medication History Form (Form 2)

Determine if the patient is taking non-prescription medications (e.g., vitamins, herbal etc.). Add the following information to Table 2 on Form 2. Table 2 is similar to Table 1 but addresses issues such as reason for use, physician awareness, and evidence of benefit to the patient.

Complete columns A-F as per patient feedback.

Q. In the past six months have you taken any non-prescription or over-the-counter medications other than the ones you have described to me? Prompt for: cough/cold, GI, analgesics, anti-inflammatories, vitamins, herbals, homeopathics, topicals.

Patient Knowledge

Column A (Name): *Tell me the name of your medication.*

Column B (Dose): *What is the dose?*

Column C (Route): *How do you use it?*

Column D (Frequency): *How often do you take it?*

Column E (Reason for Use): *Why are you taking this non-prescription medication?*

Column F (Evidence of Benefit): *Do you find that it is helping you? Please explain.*

Column G (MD Awareness): *Is your doctor aware that you are taking this medication?* Place "✓" if the physician is aware of the medication and "x" if they are not. If relevant, remind the patient the importance of sharing this information with their physician.

Column H (Storage Appropriate): *How do you store this medication?* Assess for proper storage conditions and containers.

Column I (Expiry Date): *Is this an expired or out-of-date medication*? If so, then advise patient of this and offer to dispose of them properly.

Column J (Patient Adherence): *Do you take your medications as directed (either by physician, pharmacist, packaging, or other source)?* Document any findings in Table 2 under Comments.

Column K (Adverse Effects): *Do you experience any side effects from this medication? If you do, how bad are they and how often do you get them?* Prompt for commonly reported and serious adverse effects (e.g., nausea, diarrhea/constipation, dizziness, rash, visual disturbances, respiratory effects, etc.)

Complete Documentation and Follow-Up

Address any issues that were identified and document them in the **Action Plan** (Form 3). For example, if the patient is unaware of the indication, dose, or frequency then discuss this with the patient according to your records. If they are having problems with the packaging (e.g., cannot open a dropper bottle), suggest alternatives. If patients improperly store their medications, advise them on how best to store them. If patients are experiencing side effects, tell them how to manage them or what course of action they should follow. This form is meant to be an aid to summarize actions to be taken by the pharmacist, patient, physician, or caregiver. Most actions related to medication adherence will be completed by the pharmacist (e.g., change to snap caps) or the patient (e.g., take medication regularly).

Complete the **Personal Medication Record** (Form 4) for the patient. Both the pharmacist and the patient must sign the form. The pharmacist must retain a copy of this form for the records.

Ask the patient if he is having any further questions or concerns.

Ask the patient to complete the **Personal Medication Review Satisfaction Survey.**

Follow up with the patient as necessary on issues outlined in the Action Plan. Contact their physician, if necessary. You may wish to include the Action Plan along with the Personal Medication Record (Form 4).

Document the completion of the Medication Review in the Patient Profile in your computer system.

Form 1 Patient Background Form

Patient Information		
Name:	Date:	
Address:	Caregiver (if appropriate):	
Telephone:	Pharmacist Name:	
Date of Birth:		
Consent		
Patient has received information on and consented to the review process	Yes ☐	No ☐
Patient has agreed that information may be shared with their doctor	Yes ☐	No ☐
***MedsCheck* Patient Criteria:**		
Is the patient taking 3 or more chronic prescription medications?	Yes ☐	No ☐
Has the patient had a *MedsCheck* review in the past 365 days?	Yes ☐	No ☐
Is this a "Follow-up" *MedsCheck*?	Yes ☐	No ☐
If yes, is it due to a (circle one): Hospital discharge? Pharmacist's documented decision? MD or RN (EC) request? Planned hospital admission		
Health Information		
Medical Conditions:		
Allergies (specify):		
Pregnant: Yes ☐ No ☐ If Yes, which trimester? 1st ☐, 2nd ☐, or 3rd ☐	Breastfeeding: Yes ☐ No ☐	
Other lifestyle factors (e.g., alcohol, smoking etc.):		
Background Information		
Do you administer all the medications yourself? If no, please specify:	Yes ☐	No ☐
Do you have any difficulty swallowing?	Yes ☐	No ☐
Comments:		

Form 2

Table 1 Patient Medication History Form (Prescription)

Medication				Patient Knowledge				Usage				Adverse Effects (e.g., effect, frequency, severity)	Comments
A	B	C	D	E	F	G	H	I	J	K	L	M	
Name	Dose	Route	Frequency	Name	Reason for Use	Dosage/ Frequency	Special Instructions	Labeling & Packaging Appropriate	Storage Appropriate	Expiry Date	Patient Adherence		
				✓	✓	✓	✓	✓	✓	✓	✓		

↑	↓
Step 1: Complete columns A-D prior to Review Step 2: Place "✓" to acknowledge discussing columns E-L and to verify understanding Step 3: Identify any adverse effects in column M	Step 1: Complete columns A-F as per patient feedback Step 2: Place "✓" if MD is aware of drug and an "x" if they are not in column G Step 3: Place "✓" to acknowledge discussing columns H-J and to verify understanding Step 4: Identify any adverse effects in column K

Table 2 Patient Medication History Form (OTC/Herbal)

OTC/Natural/Other				Background			Usage			Adverse Effects (e.g., effect, frequency, severity)	Comments
A	B	C	D	E	F	G	H	I	J	K	
Name	Dose	Route	Frequency	Reason for Use	Evidence of Benefit	MD Awareness ✓	Storage Appropriate ✓	Expiry Date ✓	Patient Adherence ✓		

Form 3

Medication Review: Action Plan Date of Review:

Patient Name: Doctor Name:

Address:

Pharmacist Name:

Medication Use Issue	Proposed Action	Action by	Outcome, if known, with dates

☐ **Patient**	☐ **Doctor**
This is your copy; please retain it for your personal use. You may wish to share it with other health care professionals. ☐ Please make an appointment with your doctor to discuss within ___ weeks ☐ Take this form to your next scheduled doctor appointment ☐ Follow actions agreed above	This is your copy; please retain a copy in your patient's notes ☐ For information only – no action required ☐ Please review the actions proposed above

Form 4 Personal Medication Record

Patient	Primary Physician (Phone)	Pharmacist and Pharmacy (Phone)	Date Prepared

Date of Last Meds Check:

Medication Brand (Generic)	Start Date	Dosage	Route	Times Per Day	Scheduled Time	Purpose for Use	Prescriber (If different)	Comments

Allergies: No known allergies ☐

Product	Reaction

Pharmacist Signature

Patient Signature

Pharmacy Logo

[* Adapted from Website "Drug Information and Research Centre, 2007, www.dirc.ca]

CHAPTER 5

Ward Round Participation

Objectives

After reading this chapter the student should be able to:

- Define and understand the concept of Pharmacist ward round
- Discuss the need or rationale for Pharmacist ward rounds
- Develop an idea about the goals and objectives of ward rounds
- Role of Pharmacist in ward round and the preparation needed by Pharmacist
- Classify the types of ward rounds

5.1 Introduction

The essence of any clinical practice is direct patient care. Clinical medicine involves taking care of patients and their diagnosis, whereas clinical pharmacy is taking care of patients and their treatment. This type of practice requires knowledge of patients and their health. The Clinical Pharmacist in a hospital can better understand the patient's health condition, treatment being given, dosage compliance, drug usage, etc., by meeting and interacting with the patients directly in the wards. The participation of the Clinical Pharmacist in the ward round along with the physician will promote the understanding between medical profession and pharmacist. The role of nursing in patient care is enormous and a proper interaction between the nursing staff and the pharmacy personnel will improve patient care. This interaction is possible in the ward round participation by the Clinical Pharmacist.

The Pharmaceutical Care concept empowers the pharmacists with greater responsibility and accountability in the patient care process. Pharmaceutical Care involves the process through which a pharmacist cooperates with a patient and other professionals in designing, implementing and monitoring a therapeutic plan that will produce specific therapeutic outcomes for the patient.

Pharmacy traditionally has been concerned with delivering a drug product to the patient. Since 1960's the pharmacists began incorporating 'patient-oriented' services such as unit dose with patient profiles, IV admixtures, drug monitoring, medication histories, patient education, and ward rounds into their daily practice. These clinical services have provided pharmacists with the opportunity to make recommendations concerning drug therapy.

Ward rounds is a key activity in thc total process of patient care in the hospital. When the pharmacist rounds with the physician, he can assess the patient for drug-related problems, monitor drug therapy for therapeutic or adverse effects, promote rational drug therapy, and provide drug information to the physician, patient, and other health professionals. By rounding, the pharmacist is able to meet the patient, create direct dialogue with the physician, and gain an appreciation for the real world of patient care. As a result, rounding complements other patient-oriented clinical services.

It's the pharmacist's fundamental responsibility to ensure that every patient receives the most appropriate treatment in the most convenient and cost effective form. Retrospective review of medication orders by pharmacists on the wards has been shown to maximize safe prescribing. Pharmacist's impact can be substantial if input is provided at the time of prescribing.

5.2 Definition

Medical ward round is a visit made by a medical practitioner, alone or with a team of health professionals and medical students, to hospital inpatients at their respective bedside to review and follow up the progress in their health. *The participation of the pharmacist in the ward round along with the physician or alone on his own, to assess the patient for drug related problems, monitor drug therapy for therapeutic or adverse effects, promote rational drug therapy, and provide drug information to the physician, patient, and other health professionals is called as pharmacist ward round.*

5.3 Need

The addition of pharmacist to the health care team attending ward rounds in various practice settings helps to ensure safe, effective, and economic use of drugs. The net result is a decreased number of adverse drug events, improved patient care, and reduced length of hospital stay and reduced health care costs.

Pharmacists are uniquely qualified to contribute to the prevention of drug-related problems and to assist in drug therapy decision making by the very nature of pharmacists education and training. During ward rounds, pharmacists utilize their patient assessment skills, interviewing techniques, and knowledge of pharmacology and therapeutics in order to improve the effectiveness of drug therapy. Pharmacists also help reduce drug-related expenses by keeping physicians informed regarding the formulary status of drugs, equivalent substitutions, and appropriate dosages. Hospital and patient expenses also have been reduced when pharmacists have been authorized to determine the appropriate timing of serum level sampling. Increased pharmacist satisfaction is another important benefit that comes from pharmacist involvement in rounding. Many pharmacists have evaluated the potential benefits, both to patient care and to the hospital, and have designed innovative mechanisms to assess and justify pharmacist interaction in clinical services such as rounding.

Ward round participation provides learning opportunities for pharmacist. The pharmacist gets the first hand information on how drugs are used and prescribed and to see the effects of these drugs on patients. Pharmacist also develops an appreciation of how the patient's own wishes and their social, cultural and economic circumstances may influence therapeutic choices. In addition pharmacist ward round participation strengthens interpersonal relationship and interprofessional relationship.

(a) Patient Care

The participation of pharmacist in ward rounds provides him with an opportunity to offer specialized information that directly enhances patient care. By promoting rational drug therapy and providing accurate drug information the pharmacist can directly improve the patient care.

- ***Promotion of Rational Drug Therapy:*** The pharmacist is able to contribute to the promotion of the rational use of drugs by monitoring the drug therapy. With the knowledge and training the pharmacist can evaluate the appropriateness of the selected drug, calculate the dosage in renal and hepatic dysfunction, determine the dosage interval appropriate for compliance and efficacy, and possibly prevent any drug-related adverse effects. Pharmacists can promote rational drug therapy by:
  - Evaluating the appropriateness of the selected drug
  - Calculating the dosage consistent with the renal and hepatic function of the patient

- Determining an acceptable dosage interval that will ensure therapeutic benefit and compliance.
- Preventing drug-related adverse effects.

- ***Provision of Drug Information:*** During ward round participation the pharmacist can provide both solicited and unsolicited drug information. The pharmacist can also ask questions that are necessary if he is to provide useful drug information for drug therapy selection.

(b) Education

The pharmacist on rounds is having an excellent opportunity and is in a position to educate patients and the hospital staff concerning drugs. This process provides a chance to the pharmacist to improve his own knowledge of drug therapy. During the ward rounds the pharmacists can familiarize patients and other health professionals with available pharmacy services.

- ***Educating and interacting with the Patient:*** Patients often are unaware of the clinical pharmacy services that they receive or that are available to them in the hospital. When rounding with the physician, the pharmacist meets the patient, and communication is enhanced. By rounding, the pharmacist can better coordinate utilization of appropriate pharmacy services. The pharmacist may refer a patient who is in need of in depth evaluation, to a fellow pharmacist who has a special interest in the patient's particular problem. This also could include referring patients to a nutritional support, pharmacist identifying patients for specialized drug-education classes, and identifying patients who meet the criteria for an investigational drug or study protocol.

In the ideal situation, the pharmacist sees the patients for:

- an initial medication history interview to determine drug usage patterns, problems, etc.,
- drug therapy monitoring
- evaluation of any drug-related problems and
- education about medications before discharge (this may require specific drug cards and/or drug calendars to help with compliance).

- ***Educating self:*** Pharmacists obtain a better perspective on the use of drugs when they are exposed to the direct patient care where they have an opportunity to interact with the patient and also with the other medical staff including the physician. The pharmacist gets *clinical feel* for the use of particular drugs in particular types of patients. In addition, keeping abreast of new technology and the clinical use of drugs is paramount to maintaining and/or developing competence. For example, after the evaluation of several patients with a particular problem, pharmacist feels comfortable in recommending specialized dosages and / or regimens.

- ***Educating Other Health Professionals:*** By discussing drug-related topics with the medical team, the pharmacist is educating physicians. This is done when questions are answered in relation to specific patient situations. Since physicians do not always know which questions to ask, the pharmacist, by suggesting a specific drug, dosage, serum level, etc., is also educating members of the team. The physician becomes aware of the pharmacist's role by seeing what the pharmacist has to offer.

5.4 Goals and Objectives

The participation of pharmacist in ward rounds will ensure the following:

- Provide relevant information on various aspects of the patient's drug therapy such as pharmacology, pharmacokinetics, drug availability, drug interactions, and adverse reactions.
- Optimize therapeutic management by influencing drug therapy selection, implementation, monitoring, and follow up.
- Gain an improved understanding of patient's clinical status and progress, current planned investigations, and therapeutic goals.
- Investigate unusual drug orders, or doses.
- Detect adverse drug reactions, and drug interactions.
- Participate in patient discharge planning.

5.5 Pharmacist Participation in Ward Rounds

Pre Ward Round Preparation

The pharmacist has to thoroughly equip himself before going to the ward rounds. The following guidelines will help a pharmacist for preparing for rounds.

- ***Preparing Self***

  The pharmacist on rounds should be familiar with appropriate references, knowledgeable concerning current drug therapy, able to monitor patients drug therapies according to specific and appropriate criteria, and consistent in his attendance at rounds. The pharmacist must become familiar with the reference books available in the library and the drug files, keep abreast of the latest research taking place in the medical and pharmacy fields, determine appropriate patient monitoring criteria, understand and maintain the rounding schedule. When the number of patients are more in the ward the pharmacist should select those patients most in need of clinical pharmacy monitoring services. The pharmacist should be in touch with the physician and decide the timing of the rounding. The pharmacist should have a perfect understanding of the hospital formulary, especially in hospitals that have a formulary or drug list and he should ensure that all prescriptions are in accordance with the hospital formulary.

- ***Specific Planning***

  Specific planning for rounds requires the development of appropriate forms to assist in monitoring patients and their therapies, determination of a means for communicating with the other members of the rounding team, as well as other activities by the pharmacist in order to ensure appropriate and effective pharmacist input.

  Determine the Best Method for Communicating with the Rounding Team: Some of the physicians would like to have the pharmacist's recommendations, with pertinent references, recorded in the chart while, others may prefer verbal communication. The pharmacist can record the ADRs and also the kinetic parameters in the chart. This will be helpful to the physician. Good communication skills both written and spoken and sound clinical knowledge are prerequisites for effective participation in ward rounds and clinical meetings. Knowledge of local language along with English will help the pharmacist communicate effectively.

  Develop a Monitoring Profile and/or Patient Log Sheet: The profile card should have space to record each patient's name, unit number, diagnosis/problem list, current drugs (listed beside the problems they are prescribed to treat), past drug history, IV fluids, lab tests, comments, etc. It is important to evaluate each patient daily according to the goals that have been selected for the patient's drug therapy. For example, an arthritic's pain history should be evaluated to measure the success of the non-steroidal anti-inflammatory agent used. It is helpful to record the outcomes selected for each problem.

  Periodic reassessment of the Drug Therapy: The pharmacist can assess the patient periodically to check whether the patient is improving as planned or whether another drug, dose, etc. should be ordered. Follow up and reassessment can give an opportunity to the pharmacist to watch the patient benefit from the inputs given. Talk to the physician privately if he refuses to follow the advice given and find out the reasons.

  Presentation of Lectures: Presentation of at least one drug-related lecture each month is advisable. These presentations will help establish that the pharmacist is a resource to be consulted when patients are seen with problems requiring special expertise.

Work out a System where you can be contacted readily: This may include requesting or purchasing a beeper or mobile. If the physician cannot communicate with you easily, he may not call you concerning new patients, drug information, etc.

Make certain that other Pharmacists and Supportive Personnel understand what you are doing: Communication and sharing of pertinent cases with peers is recommended.

Identify potential problems: The pharmacist should identify potential problems like drug interactions, adverse drug reactions and medication errors etc., and be prepared to suggest alternatives.

- ***Specific Monitoring Aids and Check List***

  Preparing for rounds each day involves making certain that you understand the disease state, drug therapy (mechanism, kinetics, alterations in various disease states, dosage range, etc.,) and special needs unique to each patient you are monitoring. This involves self-education on disease states, drug problems, specialized dosing considerations, etc. To be an effective clinical pharmacist, you must understand the disease process and how the disease affects various parts of the body.

  In specialized areas such as intensive care units or on specialized rounds such as oncology, pulmonary, renal, etc., monitoring criteria and protocols may be written to help determine the degree of monitoring needed. The protocol should include symptoms, laboratory tests, dosing guidelines based on patient characteristics, major adverse effects and how they present, and a monitoring flow sheet to record the needed clinical information and serum levels. On a general service, special monitoring sheets for patients receiving specific drugs such as amino glycoside antibiotics, theophylline, etc. should be considered.

5.6 Pharmacist Selection of a Rounding Team

The pharmacist has to select a rounding team in which he can participate based on certain parameters. His presence in the rounding team should benefit the patient and the department. Generally pharmacists tend to become involved with the medical specialists due to the high consumption of drugs in these areas. When there are more medical teams available to choose from, other factors should be considered.

- ***Time***

  The time available for rounding to a pharmacist will be the prime consideration when determining an appropriate team to round with. Teaching rounds, especially with interns and PG students, tend to be time-consuming since the Professor plans to educate students and residents on case presentation, diagnosis, and treatment.

- ***Compatibility with Physician***

  The pharmacist's compatibility with physician is a major consideration, especially when determining which private practice physician to round with. The opportunity for effective interaction is dependent on the mutual respect, professional competence, and communication skills of physician and pharmacist.

- ***Patient Care***

  The selection of ward by the pharmacist to round with depends on the availability of number of pharmacists, average length of hospital stay by the patients, necessity of the particular patient's stay in a ward etc., For example, special acute care units, such as ICU, ICCU, ICN, NICU etc. have rapidly changing drug needs and patients might not stay on these units for a long period of time. But the most toxic drugs are used in the acute care areas.

- ***Personal Interests***

  The strengths and interests of the pharmacist should be considered while selecting a team to round with. Often, a rounding team that admits many patients to a pharmacy area serviced by a unit dose satellite pharmacy is selected since the patient information would complement the unit dose patient-monitoring program.

- ***Acceptance by the Rounding Team***

  Physicians requesting pharmacist input on rounds are generally very supportive of the services the pharmacist provides; therefore, pharmacist should select a physician who uses pharmacy services, such as drug information, investigational drugs, etc. Likewise, physicians who have worked with pharmacists at other institutions and have learned to depend on the pharmacist should be given special consideration when selecting a rounding service.

5.7 Common Types of Rounds

The basic types of rounds are as follows:

- Medical teaching rounds with faculty or PG's and interns
- Private physician rounds
- Special unit rounds
- Interdisciplinary rounds and
- Pharmacy rounds.

Teaching Rounds

Medical teaching service rounds, found in community teaching and university teaching hospitals are headed by a supervising or attending physician. This physician may be a faculty member from the medical school or a private physician from the community. Patients without a private physician who are admitted through the emergency department and patients in the outpatient department generally are cared for on the medical teaching service. The rounding team is composed of second or third year residents, first year residents, medical students, and the attending or supervising physician. The first year resident, supervised by the second or third year resident, is primarily responsible for the clinical decisions involved in the care of the patients. The supervising physician, while ultimately responsible for the patients care, may choose to let the resident make the decisions independently as part of the resident's education.

Private Physician Rounds

In non-teaching hospitals, selecting a particular clinician for the pharmacist to round with is usually necessary since formalized teaching teams may not exist. Morning and/or afternoon rounds are usually shorter than in teaching rounds with the physician returning to his office during the day. In rounding teams having no residents or students, the pharmacist may assist with data gathering for the physician in addition to assessing each patient.

Special Rounds

Special unit teams in acute areas, such as intensive care nursery, surgical and medical intensive care, coronary care, etc., may have rounds once or twice a day. This is usually the case when the hospital employs a medical specialist to head the area. The pharmacist is able to develop specific drug protocols and monitoring criteria for the patients treated in the unit.

Interdisciplinary Rounds

Interdisciplinary teams, such as nutritional support, see patients throughout the hospital and may be composed of physicians, pharmacists, nurses, dietitians, and other health professionals. The rounding format is similar to that of other types of rounds with specialized monitoring parameters and flow sheets facilitating patient monitoring.

Pharmacy Rounds

The pharmacist makes his own rounds, independently or with fellow pharmacists/students, to evaluate the patient's drug therapy. By visiting the patient to ask specific questions and examining the chart for laboratory data, X-ray reports, symptoms, etc., the pharmacist is able to develop a monitoring plan for the patient. This usually involves filling out a monitoring card.

The Clinical Pharmacist encounters certain issues during a ward round that require some follow up like responding to queries on drug information, communicating information, completing documentation etc.,

Conclusion

Pharmacists are uniquely qualified to contribute to the prevention of drug-related problems and to assist in drug therapy decision making. Pharmacist ward rounds promote the appropriate use of drugs in the institution, to provide drug information when decisions are being made, to educate the physician and patient, to identify referrals for special pharmacy services, and to identify drug delivery concerns. Pharmacist credibility develops with appropriate recommendations, accurate drug information, and appropriate follow up. Rounding complements the other clinical services provided by the pharmacy department by increasing pharmacist's direct contact with patients, physicians and other health professionals.

Study Outline

Medical ward round is a visit made by a medical practitioner alone or with a team of health care professionals and medical students to hospital patients at their respective bedside to review and follow up the progress in their health.

The addition of pharmacist to health care team attending ward rounds in various practice settings helps to ensure safe, effective and economic use of drugs.

The reasons a pharmacist should round are to promote the appropriate use of drugs in the institution; to provide drug information when decisions regarding drugs are being made; to educate the physician and patient; to identify referrals for special pharmacy services; and to identify drug delivery concerns. In addition, the pharmacist gains first-hand experience in monitoring drugs. The pharmacist's preparation for rounds involves reading, defining monitoring criteria, and working out specific details. Pharmacist credibility develops with appropriate recommendations, accurate drug information, and appropriate follow-up.

Rounding complements the other clinical services provided by the pharmacy department by increasing pharmacist's direct contact with patients, physicians, and other health professionals.

During ward rounds pharmacists utilize their patient assessment skills, interviewing techniques, and knowledge of pharmacology and therapeutics in order to improve the effectiveness of drug therapy.

Ward round participation by pharmacist provides him with an opportunity to offer specialized information that directly enhances patient care, by promoting rational drug therapy and providing accurate drug information.

Ward round participation by pharmacists enables him to

- educate and interact with the patient
- educate self
- educate other health care professionals

Objectives

Ward round participation by pharmacists ensures fulfillment of following objectives

- provide relevant information on various aspects of drug therapy
- optimize therapeutic management
- improved understanding of patients clinical status and progress
- investigate unusual drug orders/doses
- detect adverse drug reactions and interactions
- participate in patient discharge planning

Preward Round Preparation

- preparing self by familiarizing himself with the appropriate data by making use of reference books, drug files, updating his knowledge. He should have a perfect understanding of the hospital formulary.
- Specific planning for development of appropriate forms to be filled in, communicating with rounding team, periodic reassessment of drug therapy, presentation of lectures, ready accessibility and identification of potential problems.
- Specific monitoring aids and check list.
- Pharmacists selection of a rounding team should take into consideration his time, compatibility with physician, patient care, personal interests, acceptance by rounding team.

Types of Ward Rounds

- Medical teaching rounds
- Private physician rounds
- Special unit rounds
- Interdisciplinary rounds
- Pharmacy rounds

CHAPTER 6

Monitoring Drug Therapy

Objectives

After reading this chapter the student should be able to:

- Define and understand the importance of Drug Therapy Monitoring.
- Understand the role of medical records in Drug Therapy Monitoring.
- Explain the process for Drug Therapy Monitoring.
- Develop a plan of study for Drug Therapy Monitoring.

6.1 Introduction

Definition:

Monitoring drug therapy or Drug therapy monitoring is a process which encompasses all those functions necessary to ensure appropriate, safe, efficacious, and economical drug therapy to the patient.

They include:

- Reviewing the prescriber's choice of a drug for the diagnosed condition
- Reviewing drug administration
- Assuring correct dosing (which includes amount, frequency, route, and dosage form)

- Recognizing the presence or lack of adequate therapeutic response
- Assessing the potential for and occurrence of adverse effects, and
- Recommending changes or alternatives in therapy as the particular situation dictates.

The goal of monitoring drug therapy is to ensure appropriate, safe, efficacious, and economical therapy. There are several significant problems with regard to the drug therapy. These problems occur more frequently due to the ever increasing number of available drugs. Some of these are inappropriate prescribing and dosing, adverse drug reactions and/or drug-induced disease, patient noncompliance with prescribed medication regimen, and errors in medication administration. The risk for a hospitalized patient is more as he is receiving multiple drug therapy, and this in itself has been identified as a factor in increasing drug-induced disease. The process of monitoring the drug therapy can decrease and/or prevent these problems. The pharmacist can contribute significantly to the care of medicated patients. The goal of monitoring drug therapy can be phrased as '*maximizing the benefits of drug therapy and minimizing the risks*'.

0.2 Role of Medical Records in Drug Therapy Monitoring

In the process of monitoring drug therapy, the pharmacist becomes very familiar with patients medical records. In order to monitor drug therapy appropriately, it is essential that the pharmacist has an understanding of the types of patient records and their contents.

- ***The Source-Oriented Record***: In this type of record the clinical information written or placed in the medical record has been recorded in a narrative, chronological sequence in major subsections of the chart. This is termed the "source-oriented record" (SOR). The various sections of the SOR usually are separated by some sort of index system; for instance, the major sections of progress notes, physician orders (including medication), laboratory results, and nursing notes are separated by an index tab preceding each major section. The order sheet, progress notes, laboratory results, and vital signs sheet should be monitored daily in order to assess properly the patient's clinical status.
- ***The Problem-Oriented Record:*** This system of record keeping of clinical information is in a more orderly format and provides a more organized approach to clinical data than does the SOR and allows for easy interpretation of the patient's status. The basic information found in the POR is divided into the following sections.

    Data base Section: This section essentially contains all pertinent history, physical, and laboratory information of the patient.

    Problem List: This information is usually listed on a separate problem page at the front of the chart and may include proven diagnosis, syndrome, operation, symptoms, abnormal laboratory values, allergies, and/or social or psychological problems. In short, the problem list is "what is wrong" with the patient, and the problems are dated and listed as active, inactive, or resolved.

Plan: This section spells out a plan for each problem. This section actually takes the place of the traditional order sheet and encompasses any intervention for the patient.

Progress Notes: This consists of chronological notes on the problems listed for the patient. This section may be a composite of notes from all health care personnel who need to write in the chart. Each problem is approached in a specific format called "SOAP". In this format, S = subjective or symptomatic information, O = objective information (such as lab results or specific physical findings), A = assessment of the problem, and P = plan of action. Progress notes written in this fashion helps to facilitate patient care, especially drug monitoring, since the plan or goal of therapy is clearly identified.

Discharge Summary: This section contains a problem-by-problem discharge summary utilizing the SOAP format.

6.3 Patient Selection

Those patients who are at significant risk for developing adverse effects from drug therapy should be identified. This can be done by reviewing the diagnosis and/or the types of drug therapy being used.

- ***By Disease State***

  Patients who are admitted with multiple disease states or problems may be at high risk of developing drug-related problems because they usually receive multiple drug therapy. Patients with problems that require toxic therapeutic agents (e.g., cancer patients) are at risk for drug-related toxicity. Patients with significant heart failure, renal failure, lung disease, or liver dysfunction are also at risk due to the possibility of abnormal drug metabolism and elimination in these disease states. If the patient is elderly or very young, this may also increase risk.

- ***By Drug Therapy***

  In addition to selecting patients based on their problems, the pharmacist should also screen the drug(s) prescribed for each patient. Like certain disease states, there are therapeutic agents which put a patient at high risk for adverse effects. Monitoring for these adverse effects, and thus being in a position to prevent or downgrade therapeutic problems, is obviously, a very important function. In order to begin selective monitoring, using drug therapy as the selection criterion, the pharmacist must develop an effective and efficient mechanism for this process. Computer profiles of medications that the hospitalized patients are receiving would be very valuable tools, enabling an efficient initial review and subsequent monitoring activities. In lieu of a computerized format, the pharmacist can utilize a manual system for drug review and monitoring. Obviously, patients receiving those agents with high risk of toxicity will need to be followed more closely. Such agents include antibiotics, anticonvulsants, anticoagulants, antiarrhythmics, and antineoplastics. Criteria have been published for use in selective patient monitoring that aid in risk identification with regard to drug therapy.

In general, patients with multiple problems and those treated with polypharmacy are candidates for drug therapy monitoring. Once these patients and drugs are identified, the review and monitoring process can begin.

6.4 Process of Monitoring Drug Therapy

In order to monitor drug therapy appropriately, the pharmacist should be able to perform the following functions, which are really the basis of drug therapy monitoring:

- ***Take patient data and orient the data into a problem format***

  The Pharmacist should review the patient's medical record, including all of its major sections. The patient's problem list should be reviewed and patient profile should be prepared which should be simple. The profile should consist of patient's name, age, weight, sex and location in the hospital as well as any pertinent information gained from the medication history. It also should include provisional diagnosis or the reason the patient was admitted. Once this patient profile is documented, each problem should be listed by number and under each problem the pharmacist should develop SOAP format. This will allow integration of drug therapy into the plan or goal of therapy for that problem. The pharmacist should review and re-evaluate the plan daily for any changes that may have occurred and update the same.

- ***Relate drug therapy to the specific problem or disease states in order to determine the appropriateness of the specific therapy***

  The rational for the use of any drug is determined by experience, judgment and reference to appropriate resources in the pharmacy or hospital library. This requires evaluation of the specific drug used for a given disease entity or problem, correctness of dose, dosage form and dosing interval.

  Many a times the pharmacist is not present during prescribing, so he should depend on the information given in the record to assess the correctness of the use of a particular drug. After assuring himself about the rational use of the drug he can proceed with other monitoring activities. With the application of pharmacokinetic principles of dosing the pharmacist will determine the correct dosing regimens. Certain disease states such as kidney or liver disease must be considered while determining the dose. Some agents like digoxin, amino glycoside antibiotics etc. have a narrow therapeutic index or associated with adverse drug reactions and can cause difficulty in clinical setting. The Pharmacist is expected to be familiar with the pharmacokinetic characteristics of these agents.

Frequency of administration and dosage form should be reviewed regularly for appropriateness. If dosing problems are noted at any point, the pharmacist should determine a solution or alternative. Screening should be done for drug-drug, drug-lab and drug-food interactions.

- ***Develop specific therapeutic goals***

  Generally, the goal of therapy for a disease or problem will be to cure or alleviate it. The physician will set certain goals for treatment for individual patient. These goals are included in the plan section of the SOAP format. As it is not possible to cure all the diseases, at times, other goals are required. For example, the goal for most infectious diseases is to cure the disease, where as for diseases like diabetes or heart failure, the goal is to halt the progress of the disease.

- ***Develop monitoring parameters for each drug used***

  Specific parameters to be utilized in the process of monitoring drug therapy should be prepared by the pharmacist. These parameters will be helpful to determine the therapeutic effectiveness and the occurrence of adverse effects. Each individual drug should have a set of specific parameters that are used to assess the effectiveness and adverse effects. To save time and make the process more efficient the pharmacist can enter all the information into a computer or on small index cards or on large forms for permanent filing.

  The pharmacist should review daily and routinely the nursing and physician progress notes, lab test reports and assess any changes in drug therapy.

- ***Identify problems and/or the potential for adverse drug reaction***

  Problems such as contraindications to drug use, dosing inappropriateness, drug toxicity, administration error, inappropriate therapy etc., may arise during the monitoring process. The pharmacist should identify such problems and take corrective measures. The pharmacist first must determine if this problem is drug related and then confirm. Drug information sources can be reviewed for documentation. He should then determine the clinical significance of the problem.

- ***Develop alternatives or solutions to problems***

  Alternatives or solutions must be formulated to the problems identified if they are found to be clinically significant. The pharmacist after confirming alternatives or solutions formulated by doing thorough research of drug information can recommend the same to the physician. These recommendations can be either oral or written and should include the identification and confirmation of the problem, its clinical significance and recommendation for correction.

- ***Communicate, any findings and recommendations for solutions or alternatives to the problems identified***

  Before the pharmacist communicates his recommendations for corrective action, he should identify exactly the person who should be communicated and in whose area of operations the problem lies i.e. nurse, physician or other health care personnel. For example, if the problem involves an area such as drug administration, then the pharmacist and nurse can solve the problem.

  Generally, when a pharmacist makes a decision regarding a problem's clinical significance, he is making a judgment about the importance of that problem with regard to patient safety. If there appears to be a question concerning safety or the development of an adverse drug effect (toxic response), the physician should be notified immediately and advised orally by the pharmacist as to possible solutions or alternatives to the problem. The pharmacist should then carefully monitor the patient and his course for further developments.

6.5 Developing a Plan of Study

In order to monitor drug therapy effectively, it is clear that most pharmacists need to become familiar with certain aspects of health care with which they have been unacquainted. These areas are pathophysiology, applied therapeutics, clinical pharmacokinetics, clinical chemistry and hematology, and certain aspects of physical diagnosis. The task that the pharmacist will find most time consuming will be the updating of his knowledge of disease processes, or the pathology of disease. While there is a tremendous amount of information to be processed, the pharmacist should not let this intimidate him. The pharmacist should remember that, in time, he will become comfortable with the jargon and with the common, recurring problems.

The pharmacist should begin by monitoring a few patients at a time, under supervision, and reviewing the pathophysiology of each problem of disease in an appropriate medical text (medicine, pediatrics, etc.). The same is true for drug therapy; as the pharmacist reviews the drug monographs, his knowledge base will expand. This is all self study, and the pharmacist should take advantage of continuing education programs designed to upgrade and advance clinical skills. There are many good continuing education programs being offered at national and state levels both in self-study and meeting formats. There also might be appropriate conferences offered in one's own institution. The aspiring clinical pharmacy practitioner should take advantage of these programs whenever possible.

A good reference library is essential to clinical practice. In addition, the pharmacist should make it a habit to review those journals and publications offering up-to-date information on drug and applied therapeutics. It is essential to the pharmacist's developing credibility that he be up-to-date and well read. As the pharmacist reads the journal literature, he should begin to keep a file of key articles that pertain to applied therapeutics and disease states. It is also important to get some sort of feed back regarding his self study program and direction. The pharmacist and his supervising clinical pharmacist should meet routinely to discuss any questions that arise in this new environment. In the beginning, it would be wise to have supervision of the pharmacist's monitoring activities and any recommendations that he makes. This guidance can be very helpful for a new pharmacist. If the pharmacist is without clinical supervision, he should proceed slowly and make certain his information is sound.

Conclusion

Monitoring therapy during treatment is necessary to assure continued appropriate and rational therapy. Involvement in the therapeutic process is one of the important clinical functions of the pharmacist. The pharmacist should develop his clinical skills so that he can meet the demands and responsibilities of monitoring drug therapy successfully.

Study Outline

Monitoring drug therapy is the process which includes all those functions necessary to ensure appropriate, safe, efficacious and economical drug therapy to the patient.

Patient records especially medical records play an important role in the process of monitoring drug therapy. There are two types of medical records:

- the source oriented record
- the problem oriented record

Patient Selection

Patients for monitoring drug therapy are selected based upon the severity of developing adverse effects. This can be done by reviewing the diagnosis and / or the types of drug therapy being used.

- by disease state
- by drug therapy

Process of Monitoring Drug Therapy

- Take patient data and orient the data into a problem format
- Relate drug therapy to the specific problem or disease states in order to determine the appropriateness of the specific drug therapy
- Develop specific therapeutic goals
- Develop monitoring parameters for each drug used
- Identify problems and / or potential for adverse drug reactions
- Develop alternatives or solutions to problems and
- Communicate, if necessary, to the physician or allied health personnel any findings and recommendations for solutions or alternatives to the problem identified.

CHAPTER 7

Therapeutic Drug Monitoring

Objectives

After reading this chapter the student should be able to:

- Define and understand the importance of Therapeutic Drug Monitoring
- Explain the precautions and guidelines needed for Therapeutic Drug Monitoring
- Understand the need and importance of Therapeutic Drug Monitoring
- Interpret Therapeutic Drug Monitoring and understand the economies of Therapeutic Drug Monitoring

7.1 Introduction

Therapeutic Drug Monitoring (TDM) is a means of monitoring drug levels in the blood i.e., measurement of drug concentrations in biological fluids with the purpose of optimizing a patient's drug therapy. TDM is done at specific intervals to maintain a relatively constant concentration of the medication in the bloodstream. Monitoring drug therapy by TDM is a process which encompasses all those functions necessary to ensure appropriate, safe, efficacious, and economical drug therapy to the patient.

TDM is required to be done to only those medications that have a narrow "therapeutic range". Most of the drugs have a larger therapeutic range and can be prescribed based upon established dosing schedules. The effectiveness of these treatments can be evaluated using TDM, but it is not usually necessary to determine the concentration of the drug in the bloodstream. Examples of this include high blood pressure medications and many of the antibiotics given to treat bacterial infections. If the infection resolves and the blood pressure is lowered, then the treatments have been effective.

TDM is a practical tool that can help the physician provide effective and safe drug therapy in patients who need medication. Monitoring can be used to confirm a blood drug concentration level that is above or below the therapeutic range, or if the desired therapeutic effect of the drug is not as expected. If this is the case, and dosages beyond normal have to be prescribed, TDM can minimize the time that elapses.

Therapeutic drug monitoring refers to the individualization of dosage by maintaining plasma or blood drug concentrations within a target range (therapeutic range, therapeutic window). There are two major sources of variability between individual patients in drug response. These are variation in the relationship between:

- dose and plasma concentration (pharmacokinetic variability)
- drug concentration at the receptor and the response (pharmacodynamic variability)

By adjusting doses to maintain plasma drug concentrations within a target range, variability in the pharmacokinetic phase of drug action is greatly reduced. The major sources of pharmacokinetic variability are shown in Table 1.

Table 7.1 Major sources of pharmacokinetic variability

Compliance
Age - neonates, children, elderly
Physiology - gender, pregnancy
Disease - hepatic, renal, cardiovascular, respiratory
Drug interactions
Environmental influences on drug metabolism
Genetic polymorphisms of drug metabolism

7.2 Importance of Therapeutic Drug Monitoring

Many of the drugs that are monitored therapeutically are taken for a lifetime. The blood levels of these drugs must be maintained at steady concentrations for a long period. The patient undergoes lot of changes like increasing age, occurrences of events such as pregnancies, temporary illnesses, infections, emotional and physical stresses, accidents, and surgeries. Over time, patients may acquire other chronic conditions that also require lifetime medication which may affect the processing of their monitored drugs. Examples of these conditions include cardiovascular disease, kidney disease, thyroid disease, liver disease, and HIV/AIDS.

Therapeutic drug monitoring follows these changes and accommodates them. It identifies patient noncompliance (when the patient does not take the medication regularly as prescribed), identifies the effect of drug interactions (may cause drug concentrations that are higher or lower than expected at a given dosage), and helps to tailor dosages to fit the current needs of the specific patient. Along with tests such as BUN, creatinine, and liver panel to check kidney and liver function, monitoring can help identify decreases in the efficiency of and dysfunctions in the body in metabolizing and eliminating therapeutic drugs.

TDM is important for patients who have other diseases that can affect drug levels, or who take other medicines that may affect drug levels by interacting with the drug being tested. As an example, without drug monitoring, the physician cannot be sure if a patient's lack of response to an antibiotic reflects bacterial resistance, or is the result of failure to reach the proper therapeutic range of antibiotic concentration in the blood. In case of life-threatening infections, timing of effective antibiotic therapy is critical to success. It is equally crucial to avoid toxicity in a seriously ill patient. Therefore, if toxic symptoms appear with standard dosages, TDM can be used to determine changes in dosing.

Drawn blood used for TDM, demonstrates a drug action in the body at any specific time, whereas drug levels examined from urine samples reflect the presence of a drug over many days (depending on the rate of excretion). Therefore, blood testing is the procedure of choice when definite data are required. However, for adequate absorption and therapeutic levels to be accurate, it is important to allow for sufficient time to pass between the administration of the medication and the collection of the blood sample.

Blood specimens for drug monitoring can be taken at two different times: during the drug's highest therapeutic concentration ("peak" level), or its lowest ("trough" level), occasionally called residual levels, trough levels show sufficient therapeutic levels; whereas peak levels show poisoning (toxicity). Peak and trough levels should fall within the therapeutic range.

The timing of blood collection is an important part of therapeutic drug monitoring. When a person takes a dose of a drug, the amount in the blood rises for a time period, peaks, and then begins to fall, usually reaching its lowest level (trough) just before the next dose. To be effective, peak levels should be below toxic concentrations and trough levels should remain in the therapeutic range. Through experience and studies, the physician can know when to expect peaks and troughs and will request blood sample collections as either trough levels (usually drawn just before the next dose), peak levels (timing varies depending on the drug), or sometimes will request a random level. Consistent and accurate interpretation of the results depends on the timing of sample collection.

While measuring the TDM following factors are to be considered:

- age and weight of the patient
- route of administration of the drug
- the drug's absorption rate
- excretion rate
- delivery rate
- dosage
- other medications the patient is taking
- other diseases patient has
- the patient's compliance regarding the drug treatment regimen
- lab methods used to test for the drug

7.3 Need for Therapeutic Drug Monitoring

The goal of TDM is to achieve a drug concentration which is known to be effective, without toxicity, in majority of the people. It also ensures appropriate, safe, and economical therapy. TDM is employed to measure blood drug levels so that the most effective dosage can be determined, and toxicity prevented. TDM is also utilized to identify noncompliant patients (those patients who, for whatever reason, either cannot or will not comply with drug dosages as prescribed by the physician). TDM is not used if the response to drug therapy can be directly and easily measured. e.g., anti-hypertensive drugs and patient's blood pressure measurement.

TDM is important for drugs with narrow therapeutic index, non linear pharmacokinetics or drugs with large inter individual variation in pharmacokinetics.

For TDM to be useful there must be a relationship between dose, plasma or blood drug concentrations and pharmacodynamic effects. The greatest benefits of TDM are in targeted patient populations e.g., in children or elderly patient's or in patient's with renal impairment.

Therapeutic drug monitoring is useful to,

- Assist the optimization of drug therapy, including minimizing the risk of serious drug toxicity and assessment of the appropriateness of dosing for drugs used as prophylactic therapy
- Identify a drug or substance which may be contributing to the presentation of a medical emergency (clinical toxicology).

The common clinical situations where TDM is useful are,

- To confirm adequate serum concentrations where clinical response is inadequate, e.g., lithium in bipolar disorder
- To avoid drug toxicity e.g., amino glycoside antibiotics such as gentamicin causing nephrotoxicity or ototoxicity
- To assist dose adjustments in various disease states where individual variations in drug absorption, distribution, metabolism, or elimination may be important, e.g., hepatic or renal impairment
- To individualize dosing for some drugs with an unpredictable dose response curve, e.g., phenytoin which is having non linear kinetics. Increasing the dose may lead to disproportionately large increase in the serum drug concentration
- To minimize the time period needed for dosage adjustment
- To identify poisons and to assess the severity of poisoning on an emergency basis in a poisoned patient.

7.4 Preparation

In preparing for this test, the following guidelines should be observed:

- Depending on the drug to be tested, the physician should decide if the patient is to be fasting (nothing to eat or drink for a specified period of hours) before the test
- For patients suspected of symptoms of drug toxicity, the best time to draw the blood specimen is when the symptoms are occurring
- If there is a question as to whether an adequate dose of the drug is being achieved, it is best to obtain trough (lowest therapeutic concentration) levels
- Peak (highest concentration) levels are usually obtained one to two hours after oral administration, approximately one hour after intramuscular (IM) administration and approximately 30 minutes after intravenous (IV) administration. Residual or trough levels are usually obtained within 15 minutes of the next scheduled dose.

7.5 Factors Affecting Serum Drug Concentration

The following factors influence the serum drug concentrations:

- patient demographics - age , sex, body weight and ethnicity
- dosage regimen and duration of therapy
- sampling time – for drugs with short half life the samples should be drawn immediately before the next dose i.e., a trough level and for drugs with long half life the samples may be drawn at any time during the post distribution phase once the steady-state levels are achieved
- Patient compliance – patient non compliance can cause a decrease in the serum concentration
- Genetic factors - individual capacity to distribute, metabolize and excrete the drug
- Altered protein binding due to malnutrition or nephropathy may reduce the concentration of plasma proteins. e.g., any decrease in protein concentrations can cause high concentration of the unbound drug as in the case of phenytoin
- Drug interactions – digoxin concentration increases if other drugs such as amiodarone, quinidine or verapamil are commenced with out a reduction in the digoxin dose
- Pathological factors
- Alcohol and tobacco use – chronic alcohol use can cause non specific hepatic microsomal enzyme induction, resulting in increased clearance and decreased serum concentrations of hepatically cleared drugs such as phenytoin

7.6 Drugs that Require Monitoring

The characteristics of drugs which make them suitable for, or make them require TDM are those

- showing marked pharmacokinetic variability
- which have concentration related therapeutic and adverse effects
- having narrow therapeutic index (TI)
- defined therapeutic concentration range
- in which desired therapeutic effect is difficult to monitor

Table 7.2 Drugs that can be monitored by TDM Technique

Drug Category	Drugs in the Category	Treatment / Use
Cardiac drugs	Digoxin, Digitoxin, Quinidine, Procainamide, N-acetyl-procainamide (a metabolite of procainamide)	Congestive heart failure, angina, arrhythmias
Antibiotics	Aminoglycosides (gentamicin, tobramycin, amikacin), Vancomycin, Chloramphenicol	Infections with bacteria that are resistant to less toxic antibiotics
Antiepileptics	Phenobarbital, Phenytoin, Valproic acid, Carbamazepine, Ethosuximide, Gabapentin, Lamotrigine	Epilepsy, prevention of seizures, sometimes to stabilize moods
Bronchodilators	Theophylline, Caffeine	Asthma, Chronic obstructive pulmonary disorder (COPD), neonatal apnea
Immunosuppressants	Cyclosporine, Tacrolimus, Sirolimus, Mycophenolate mofetil, Azathioprine	Prevent rejection of transplanted organs, autoimmune disorders
Anti-cancer drugs	Methotrexate	Psoriasis, rheumatoid arthritis, various cancers, non-hodgkin's lymphomas, osteosarcoma
Psychiatric drugs	Lithium, Valproic acid, some antidepressants (imipramine, amitriptyline, nortriptyline, doxepin, desipramine)	Bipolar disorder (manic depression), depression
Protease inhibitors	Indinavir, Ritonavir, Lopinavir, Saquinavir, Atazanavir, Nelfinavir	HIV/AIDS

Table 7.3 TDM values for commonly monitored drugs

Drug	***Therapeutic range mg/L***
Digoxin	0.5 – 2.1
Amiodarone	1.0 – 2.5
Lignocaine	2.0 – 5.0
Quinidine	2.0 – 5.0
Flecainide	0.2 – 0.9
Mexilitine	0.5 – 2.5
Salicylate	150 - 300
Perhexiline	0.15 - 0.6
Theophylline	10 – 20
Phenytoin	10 – 20
Carbamazepine	5.0 – 12
Sodium valproate	50 – 100
Phenobarbitone	15 – 40
Gentamicin, Tobramycin, Netilmicin	trough <2; peak >5
Amikacin	trough <5; peak >15
Vancomycin	trough <10; peak 20 - 40
Lithium	0.6 – 1.2

(1) microgram/L

(2) for 8-hourly dosing

(3) mmol/L

7.7 Information Required for Interpretation of TDM Values

Drug concentrations need to be interpreted in the context of the individual patient without rigid adherence to a therapeutic range.

The basic information about the sample and the patient, required for adequate interpretation of a drug concentration is shown in Table 4. Besides this, a good knowledge of the disposition of the drug is needed.

There are two important factors which can make interpretation of a result difficult in some cases. These are changes in protein binding and active metabolites.

Table 7.4 Information required

Time of sample in relation to last dose
Duration of treatment with the current dose
Dosing schedule
Age, gender
Other drug therapy
Relevant disease states
Reason for request e.g. lack of effect, routine monitoring, suspected toxicity

Protein Binding

Assays are done using plasma or blood and thus measure bound and unbound drug, whereas it is the unbound drug that interacts with the receptor to produce a response. If binding is changed by disease states, displacement by another drug or non-linearity in protein binding, the interpretation of total plasma or blood drug concentrations must be modified. For example, the therapeutic range for phenytoin based on total drug concentration is 10-20 mg/L which corresponds to an unbound drug concentration of 1-2 mg/L (fraction unbound, f_u is normally 0.1). If f_u is increased to 0.2, as, for example, in renal disease, the target unbound concentration is still 1-2 mg/L, but the therapeutic range for total drug is 5-10 mg/L. Unless this is realized, inappropriate dose adjustments may be made, resulting in toxicity.

Sodium valproate and salicylate show non-linear binding in the therapeutic range making interpretation of total drug concentrations difficult.

Active Metabolites

Metabolites which may not be measured can contribute to the therapeutic response. Examples include carbamazepine (carbamazepine-10, 11-epoxide), and procainamide (N-acetylprocainamide). Theophylline in neonates (but not in adults) is converted to caffeine, so the therapeutic range for theophylline in neonatal apnoea is 6-12 mg/L (allowing for the contribution of caffeine), whereas it is 10-20 mg/L for obstructive airways disease in adults. The therapeutic ranges for imipramine and amitriptyline are based on the combined concentrations of parent drug and active metabolite (desipramine and nortriptyline respectively). Finally, primidone treatment is monitored by measuring the concentration of the active metabolite phenobarbitone, but primidone itself and another metabolite, phenylethylmalonamide, are also active.

7.8 Economies

The cost effectiveness of TDM is demonstrated when total cost of performing the drug analysis is less than the financial savings realized in terms of reduced stay, the use of other medications and decreased side effects. Cost-benefit analysis attempts to quantify this effectiveness in terms of real money. For any drug it must be demonstrated that monitoring of the blood concentration leads to improved patient care and that there is an overall cost saving associated with use/monitoring of the drug. Studies have shown that TDM significantly reduced mortality and exhibited favourable cost-benefit as a result of reduction in length of stay, cost of patient care, decreased number of febrile episodes and improved patient survival.

7.9 TDM Details on Some Drugs

Amitriptyline: Steady-state plasma concentrations generally obtained within 7-10 days of starting treatment, although maximum clinical benefit may take up to 4-6 weeks to be achieved. The main active metabolite, nortriptyline is also measured. Blood specimens should be taken just prior to dosing (trough concentration).Target range 100-250 μg/L.

Caffeine: When used to treat apnoeic attacks in neonates, plasma caffeine concentrations appear to correlate with clinical effects. In addition to plasma concentrations, clinical symptoms of toxicity (irritability and tachycardia) should be monitored during treatment. Target range 12-36 mg/L.

Carbamazepine: Induces its own metabolism so that following the initiation of therapy, it takes 2-4 weeks to obtain a steady state. Treatment should, therefore, commence with low doses, increasing at weekly intervals for the first month. Target range 4-12 mg/L. There is no clinical value in quantifying the epoxide or other metabolites of carbamazepine.

Clomipramine: Steady-state plasma drug concentrations may take up to 4-6 weeks to be achieved. Blood specimens should be taken just prior to dosing (trough concentration).

Desipramine: Steady-state plasma concentrations are generally obtained within 7-10 days of starting treatment, although maximum clinical benefit may take up to 4-6 weeks to be achieved. Blood specimens should be taken just prior to dosing (trough concentration).

Digoxin: The low therapeutic index of digoxin means that dose adjustment must be performed with caution. Results can only be interpreted correctly if samples are taken at least 6 h post-dose to ensure that distribution of digoxin is complete. Digoxin elimination is strongly influenced by renal function. Hypokalemia and hypo magnesia may influence (increase) myocardial sensitivity to digoxin.

Dothiepin: Steady-state plasma concentrations are generally obtained within 7-10 days of starting treatment, although maximum clinical benefit may take up to 4-6 weeks to be achieved. The active metabolite, nordothiepin, is also measured. Blood specimens should be taken just prior to dosing (trough concentration).

Ethosuximide: There is good correlation between dose and plasma concentration, and a high therapeutic index for this drug. Steady-state in children is achieved in 5-7 days, compared with 10-14 days in adults.

Fluoxetine: This is the most widely prescribed of the SSRI group of antidepressants. Achieving steady-state plasma drug concentrations may take between 4-6 weeks. The main active metabolite, norfluoxetine, is also measured. This drug is also a potent inhibitor of drug metabolizing enzymes and may cause an increase in plasma drug concentrations of other drugs if prescribed at the same time. Blood specimens should be taken just prior to dosing (trough concentrations).

Gabapentin: Absorption of gabapentin is very rapid with peak concentrations occurring at 2-3 hours. The elimination half-life of 5-7 hours necessitates dosing three times daily, but steady state is achieved within 1-2 days. The drug is eliminated entirely via the kidneys as unchanged compound, resulting in the clearance being proportional to renal function.

Imipramine: Steady-state plasma drug concentrations are generally obtained within 7-10 days of starting treatment, although maximum clinical benefit may take up to 4-6 weeks. The main active metabolite, desipramine, is also measured. Blood specimens should be taken just prior to dosing (trough concentration).

Lamotrigine: Concomitant therapy with other anticonvulsants has a marked effect on clearance. Valproate doubles the half-life from 25 to 48 hrs, whilst carbamazepine and phenobarbitone reduce the half-life to around 12 hrs. There is some evidence that adverse effects of lamotrigine may be concentration dependent.

Nortriptyline: Steady-state plasma concentrations generally obtained within 7-10 days of starting treatment, although maximum clinical benefit may take up to 4-6 weeks. Blood specimens should be taken just prior to dosing (trough concentration).

Phenobarbitone: Results on samples taken before steady-state has been achieved (1-2 weeks in children; 2-4 weeks in adults) will not be helpful, except to confirm a diagnosis of toxicity.

Phenytoin: Monitoring is imperative as a guide to dosage adjustment, since phenytoin has a low therapeutic index and exhibits saturation kinetics (i.e. small increases in dose result in large increases in concentration).

Theophylline: Plasma concentrations are related predictably to both bronchodilator and toxic effects. Theophylline can be metabolized to caffeine in neonates, and in some adults where there is impairment of hepatic drug metabolism.

Valproic acid: The anticonvulsant activity and toxicity of valproic acid show no simple relationships to its plasma concentration. Hence there is generally little clinical value in the measurement of valproic acid. The short plasma half-life results in large variations in plasma concentrations between doses.

Vigabatrin: Vigabatrin irreversibly inhibits the enzyme GABA-Transaminase thereby increasing the concentration of GABA in the brain and decreasing the propagation of abnormal discharges.

Conclusion

The appropriate use of TDM ultimately leads to effective patient care management. Optimization of pharmacological therapy leads to decreased incidence of drug/drug related toxicity and decreased disease exacerbation. To ensure optimal effectiveness of TDM, good laboratory practices and use of high quality laboratory methodologies must be employed.

The cost effectiveness of TDM is demonstrated by showing that the total cost of performing the drug analysis is less than the financial savings realized in terms of reduced hospital stay, use of other medications and decreased side effects.

Thus TDM can be described as a reliable, valuable and efficient surveillance tool of patient compliance and management of therapy in patients receiving complex co-medication or suffering from other diseases.

Study Outline

Therapeutic Drug Monitoring (TDM) is a means of monitoring drug levels in the blood or any other body fluid to optimize the patient's drug therapy.

TDM is required to be done to only those drugs that have a narrow therapeutic range like cardiac glycosides, antiarrhythmic drugs, antibiotics, and immunosuppresants.

Factors to be considered during TDM

- Age and weight of patient
- Route of administration
- Absorption rate / excretion rate
- Delivery rate
- Dosage
- Other medications taken by patients

- Other diseases that patient has
- Patient compliance
- Lab methods to analyze drug concentration

Drugs that require TDM

- Which show marked pharmacokinetic variability.
- Which have concentration related therapeutic and adverse effects
- Which have narrow therapeutic index.
- Which have defined therapeutic concentration range.
- Whose desired therapeutic effect is difficult to monitor

Need for TDM

- To achieve a drug concentration which is effective without toxicity.
- To ensure appropriate, safe, and economic therapy
- To identify non compliant patients
- To identify drugs which may contribute to presentation of medical emergency.

CHAPTER 8

Drug Utilization Review

Objectives

After reading this chapter the student should be able to:

- Define and understand the concept of Drug Utilization Review (DUR) / Drug Use Evaluation
- Identify the elements for DUR
- Define the framework of the DUR program
- Understand the problems of drug use and suggest solutions

8.1 Introduction

Drugs can allay human suffering, stabilize the progression of chronic disease, and cure and control the spread of infectious disease. Conversely, drugs can cause human suffering through uncomfortable side-effects, produce iatrogenic disease states, favor the development of drug-resistant bacteria, and result in fatal outcomes. Optimal benefits of drug therapy may not be achieved because of the underutilization, overutilization, or misuse of drugs in patient care.

Given the important place that drugs have in medical treatment plans and their potential for effecting both very positive and very devastating outcomes, assuring optimal drug use merits high priority in the health care setting. Clinically oriented pharmacists can serve an important function in evaluating and improving the quality of drug therapy within their institutions.

8. 2 Definition

The *Drug Utilization Review (DUR) / Drug Use Evaluation* (*DUE*) process involves the development, use, monitoring, refinement and adjustment of objective, measurable criteria that describe the appropriate use of a drug.

The DUR may be applied to any drug; the drugs given the highest priority for evaluation are those with therapeutic problems and those with high costs.

A *Drug Use Review* (*DUR*) program, simply stated, is a quality assurance program for drug therapy. Achievement of optimal drug therapy within a health care setting is predicated on the existence of an organized, ongoing program to assess important aspects of drug use and to correct identified problems.

Prospective DUR (*PDUR*) is the review that a pharmacist conducts prior to dispensing a new prescription order. The new prescription order is reviewed with the intention of maximizing therapy, detecting problems caused by incorrect dosage, route of administration, duration of therapy, therapeutic duplication, drug-allergy or drug-disease contraindications, undesirable drug-drug interactions, inappropriate therapeutic use, and over or under utilization of medication. To conduct the Prospective DUR pharmacist should have access to information about the patient's life style, medical history, current diagnosis, past and present medication use, and laboratory values.

Retrospective DUR (*RDUR*) is a review generally involving a large number of prescription orders that have already been dispensed. This large data base is examined for potential problems, such as fraud, abuse, gross overuse, or inappropriate or medically unnecessary care among physicians, pharmacists and patients. The goal of RDUR is to maximize cost-effective, rational therapy.

8.3 Elements of DUR

The following basic elements are considered essential for Drug Utilization Review:

- Identify important or potential problems
- Determine priorities for investigating and resolving problems
- Objectively assess the cause(s) and scope of problems using clinically valid criteria
- Plan and implement actions to correct or eliminate problems

When a new or renewal prescription order is presented to the pharmacist, the following DUR elements should be considered.

- Accuracy and completeness of the prescription order
- Appropriateness of dose, route of administration, dosage schedule, and dosage form
- Previous allergic reaction or adverse effect with the prescribed drug or with a drug that is similar structurally or therapeutically, so that a similar undesired reaction could possibly occur if a new prescription is dispensed.
- Undesired change in dose and schedule with a new prescription order for a currently used medication
- Quantitative misuse of current medications by the patient i.e., over utilization or under utilization
- Undesired duplication of ingredients or therapeutic class
- Undesired additive effects from multiple medications
- Adverse effects from current medications
- Drug-drug interactions
- Drug-disease interactions
- Irrational therapeutics

8.4 Frame Work

Pharmacists and Physicians need to work together in collaboration to assure optimal drug use. The responsibility for drug review processes is generally delegated to a committee of the medical staff. The committees which may be given this authority are as mentioned below.

- ***Pharmacy and Therapeutics Committee:*** As the Pharmacy and Therapeutics Committee is responsible for overseeing all aspects of the drug cycle in the hospital, from procurement to evaluation, and also it contains the necessary mix of health care professionals, this committee is frequently responsible for directing drug review.
- ***Infection Control Committee:*** Because of its focus on surveillance and control of infections, this committee is sometimes given responsibility for antibiotic review.
- ***Medical Department Committee:*** Some hospitals choose to work through existing medical department committees (e.g., Pediatrics, Surgery, Internal Medicine, etc.) in conducting drug use review.
- ***Drug Use Review Committee:*** Some institutions may appoint a special committee with specific responsibility for drug review.

- ***Medical Audit Committee:*** This committee is delegated with the authority and accountability for evaluation of medical care services. Medical Audit Committee is standing committee of the organized medical staff. Review of medical care by other physicians is commonly referred to as peer review.
- ***Quality Assurance Committee:*** Quality Assurance Committee constituted by many institutions is a centralized committee and is responsible for integrating all of the quality assurance processes occurring throughout the institution. This committee rarely participates directly in the problem assessment and action phases of DUR, but oversees program effectiveness.

8.5 Drug Use Problems

(a) *Identification Phase*

The goal of achieving quality patient care needs us to focus on the problems associated with the use of drugs. By recognizing and identifying the problems in drug use by reviewing multiple data sources and selection of problems for assessment we can solve the problems in working towards the achievement of goals for quality patient care.

Multiple Data Sources

The pharmacist need to take the assistance of various data sources in order to identify and delineate the potential or real drug problems that might be present in a health care setting. These problems may impede the optimal drug therapy if not attended to and solved. The data sources that can be of use to a pharmacist in the process of identifying such problems are

- Medical/Pharmaceutical literature
- Adverse reaction reporting
- Clinical Pharmacist monitoring
- Incident reports
- Drug Information queries
- Medication orders
- Medical records
- Pharmacy drug use statistics
- Medication profiles

The medical or pharmaceutical literature may expose a potential problem worthy of investigation. Incident reports may provide documentation for a needed change in drug dispensing/administration systems or responsibilities. Review of a clinical pharmacist's monitoring notes or adverse reaction reporting forms may show recurrent problems and interventions, signaling the need for comprehensive assessment and action. Review of pharmacy-generated drug use statistics, medication profiles, and orders may demonstrate trends that give reason for concern. Drug information questions may expose problems or concerns.

Setting priorities in the selection of a problem

By following the above described process several drug problems may be identified in the hospital. Each identified problem may not be immediately solved due to limited personnel and financial resources for such activities. We need to set the priorities for reviewing and assessing these problems.

While establishing priorities, the problems selected should meet two essential criteria - they should be clinically significant, and they should be correctable.

1. *Clinical Significance*: Clinical Significance can be assessed by identifying the problems which have the most immediate and potentially adverse impact on patient care and patient outcome. Certain points like frequency of drug use, frequency and severity of adverse effects and severity of harmful effects resulting from inadequate or inappropriate treatment need to be considered.
2. *Correctability*: Problems which can potentially be resolved, depending on the situation of the hospital, need to be identified. There is no benefit either to the hospital or the patient in identifying a problem and documenting it which cannot be resolved. Certain issues to be considered while identifying a resolvable problem are - motivation to solve the problem, length of time the problem has existed, time and effort to complete an assessment, cost, impact on cost containment efforts, complex political realities.

The problem chosen for review should be defined clearly and specifically so that objectives can be determined to focus the review. Once the problem and objectives are set, the assessment phase can begin.

(b) *Assessment Phase*

In the assessment phase we can verify the existence of a problem and find out the cause. Also we can develop an action plan to resolve the problem.

For some problems, the nature and scope can be immediately recognized and action can be planned to resolve them without any detailed study. However, many drug use problems require further study in order to determine their cause and scope. Assessment of such problems involves verification of the following issues like -

- Whether any patient care deficiency is existing
- Identifying the person responsible for the deficiency (individual practitioner, department, or entire staff), and
- If possible, determining why the problem occurred (knowledge-gap, performance, or system deficiencies).

To answer these questions, criteria for drug use must be established, a time frame for problem assessment selected, and the patient sample or census reviewed.

Establishing Criteria

Criteria are statements of tangible elements that are deemed critical to the optimal use of a drug. The use of explicit or written criteria allows objective comparison of actual drug therapy to optimal drug use characteristics. Criteria for drug review must be clinically valid. Criteria can be developed with citations from the current literature. In developing criteria the professional experience and judgment of a local expert can be taken and will be invaluable. The criteria developed based on the literature can be needed to be amended due to differences in availability of diagnostic and laboratory procedures, variations in clinical judgment, or cost considerations.

Clinically valid criteria should be agreed upon prior to use in the assessment phase. Criteria must also be measurable. The data necessary to measure compliance to optimal drug use standards should be available to the reviewer.

By identifying important problems or potential problems in drug use and defining specific objectives of the review, it is possible to focus drug review activity on a specific facet of drug use. If the problem identified is narrow enough in scope, there may be only one criterion for review. By carefully defining the problem and the objectives the criteria can be limited to a few areas only. Managing the review of patient care based upon these limited criteria would be easy.

With problem, objectives, and criteria defined, the next step is selection of a time frame for investigation.

(c) ***Investigation Phase***

Selecting the time frame

Several time frames for drug use review might be considered.

Retrospective Review: Retrospective review entails review of drug use after it has been administered i.e., retrospective review occurs after a patient has completed a course of therapy. Retrospective review generally uses the medical record as a major resource since this record is the composite documentation of the care prescribed by the physician, including the subsequent results. Retrospective review, then, is a review of the past care provided to the patient.

The major strength of retrospective review lies in its use as a mechanism for exploring problems in depth. By applying the criteria developed to indicate quality drug use, the retrospective review depicts overall patterns of care being provided at the health care institution and identifies any deficiencies present.

The validity of patient care assessment with retrospective review is dependent upon the completeness and accuracy of the records being examined. All the information needed for comparing patient care to the established criteria must be present.

Concurrent Review: Concurrent review is the review that occurs during the course of treatment. Concurrent review is a review of contemporary or present care being provided to the patient.

Prospective Review: Prospective Review is a system in which the review is done prior to prescribing, dispensing, or administering the drug, and it anticipates the results of those actions. Prospective review is a review of the potential implications of the future care planned for the patient.

Prospective and concurrent reviews focus on individual patient care situations. Their assessment strength lies in their ability to isolate a problem for timely and relevant intervention. The assessment phase can be tied in with the action phase. The requirement of medical records in concurrent and prospective review is not much and to a lesser extent than the retrospective review.

Selecting the appropriate sample

The time and expense involved can be a prohibitive factor to review every patient during problem assessment. Therefore, a decision must be made on the selection of an appropriate population for review through census or sample techniques.

Census: A population that includes all relevant patients is a census. A census-based review would provide the true description of patient care since every patient affected would be reviewed (e.g., all patients receiving digitalis). A census may be necessary for the study of problems that occur infrequently (but which, because of their potential for serious consequences, have been selected for review). Prospective and concurrent review processes may use a census so that each patient's drug therapy can be assessed. A census is particularly important in prospective or concurrent review.

Sample: The purpose of sampling is to obtain reasonable conclusions about drug use characteristics in a health care institution from the therapy of a representative group of patients. To make valid inferences from the sample about the quality of drug use within the institution, it is important to select an appropriate sample. Two common sampling techniques used in reviewing patient cases include chunk sampling and systematic sampling. These are defined below.

- Chunk sampling: selection of a pre-determined section of the population (e.g., all patients receiving albumin during a particular month).
- Systematic sampling: random selection of the first patient and then every patient at a fixed interval (e.g., every fifth patient receiving lidocaine after random selection of the first patient).

Collecting Information

There is no standardized method for documenting or displaying drug use data. Worksheets that organize information to be used in the review process may be formatted to suit the unique needs of each review.

With a few well-defined criteria, it is a relatively simple and quick process to extract the appropriate patient care data. Though almost any category of allied health care personnel can be delegated to gather the information, there are certain advantages in involving the pharmacist in this process, particularly with prospective and concurrent time frames. The pharmacist is familiar with the physical and pharmacological properties of the drug, patient factors that might interfere with the drug's activity, and disease states. Further, it is expected that a pharmacist would have the professional motivation to identify and resolve drug use problems.

8.6 Drug Use Problems-Solutions

The process of problem identification and assessment is exhaustive and expensive. The value of this is limited unless appropriate corrective action is taken.

Corrective action depends to some extent upon the time frame selected to assess problems in drug therapy.

Retrospective review has a historical focus. By the time committees convene, review, deliberate, and recommend action, the opportunity to help the patients involved is past. Dosages cannot be modified, therapies cannot be changed. The purpose of reviewing past performance is to detect patterns of care which can be improved by developing new routines in the care of future patients.

In concurrent and prospective review, when problems in the patient care are identified, timely, relevant, and individualized feedback can be given to improve care. Initiating action prior to prescribing, dispensing, and/or administering a drug, as in prospective review, may prevent inappropriate therapy from occurring. (Inherently, this is the most effective type of assessment and action.) Initiating corrective action while the patient is receiving a drug, as in concurrent review, could lead to a better monitoring or beneficial changes in the patient care.

Action Plan - Strategies

Several methods may be useful in corrective action plans; some are discussed below and presented in Table 8.1.

- *Education:* One of the most common action plans in quality assurance is the presentation of a continuing education program which focuses on identified problems. Such programs typically include the results of recent drug reviews and are directed to those responsible for any deficiencies which may have been detected. Instances of drug use which deviate from established criteria are cited.

The desired outcome of reporting such problems is that the practitioner will apply this knowledge effectively in future patient care.

- *Restriction of Drug Usage:* Another action plan to effect compliance to drug use standards is to restrict usage of the drug. This has been a common action plan for improving antibiotic usage within an institution. Consultation with an infectious disease specialist is required in some hospitals before certain antibiotics may be used; in other cases, antibiotics have been withdrawn from the formulary. Such control systems have been shown to alter prescribing practices.
- *System Changes*: When the assessment phase indicates that inappropriate drug use arises from organizational or environmental problems, actions to implement changes in systems would be appropriate. Examples of system changes may include extending pharmacy services to twenty-four hours, purchasing equipment to perform serum drug assays and developing or revising certain policies and procedures. Implementation of new services to support quality drug usage may also be an appropriate action (e.g., initiating drug information, clinical, pharmacokinetic, or nutritional support services).
- *Prospective or Concurrent Intervention:* Another strategy for action is to identify and correct the deviation from optimal drug use prospectively or concurrently.

Table 8.1 Strategies for Corrective Action

Method	Example
Education	Teaching conferences Pharmacy newsletter Report of DUR results Memorandum to individual practitioner
Restriction of drug usage	Withdrawal of drug from formulary Require consultation prior to prescribing Report susceptibility test result for selected antimicrobial.
System changes	Add personnel Purchase equipment Revise policies and procedures Implement new service(s)
Prospective or concurrent Intervention (s)	Identify deviation(s) from optional drug use Recommend changes in drug therapy

The clinical pharmacist is uniquely qualified to conduct prospective and concurrent review. Since the advent of clinical pharmacy, monitoring patient drug therapy has been an important part of the clinical pharmacist's activities. The prospective and concurrent review processes use written, clinically valid criteria to assess therapeutic regimens. In order to contribute to improvement in the quality of patient drug therapy, the pharmacist would need to intervene to recommend change or request information supporting the value of the present regimen.

Prospective and concurrent assessment and action have exciting implications for clinical pharmacy. Participation in such reviews augments and expands our professional role as drug therapy advisors. It adds a new dimension to patient care by developing a program to prevent or correct problems related to drug therapy and to improve the quality of drug therapy by application of optimal drug use standards to daily care of patients. It also introduces the non-clinically trained pharmacist to patient care evaluation through physician-endorsed, written criteria.

A drug review program employing all types of review — retrospective, concurrent, and prospective, would probably provide the most comprehensive and productive evaluation of drug use. Thorough retrospective studies are useful in identifying aspects of care that could be improved by immediate action through prospective or concurrent intervention.

8.7 Role of Computers in DUR

Computer technology has permeated the medical environment, providing data management for administrative, financial, and patient care needs. Computers can provide quantitative and qualitative assistance in DUR, depending on the comprehensiveness of the system. They can be used to profile drug consumption data, isolate patients for review, provide specialized monitoring functions, or automate the assessment and assurance of optimal drug therapy.

- *Drug Consumption.* Several types of statistical reports can be generated by computers that are useful for characterizing drug prescribing frequencies. Programs for retrieving, sorting, and statistically describing drug use have been developed and are now in use. Because the resultant reports primarily focus on distribution and cost aspects of drug usage, the reports have limited potential for identifying and evaluating specific prescribing problems. However, such reports may prove useful in formal DUR studies.
- *Patient Identification.* Computerized records are also important in identifying patients for assessment or action. In retrospective review, reports can be generated to identify patients who meet the desired sample characteristics. Depending on the scope of the computer services, these reports can be sorted by multiple variables including date, medical service, drug, therapeutic class, diagnosis, patient age, sex, and inpatient/outpatient status.

- *Specialized Computer Functions*. In recent years we have witnessed a growth in the application of computer technology in a number of ways related to drug therapy.

  Certain computer programs are developed which recommends therapeutic regimens, customizes dosing specific to a patient's age and renal function, and generates graph depicting the expected blood level of each drug as a function of time.

  Pharmacokinetic dosing services supported by computer have been reviewed in the literature. Computers have also been used for the iterative process of checking drug-drug interactions, drug-lab interactions, and allergies in each patient, alerting the pharmacist to potential problems. These drug interaction screening programs, pharmacokinetic services, and consultation programs all support the goal of optimal drug use and can be integrated into a quality assurance program as a mechanism to identify problems, thereby permitting immediate intervention.

- *Comprehensive Clinical Computer System*. The clinical computer system has the potential for reaching all patients to assure quality drug use. Essential characteristics of this system include: 1) integration into one shared data base of all elements of information related to patient care, and 2) a system programmed to monitor the content of the medical information and provide relevant feedback when it detects deviations from optimal care.

  Some of the computer programs use the patient's complete medical record to provide alerts on potential drug-related problems. It monitors drug-drug, drug-laboratory, and drug-disease interactions, drug allergies, and therapy with aminoglycosides, digitalis, and anti-coagulants. The criteria set developed by pharmacologists, pharmacists, and physicians, is applied automatically to all patient drug orders. It alerts the pharmacist to potential problems with a warning message displayed on the terminal screen and simultaneously printed as hard copy. The pharmacist then investigates the problem, serving as the informational interface between computer and physician, recording the alert and its effect on patient care.

Conclusion

Drug utilization review is a quality assurance program for drug therapy. Drug utilization review or drug use evaluation has the potential for achieving optimal drug therapy and to maximize the professional role as clinical pharmacists. Clinical pharmacy and quality assurance have a symbiotic relationship, and this union provides considerable advantage for the patient.

Study Outline

Drug use review (DUR) program is a quality assurance program for drug therapy. The DUR process involves the development, use, monitoring, refinement and adjustment of objective, measurable criteria that describe the appropriate use of a drug.

The following basic elements are considered essential for DUR.

- identify important or potential problems
- objectively assess the causes(s) and scope of problems using clinically valid criteria.
- plan and implement actions to correct or eliminate problem.

Pharmacists and Physicians need to work together in collaboration to assure optimal drug use. Several committees in the hospital are involved in this process like Pharmacy and Therapeutics Committee, Infection Control Committee, Medical Department Committee, Drug Use Review Committee, Medical Audit Committee, Quality Assurance Committee.

There are 3 phases in identifying the drug use problems

- Identification phase
- Assessment phase
- Investigation phase

Corrective action need to be undertaken for the problems after extensive, exhaustive and expensive studies. There are several methods useful in corrective action plans like education, restriction of drug usage, system changes, prospective or concurrent intervention.

Computers can play an important role in DUR

CHAPTER 9

Drug Information Services

Objectives

After reading this chapter the student should be able to:

- Identify drug information questions from various practice settings
- Respond to requests for drug information in a timely manner
- Obtain accurate and thorough background information necessary to respond to the drug information question
- Systematically and efficiently search appropriate drug information sources
- Use appropriate primary, secondary and tertiary reference sources in providing answers to drug information questions
- Critically analyze and synthesize information from primary, secondary, and tertiray sources as appropriate
- Formulate clinically relevant drug information responses to optimize patient care and outcomes
- Document in an understandable and accurate manner all appropriate information from drug information questions in an electronic method designed for this purpose
- Evaluate primary literature, such as a randomized, controlled trial, and determine its application to clinical practice
- Effectively communicate drug information to other health professionals and/or patients verbally and in writing

9.1 Introduction

Drug information refers to the provision of unbiased, well referenced and critically evaluated up-to-date information on any aspect of drug use. The information asked may be

- specific to an individual patient
- relative to a group of patients
- for academic or research purposes.

Drug information service is the most fundamental responsibility of the Pharmacist. Pharmacist can also serve as a resource for issues regarding cost effective medication selection and use, medication policy decisions (drug benefits), medication information resource selection or practice related issues.

Drug information service refers to activities that are part of the overall pharmacy service or Pharmaceutical Care process.

Drug information centre refers to the specialized facility that provides drug information to those who need it.

Poison information refers to a specialized area of drug information that provides information on the toxic effects of an extensive range of chemicals, including plant and animal toxins.

The term Drug information was first developed in the early 1960's. In the year 1962 the first Drug information centre was established at the University of Kentucky. In the year 1963 a survey was conducted in the United States of America by the National Library of Medicine to identify the availability of drug literature and the complexities involved in accessing drug information. The results of the survey which came out in the year 1965 clearly justified the implementation of Drug Information Center's in health care delivery.

The term *drug information* may have different meanings to different people depending on the context in which it is used.

In many cases individuals put this term in different contexts by associating it with other words, including

- Specialist / Practitioner / Pharmacist / Provider
- Center / Service / Practice
- Functions / Skills

The first group of words implies a specific individual, the second a place, and the third activities and abilities of individuals. The term *drug information* will be used in these different contexts to describe the beginnings and evolution of this area of practice. The term *medication information* is used in place of *drug information* to convey the management and use of information on medication therapy and to signify the broader role that all pharmacists take in information provision. Drug informatics is another term used to describe the evolving roles of the drug information specialist.

9.2 Services

A drug information centre or service provider can give all or some of the services as listed below.

- Support for clinical services
  - Answering questions
  - Developing criteria/guidelines for medication use
- Pharmacy and therapeutics committee activity
  - Development of medication use policies
  - Formulary management
- Publications – newsletter, journal columns
- Education – Patient education, health care professionals and students
- Medication usage evaluation
- Investigational medication control
  - Institutional Review Board activities
  - Information for practitioners
- Coordination of reporting programs – e.g., adverse drug reactions
- Poison information

9.3 Poison Information

Poison information is a specialized area of medication information with the practitioner typically practicing in an accredited poison information center or an emergency room. Similar to the mission of traditional drug information centers, poison information centers exist to provide accurate and timely information to enhance the quality of care for patients. However, there are several differences between a traditional drug information center and poison control center. Health professionals generate most consultations received in drug information centers, whereas in a poison control center most are generated from the public. Poison information centers must be prepared to provide information on management of any poison situation including household products, medications, and other chemicals. Because of the type of information that the specialist provides, nearly all requests for information to a poison control center are urgent, with an average response time of 5 minutes, compared to anywhere from 30 minutes to days for drug information centers, depending on the urgency of the call and complexity of information required. A specialist in poison information therefore requires expertise in clinical toxicology, as well as an ability to obtain a complete history that correctly assesses the potential severity of exposure, an understanding of where to search for this type of information, and the ability to communicate the information and plan in a comprehensive, concise, and accurate manner to a consumer at all levels of education.

9.4 Drug Information - Health Professionals Requirements

Health professional may ask a question from any of the above categories, the particular needs of each group may vary. The needs of physicians, nurses, and pharmacists only will be discussed in this chapter

- *Physicians:* When physicians prescribe drugs, they are required to make decisions regarding drug therapy in a wide range of patient types and disease states. Many times, the ability to make a rational decision will require some drug information. Most of the times, the questions of physicians are directly related to prescribing or monitoring drug therapy. As physicians are busy with their practice, they find it difficult to research questions on their own. Pharmacists have greater access to current drug literature because of their education and experience.
- *Nurses:* In many hospitals, nurses are responsible for administering drugs to patients, the majority of nurses drug information questions are concerned with drug administration. Nurses are often confronted with the problem of giving multiple parenteral drugs which need to be given at the same time to patient with only one intravenous line. Nurses are also the health professionals who have the most patient contact; therefore, they are generally the first ones to observe adverse drug reactions or to hear patients complain of them. Pharmacist is the right person to serve as primary source of drug information for nursing personnel.
- *Pharmacists:* Pharmacists have drug information questions of their own. In their drug-dispensing capacity, pharmacists encounter numerous questions from each of the eight categories described above. In order for pharmacists to be able to answer their own questions and act as the primary source of drug information for other health professionals, they must have access to an adequate reference library and knowledge of alternative sources of drug information.

9.5 Drug Information Resources

While obtaining the drug information generally, a stepwise approach is used which involves consulting tertiary and secondary (e.g. indexing and abstracting services, which can be computer based or hard copy) resources followed by primary (e.g., research articles from biomedical journals) resources.

1. ***Tertiary Resources / Literature***

Tertiary literature is sometimes referred to as general literature, and full-text computer data bases (e.g., *MICROMEDEX*, *Computerized Clinical Information System* [CCIS]. Tertiary references can be divided into five basic types:

- Product oriented
- Drug oriented
- Disease oriented
- Specific topic and
- Specialty

The basic library must contain representative references from the first four types. In addition, review articles in biomedical journals are sometimes classified as tertiary literature.

Types of Tertiary Literature

- Textbooks
- Compendia
- Full-text computer databases (including the Internet)
- Review articles

(a) ***Product-oriented references:*** This type of reference is generally the best information source for availability and identification questions. Some examples are described below.

- *American Drug Index:* (Billups, N.F., ed. J.B. Lippincott Co.Published annually). Alphabetical listing of products giving manufacturer, chemical name, and dosage forms, strengths, category of use. Cross-indexed by generic and trade name. Also includes manufacturer's addresses and phone numbers.
- *American Druggist Blue Book* (Hearst Corporation) and Drug Topics Red Book. (Medical Economics Co. Published annually). Alphabetical listing of products giving manufacturer, dosage forms, package sizes, and costs. Also include product identification guide and manufacturer's addresses and phone numbers.
- *Facts and Comparisons:* (Kastrup , I.K., ed J.B Lippincott Co. Updated monthly). Provides product monographs, comparative information on similar products, and cost index. Includes section on investigational drugs.

- *Handbook of Nonprescription Drugs*. (American Pharmaceutical Assn. Published about every two years). Contains monographs on various classes of nonprescription drugs. Compares contents of products in similar classes.
- *PharmIndex*. (Skyline Publishers, Inc. Updated monthly). Contains brief descriptions of new products, changed products, discontinued items, investigational products, and costs. Also contains a review article in each update.
- *Physicians Desk Reference*: (Medical Economics Co. Published annually). Product package inserts arranged by manufacturer. Also includes product identification guide and manufacturer's addresses and phone numbers.

(b) ***Drug-oriented references:*** These references have a stronger emphasis on the particular drug class than on the product. Types of questions which can generally be answered with these references are listed in their description. Some examples are presented below.

- *American Hospital Formulary Service*: (McEvoy, G.K., ed. American Society of Hospital Pharmacists. Updated bi-monthly). Contains extensive monographs on drugs and drug classes. Excellent source for the following categories: adverse drug reactions, drug interactions, pharmacokinetics, therapeutics and pharmacology.
- *Martindale, the Extra Pharmacopoeia*. (Blacow, N.W.ed. The Pharmaceutical Press [London]. Published every five years). Contains extensive referenced monographs on drugs and drug classes with international coverage. Excellent source for the following information categories adverse reactions, drug interactions, foreign drugs, pharmacokinetics, therapeutics and pharmacology.
- *Pharmacological Basis of Therapeutics:* (Gilman, A.G., Goodman, L.S., Gilman, A., eds. Macmillan Publishing Co. Published every five years). An extensive pharmacology textbook. Excellent source for the following categories: adverse drug reactions, pharmacokinetics, therapeutics and pharmacology.
- *Remington's Pharmaceutical Sciences*. (Osol, A., ed. Mack Publishing Co. Published every five years). Excellent pharmacy textbook includes chapters on drug classes with individual drug monographs and several other chapters useful in providing drug information. Excellent source for the following categories: drug interactions, pharmaceutical calculations, pharmaceutical compatibility and stability, therapeutics and pharmacology.

- *United States Pharmacopoeia Dispensing Information*: (United States Pharmacopoeia Convention, Inc. Published annually with updates). Contains drug monographs and drug or drug class patient consultation guidelines. Excellent source for the following categories: adverse drug reactions, drug interactions, therapeutics and pharmacology.

(c) ***Disease – oriented references:*** These references generally contain chapters on disease states. They are very useful for questions in therapeutics and pharmacology category when asked from the disease perspective, i.e., how you treat a given disease state. Some examples are given below.

- *Current Medical Diagnosis and Treatment*. (Krupp, M.A., Chaton, M.J., eds. Lange Medical Publications. Published annually).
- *Current Therapy*. (Conn, H.F., ed. W.B. Saunders Co. Published annually).
- *Applied Therapeutics for Clinical Pharmacists*. (Koda-Kimble, M.A., Katcher, B.S., Young, L.Y., eds. Applied Therapeutics, Inc. Published approximately every three to four years).
- *Cecil Textbook of Medicine*. (Wyngaarden, J.B., Smith, L.H., eds. W.B. Saunders Co. Published every four years).

(d) ***Specific topic references***: Compatibility of intravenous drugs, drug interactions, and poisonings are topics which require entire books to answer. Some examples are listed below.

- *Handbook of Injectable Drugs*. (Trissel, L.A. American Society of Hospital Pharmacists).
- *Guide to Parenteral Admixtures*. (King, J.C. Cutter Laboratories, Inc).
- *Drug Interactions*. (Hansten, P.D. Lea and Febiger).
- *Evaluations of Drug Interactions*. (American Pharmaceutical Association).
- *Clinical Toxicology of Commercial Products*. (Gosselin, R.E., *et al.* Williams and Wilkins C.)
- *Handbook of Poisoning*. (Dreisbach, R.R. Lange Medical Publications).
- *Applied Pharmacokinetics*. (Evans, W.E., Schentage, J.J., Jusko, W.J., eds. Applied Therapeutics, Inc.)

To summarize the above, a typical pharmacy library must contain the following textbooks:

- American Druggist Blue Book
- Facts and Comparisons

- Physicians' Desk Reference
- American Hospital Formulary Service
- Martindale, the Extra Pharmacopoeia
- Pharmacological Basis of Therapeutics
- Remington's Pharmaceutical Sciences
- Current Therapy
- Handbook of Injectable Drugs
- Drug Interactions
- Handbook of Poisoning
- Applied Pharmacokinetics

With only these twelve reference books, large majority of drug information questions could be answered.

2. *Secondary Literature*

Secondary literature consists of indexing and abstracting services of the primary literature. An indexing system provides only bibliographic information that is indexed by topic, whereas an abstracting service also provides a brief description (abstract) of information contained in a specific citation. Although most of these resources provide access to primary literature, each covers different biomedical journals, meeting abstracts, newsletters, textbooks, and other publications; therefore, use of more than one of these resources often allows for more thorough information retrieval.

Some Sources:

- *Anti-infectives Today* (Published monthly) – An indexing and abstracting service that summarizes current literature on drug therapy and management of infections.
- *BIOSIS Previews*: A major comprehensive resource that covers all areas of biological research, including the biomedical sciences.
- *Cancer Today*: An indexing and abstracting service that summarizes current literature on the use of drugs in the management of cancer.
- *ClinAlert*: A secondary system of adverse reaction case reports including herbal products and literature citations.
- *Index Medicus*: An index to the biomedical literature that contains references from over 3000 journals.
- *International Pharmaceutical Abstracts*: The most comprehensive abstracting service for international information relevant to pharmacy and pharmaceutical sciences.

- *Iowa Drug Information System (IDIS):* An indexing service that allows retrieval of complete articles from over 180 biomedical journals.
- *Journal Watch:* An abstracting service by the publishers of *New England Journal of Medicine* that includes recent citations from general medicine literature.
- *MEDLINE:* One of the most expansive databases of biomedical information containing approximately 370,000 references. Citations from 1966 to the present can be searched from approximately 3500 journals.
- *LEXIS-NEXIS:* This indexing and abstracting service with some full-text features provides access to wide range of news, business, legal and reference information.

3. ***Primary Literature***

Primary literature consists of research studies published in biomedical journals. Primary literature is usually the most current resource for information. Unlike tertiary or secondary resources, primary literature provides details of research methodology and scientific results that lead to therapeutic conclusions. Users of primary literature are, therefore, able to determine whether the study conclusions are sound based, on the strength of the research techniques and scientific results of the study. Tertiary and secondary resources consist of a review of published primary literature that may be biased or inaccurate.

The primary literature is growing at an exponential rate. Over 20,000 biomedical journals are published annually.

Some Sources:

- *Alternative Medicine Alert:* A news letter dealing with alternative medicines. Published monthly.
- *American Druggist:* A pharmacy magazine with a community pharmacy focus that provides information on issues relevant to this practice setting. Published monthly.
- *American Journal of Cardiology:* A journal dedicated to the specialty of Cardiology. Published weekly. Website: www.cardiosource.com
- *American Journal of Health System Pharmacy:* A journal focused on clinical and managerial aspects of pharmacy practice in health systems.

  Website: www.ashp.org
- *American Journal of Therapeutics:* A journal that provides clinical and pharmacoeconomic perspectives on pharmacotherapeutic advances.
- *America's Pharmacist:* The official journal of the National Community Pharmacists Association. Published monthly.

- *Annals of Internal Medicine:* A highly regarded medical journal of the American College of Physicians that focuses on internal medicine.

  Website: www.acponline.org/journals/annals

- *The Annals of Pharmacotherapy:* A well respected journal pertaining to safe, effective, and economical use of pharmacotherapeutic agents. Published monthly.

- *Archives of Internal Medicine:* A journal specializing in the practice of internal medicine including diagnosis and treatment of diseases. Published monthly. Website: www.ama-assn.org

- *Clinical Pharmacokinetics:* A journal that provides review articles in the area of clinical pharmacokinetics

- *The Community Pharmacist:* A journal published to meet the professional and educational needs of today's practitioner. Published bimonthly.

- *The Consultant Pharmacist:* The official journal of the ASCP devoted to pharmacists who provide consultative services in various environments. Published monthly. Website: www.ascp.org

- *Drugs:* A journal that publishes review articles on pharmacotherapeutic aspects of both new and established drugs. Published monthly.

- *F-D-C Reports (The Pink Sheet):* A news letter aimed at executives in the pharmaceutical industry that provides information pertinent to the pharmaceutical industry. Website: www.fdcreports.com

- *F-D-C Reports (The Tan Sheet):* A news letter aimed at executives in the pharmaceutical industry that provides information pertinent to the over-the-counter and herbal products. Website: www.fdcreports.com

- *Hospital Pharmacy:* A journal devoted to the practice of pharmacy in institutional settings. Published monthly.

- *JAMA. The Journal of American Medical Association:* One of the premier medical journals that publishes investigations and review information of key importance to health care. Published weekly. Website: www.jama.ama-assn.org

- *Journal of the American Pharmaceutical Association:* The official journal of the American Pharmaceutical Association that publishes news, information, and research in the areas of pharmacotherapeutic management of diseases, trends in pharmacy practice and the provision of pharmaceutical care.

- *Journal of Pharmaceutical Sciences:* A journal that focuses on the application of physical and analytical chemistry to the pharmaceutical sciences and technologies. Published monthly. Website: interscience.wiley.com

- *The New England Journal of Medicine:* One of the premier medical journals that publishes original investigations and review information considered of significant importance to physicians and other health care professionals. Website: www.nejm.org
- *Pharmacy Times:* A pharmacy magazine with a community practice focus that provides information on new drug therapies, patient counseling and management, and issues relevant to pharmacy practice. Published monthly.
- *U.S.Pharmacist:* A Pharmacy magazine focused on the practice of community pharmacy and issues pertinent to this setting. Published monthly. Website: www.uspharmacist.com

Alternate Sources of Drug Information:

- Internet, list servers and USENET news
- Local and national professional organizations
- Pharmaceutical Manufacturers
- Drug Information and poison control centers

9.6 Formulating Response

Most queries the pharmacists receive are not purely academic or general in nature. Often they get specific questions on patients and unique circumstances. Requestors for information are generally vague in verbalizing their needs and provide specific information only when probed further. The requestor, regardless of their background, is often uncertain about what the pharmacist needs to know to assist them in a reasonable manner. The pharmacist must expertly elicit the critical information that is required to answer a query, as many times requestors do not volunteer this information irrespective of their background.

Before attempting to formulate responses, pharmacists must consider several important questions to ensure that they understand the context of the query and scope. Drug information services may use the systematic approach, or an adaptation of it, as the basis for responding to drug information inquiries.

Factors to be considered when formulating a response

Patient Specific Factors:

- Demographics (e.g., name, age, height, weight, gender, race/ethnic group, setting)
- Primary diagnosis and medical problem list
- Allergies / Intolerances
- End-organ function, immune function, nutritional status

- Chief compliant
- History of present illness
- Past medical history (including surgeries, radiation exposure, immunizations, psychiatric illnesses, etc.).
- Family history
- Social history (e.g., alcohol intake, smoking, substance abuse, exposure to environmental or occupational toxins, income, education, religion, travel, diet, physical activity stress, risky behavior)
- Review of the body systems
- Medications (prescribed, over-the-counter)
- Physical examination
- Laboratory tests
- Diagnostic studies or responses

Disease Specific Factors:

- Definition
- Epidemiology
- Etiology
- Pathophysiology
- Clinical findings (signs and symptoms etc.)
- Diagnosis
- Treatment (medical, surgical, radiation, biological, gene therapies and others)
- Prevention and control
- Risk factors
- Complications
- Prognosis

Medication Specific factors:

- Name of the medication or substance
- Status and availability (investigational, OTC, prescription etc.)
- Physicochemical properties
- Pharmacology and Pharmacodynamics
- Pharmacokinetics

- Uses (FDA approved and unlabeled)
- Adverse effects
- Allergy / Cross reactivity
- Contraindications and precautions
- Effects of age, organ system function, disease, pregnancy, etc.
- Mutagenicity and Carcinogenicity
- Effect on fertility, pregnancy, and lactation
- Acute or Chronic toxicity
- Drug Interactions (drug-drug, drug-food, drug-lab)
- Administration (routes and methods)
- Dosage and schedule
- Dosage forms, formulations, preservatives, excipients, product appearance, delivery systems
- Monitoring parameters (therapeutic or toxic)
- Product preparation (procedures , methods)
- Compatibility and stability

Formulating Response - Step wise Approach

Step I. Secure demographics of requestor

Step II. Obtain background information

Step III. Determine and categorize ultimate question

Step IV. Develop strategy and conduct search

Step V. Perform evaluation, analysis, and synthesis

Step VI. Formulate and provide response

Step VII. Conduct follow-up and documentation.

Step I: Securing demographics of requestor

The first step in the step wise approach is to accept the initial question and secure requestor demographics. Determining what a drug information requestor actually wants to know is the first step in answering a question. This is done by classifying the type of requestor (i.e., physician, pharmacist, nurse) and obtaining the necessary background information.

Knowing the type of requestor will aid the pharmacist in determining the type and amount of information necessary to answer the question.

When a question involves a patient, it is important to obtain background information about the patient before responding to the query. The extent of the background information necessary to answer a question varies with the type of question. The patient's age, weight, and sex are usually needed. Specifics about the patient's medical condition, such as current diagnosis, kidney and liver function, are often important. In some cases, it may be necessary to obtain a complete medication history.

Step II: Obtaining background information

The following background information need to be collected

- Requestor's name
- Requestor's location and/or mobile number
- Requestor's affiliation (institution or practice), if a health care professional
- Requestor's frame of reference (i.e., title, profession or occupation, rank)
- Resources that the requestor already consulted
- Whether the request is patient specific or academic
- Patient's diagnosis, other medications, and pertinent medical information
- Urgency of the request (i.e., negotiate the time response)

Step III: Categorization of the question

The determination of the ultimate question is important for effective use of the modified systematic approach. If background information is obtained in an open, productive exchange, the ultimate question is easily unveiled; if adequate background information is not obtained, the determination of the ultimate question may not be possible. The ultimate question may essentially be the same as the original question, particularly if the question is truly not patient specific.

Step IV: Search Strategy

The categorization of the ultimate question prompts the resource selection process. For example, the categorization of a question as 'adverse effect' suggests the use of adverse effect oriented resources. Once resources have been selected, they are prioritized based on the probability of containing the information or data desired. Without prioritization, resources may be utilized based on ease of access or degree of comfort, instead of probable efficiency.

Once the background information has been obtained, the question can be classified in one of the categories discussed earlier (adverse reactions, availability, drug interactions, etc). With this classification in mind, the pharmacist should determine which type of reference would be the best to obtain the needed information (product oriented, drug oriented, etc). Reaching for the right reference first greatly adds to the efficiency of the process. Another important consideration which will help the pharmacist reach the right book first knows how often the reference is updated or when a particular edition was published. Basically, in a systematic search, the pharmacist should attempt to find the answer in tertiary references first. Answers usually can be found, but if they cannot, the pharmacist moves on to the next step. The next steps depend on the extent of the pharmacy library. If it includes secondary sources or drug information retrieval systems, these should be utilized. They provide a mechanism to obtain information from the primary literature and sometimes provide sufficiently detailed information to serve as a reference. Next, the primary literature is consulted, i.e., the pharmacist refers directly to journals which may contain the desired information.

If primary and secondary sources are not available in the pharmacy library, or if no answer can be found utilizing them, a drug information center or pharmaceutical manufacturer should be called for assistance.

Step V: Data evaluation, Analysis, and Synthesis

The information retrieved must be objectively critiqued at this stage.

Step VI: Formulation and provision of response

Answers to drug information questions should be communicated in a timely and professional manner. Consideration should be given to the time requirements of the individual requesting information. For example, if a nurse makes a "stat" request for information on the proper administration of a drug, even the most complete and accurate answer available will be useless if communicated six hours later.

The majority of questions will be answered verbally. Pharmacists should present their findings, with confidence and in a professional manner; responses should be brief, concise, and accurate.

Sometimes, questions need to be answered in a written form. The writing should be well organized, grammatically correct, and delivered in a timely manner.

Step VII: Follow up

Whenever possible, follow-up should be provided on certain types of questions, especially questions that are directly related to patient care. For example, a patient has an adverse reaction to a particular drug, and the physician asks for an alternative therapy. After a systematic literature search, the pharmacist can make his recommendation. He should utilize this opportunity to go to the floor, see how the patient is responding to his recommendation, and offer additional consultation. Consistent follow-up of this type increases interaction with other health professionals, which may promote increased pharmacist participation in direct care, including clinical rounds.

9.7 Drug Information Presentation

Drug Information can be provided using various vehicles like, pharmacy newsletters and verbal presentations, formal lectures etc.

Pharmacy Newsletter: Pharmacy newsletter can be a valuable service to health care professionals. The newsletter serves as a vehicle for providing drug information, and also helps the pharmacist become recognized as an excellent source of drug information. The following are guidelines for designing a pharmacy newsletter.

- Selecting Topics: Selecting appropriate topics for publication in a pharmacy newsletter is probably the most important consideration. Methods for selecting topics which will be useful are discussed below.

  Drug Information: The drug information questions received in the pharmacy are often a big help in selecting a topic. A particular question or type of question asked on numerous occasions signals the need for information on the subject. A newsletter could provide this information in an efficient manner to a large number of people.

  Pharmacy and therapeutics committee actions: A newsletter is an excellent means of communicating the actions and decisions of the pharmacy and therapeutics committee to an institution's professional staff. Information on new formulary additions can be communicated with little additional work for the pharmacist by utilizing the drug information reports presented to the committee. Policy changes affecting the use of drugs such as dosage standardizations, restricted drugs, method of handling controlled substances, etc., would be useful topics. A discussion of the formulary system, including how drugs are admitted to the formulary, can be presented periodically to reinforce the concept.

  Drug use review program: A pharmacy newsletter can be an educational tool to combat inappropriate use of drugs uncovered by drug use review studies. For example, if a drug use review finds that surgeons are not ordering prophylactic antibiotics properly, an article in the newsletter could outline how the agents should be used.

Journal articles: The articles in journals received by the pharmacy will give the pharmacist insight into topics of current interest. This includes review articles on therapeutic classes, clinical drug trials, adverse drug reaction reports, and descriptions of drug interactions.

- Writing for a Particular Audience: The drug information specialist should consider the audience and accordingly select topics and decide what to write. The pharmacist may choose to write one newsletter for physicians and another for nurses or include topics of interest to both in a single newsletter. Pharmacists will benefit from articles written for either group.

  Physicians: Topics from any of the four areas-drug information, pharmacy and therapeutic committee actions, drug use review program, and journal articles, are appropriate and useful for physicians. The content of any article should be geared to promoting rational therapeutics. The content of any articles should contain information brought together from several sources and put into a useful format.

  Nurses. Nurses can benefit from articles from any of the topics mentioned above. Content of any topic should be geared to drug administration and monitoring.

  Newsletter articles for any group should be written in brief and concise style. Neither physicians, nurses, nor pharmacists will take the time to read a ten page newsletter, even one which is well written.

- Publication and Distribution: The pharmacy newsletter must project a professional image. Proper appearance will greatly add to the newsletter's credibility and acceptance. The heading should be attractive, with the source of the newsletter clearly defined.

  A distribution list must be maintained and updated, and it should include the hospital administrator.

9.8 Oral / Verbal Presentations

Oral or verbal presentations either as formal or informal lectures, in service presentations etc., are another vehicle for providing drug information. Pharmacy involvement in verbal presentations begins when the pharmacist offers to participate. Once the health professionals in an institution see what a pharmacist has to offer, invitations become more and more frequent.

- *Selecting Topics:* Methods for selecting topics for presentation are identical to those for selecting newsletter topics. Topics that require demonstration, for example, proper administration or preparation of drugs, are especially suited to verbal presentation. Topics which are likely to generate discussion, such as the appropriate use of a new class of antibiotics or a comparison of the efficacy of an old inexpensive drug to a new expensive drug, are excellent choices.

- *Presenting to a Particular Audience*: The pharmacist should project a self-confident and professional image while making a presentation. This will enhance the pharmacist's credibility and acceptance, particularly with physicians. .
- *Teaching Techniques and Strategies*: There are several teaching techniques and strategies like length of the presentation, objectives of the presentation, instructional aids, handouts etc., which will aid in the presentation. The pharmacist should be brief in his presentation, inform the objectives of the presentation in the beginning, use instructional aids like transparencies, slides, charts, chalkboard etc., for the presentation.

9.9 Role of Drug Information in Hospital Committees

One of the important functions of the pharmacist is to involve in hospital committees. The Pharmacy and Therapeutics committee and the committee on drug use review have strong need for a pharmacist with drug information skills. Participation in these groups increases one's exposure and aids in recognition of the pharmacists as the best source for drug information.

Pharmacy and Therapeutics Committee

The pharmacy and therapeutics committee is the policy recommending body to the medical staff and hospital administration on matters related to the therapeutic use of drugs. Several functions of this committee can be supported by drug information from the pharmacist.

- *Evaluating Drugs for Inclusion in the Hospital's Formulary.* The pharmacist should take a leadership role in evaluating drugs requested for addition to the hospital's formulary. The pharmacist writes an informational and evaluative report on the drug. Reports on all requested drugs are then sent to all committee members in time for review before a meeting.

  In preparing these reports, the pharmacist must keep in mind that the formulary should strive to be sufficiently broad to meet the usual clinical problems, and, at the same time, minimize duplication within given therapeutic categories. The following sections should be included in the report.

  - general description (including indications)
  - pharmacology and pharmacokinetics
  - efficacy (documented by clinical trials)
  - adverse effects

- dosage and administration
- cost
- recommendation
- references

Making a recommendation will probably be the most difficult component of the report. This can be made easier by following a basic principle. For a drug to be recommended for addition to the formulary, it should meet at least one of the criteria listed below.

- a drug in a new class
- a drug with fewer side effects than similar formulary drugs.
- a drug with pharmacokinetic advantages over similar formulary drugs
- a drug which is more efficacious than similar formulary drugs
- a drug equal in every respect to similar formulary agents but that costs less

The recommendation section should also include any drugs which can be considered for deletion from the formulary if the requested drug is added.

- *Educational Function*. Another primary function of the pharmacy and therapeutics committee is to serve as an educational body for the professional staff of the hospital. The pharmacist can play an important role here by publishing a newsletter or therapeutic bulletin and presenting lectures, seminars, and grand rounds in his institution.

Drug Use Review Committee

Drug use review programs may be a part of either the pharmacy and therapeutics committee or the medical audit committee, or it may be a separate entity. Irrespective of what group is responsible, a pharmacist who provides drug information can be invaluable. Drug information skills would be useful in the establishment of audit criteria in such studies.

Other Committees

Ethics Committee, the Infection Control Committee and The Nutrition Committee are the other committees where the drug information skills of a pharmacist can be utilized.

9.10 Drug Information – Literature Evaluation

(A) *Basics*

Literature evaluation skills are essential in many areas of pharmacy practice. Pharmacists are faced with an increasingly literate patient population who educate themselves about drug therapy by consulting various individuals (e.g., health care professionals, surveyors of alternative medicine, family, and friends), searching the Internet, and reading both the medical literature and lay press. Such patients often seek the advice of a pharmacist to interpret information they have obtained. Likewise, physicians and other health care professionals often contact pharmacists for opinions regarding various aspects of therapy. Unbiased responses to these inquires can only be provided after careful analysis of available studies. In addition, decisions on drug policy management, such as whether to add or delete a drug from the formulary, should be based on careful review of the literature.

Currently there are more than 25,000 biomedical journals which are published annually. With such a vast number of medical literatures available the job of the Drug Information Specialist is too demanding and requires lot of skill to evaluate the available drug information. Continuing education programs and symposia help pharmacists keep up with this information; however, these resources may be subject to the bias of the author, sponsor of the program, or the literature used to prepare the programs or symposia. Pharmacists, therefore, must learn to systematically review and critique the biomedical literature. Skills in literature evaluation enable pharmacists to efficiently and effectively determine which treatment options represent therapeutic advances and which lack the potential to improve patient care and perhaps may even be harmful.

(i) *Evaluating Controlled Clinical Trials (True Experiments)*

In a clinical trial or true experiment, researchers administer a drug or treatment and follow the subjects forward in time (prospectively) to determine the effects of such treatment. Randomized controlled clinical trials, a type of true experiment, are the gold standard for determining cause and effect relationships.

(a) *Journal, Investigators, Research site and Funding*

The first step in the literature evaluation process begins by briefly scanning the article. The study should be published in a reputable journal where manuscripts undergo peer review before publication. Studies that fail the peer-review process may be submitted to alternate journals for consideration. If the research topic seems out of place for a particular journal, this may be an indication that the study was initially rejected for publication by peer reviewers from more pertinent journals.

Clinical studies are rarely, if ever, published in "throw-away" journals. Throw-away journals are characterized by being free to readers, having a high advertisement-to-text ratio, not being owned by professional societies, having a variable peer-review process, and not having a section for critical correspondence. Article published in such journals are of little benefit in clinical decision making.

(b) *Title /Abstract*

The title of the article should be brief and catch the attention of readers interested in the topic. The title should also be unbiased and should not indicate author's preferences for any particular drug treatment.

The abstract briefly describes the purpose, methods, results, and conclusion of an investigation. By scanning the abstract, readers should be able to determine whether the study is of interest and deserves further review. Abstracts should be clearly written.

(c) *Introduction*

The introduction part of a clinical study contains background information for the study; states study objectives and hypotheses, and indicate any planned subgroup or covariate analyses. This part also addresses ethical issues related to conduct of the study.

Sufficient background information should be provided to demonstrate that the study is important and ethical. Current treatment paradigms for the disease state being studied; limitations of these treatments, and reasons why the treatment under investigation may offer benefits should be discussed. Data from completed preclinical and / or clinical studies should be summarized to justify that further study in the area is needed. Background information should indicate that potential benefits outweigh risks to subjects entering the study.

(d) *Methods*

Study methodology is the most important section of a clinical study. The methods section contains information on the design, study population, instrumentation, and statistics used for the investigation. Results of studies with serious methodological flaws may be unreliable. The methods section should be sufficiently detailed to allow investigators to reproduce the study. Additionally, authors should state that the protocol is available upon request in case readers have additional questions regarding study methodology.

Parallel Versus Cross-Over Studies

In a parallel study, subjects receive only one treatment, while during a cross-over study; subjects receive all study drugs during the course of the study. Parallel studies are most appropriate when therapies are definitive or when disease states are self-limited (e.g., antimicrobials for infectious diseases). When disease states are chronic and / or highly variable (e.g., glaucoma, migraine headache), cross-over designs are more appropriate.

Important points to be considered in Cross-Over Studies:

- Wash out period must be of sufficient duration to prevent carry-over effects
- Multiple cross-over periods are useful when studying diseases with exacerbations and remissions.
- Subjects should be randomized to treatment order.
- Both investigators and subjects should be blinded to time when cross-over occurs.
- Subject drop-outs and deaths should be minimized.

Inclusion and Exclusion Criteria

Inclusion and exclusion criteria describe the study patients. Inclusion criteria list subject characteristics that must be present for enrollment into the study and exclusion criteria list characteristics that, if present, preclude enrollment into the study. Study inclusion and exclusion criteria must be carefully stated so readers can assess whether the study sample is representative of the population to which the results are intended to be generalized. Diagnostic criteria for disease states should be clearly defined.

Sample Size

A sample is a subgroup from the entire population of patients with a particular disease state who would be eligible to enter the study. Samples are used because of logistic, financial, and resource constraints that prohibit studying entire population. Sample size is very important while evaluating clinical studies. Sample size varies from study to study based on the factors discussed below.

If the sample size is too small type II error can occur i.e. false negative result is likely. The sample may not represent population. If the sample size is too large, the results may lack clinical significance.

Determinants of Sample Size

- Alpha or level of significance (i.e., probability of false-positive result)
- Beta (i.e., probability of false-negative result)
- Delta (i.e., amount of difference to be detected)
- Standard deviation (i.e., variation)

Controls

A drug may exert psychological benefits even if it is pharmacologically inactive. Factors such as the natural history of the disease, extensive monitoring and ancillary care, chance, or bias can influence the efficacy and safety outcomes of clinical trials.

Two types of controls are utilized in a clinical trial, placebo and active. In placebo-controlled trials, the control group receives a placebo that is identical to the study drug in terms of appearance, taste, smell, and other characteristics, but does not contain the active ingredient. Active controls are used when efficacy and safety of two or more drugs need to be compared or when it would be unethical to administer a placebo.

Outcome variables

The clinical outcomes should be relevant, clearly defined, objective, and clinically and biologically significant. The researcher / investigator should define variables to be measured and the amount of difference between treatment and control groups that the study is designed to detect. Variables should be measured at appropriate intervals and for an appropriate length of time to ensure that both positive and negative aspects of a therapy are adequately assessed. Both the treatment and placebo groups should be followed with the same intensity.

Randomization

Randomization is an important aspect of study design. When studies are randomized, subjects have an equal and independent chance of receiving any of the treatment modalities. Randomization is equivalent to flipping a coin and helps ensure that treatment groups are similar in regard to clinical and socio-economic factors that may affect treatment outcome. Randomization helps diminish patient and investigator bias by prohibiting investigators from assigning drug treatments. Randomization requires that an unpredictable treatment sequence be generated that remains concealed until subjects are allocated to treatment. Proper methods of randomization include use of random number tables, computer-generated random numbers, or lotteries.

Randomization can be simple (unrestricted) or balanced (restricted). Simple randomization is accomplished by referring to a list of random numbers. Balanced randomization is sometimes used. For balanced randomization, blocks of patients (e.g., every 10 consecutively enrolled patients) are randomized to ensure that similar numbers of patients are allocated to each treatment group.

Blinding

The investigators and subjects who are involved in a clinical study usually have an opinion about the therapy undergoing investigation. The response of the subject and researcher evaluation may be affected by these views.

Blinding helps prevent these biases from influencing study results and ensures that monitoring and ancillary care is applied equally to both treatment and control groups. Mechanisms for blinding the study and similarities between the treatment and control (e.g., appearance, taste, smell) should be described in clinical trial reports. The location of the code and whether or not the blind was broken during the clinical trial should also be discussed.

In a single-blind study, either patient or investigators are unable to identify the treatment (active or control) assigned; the alternate group (i.e., patient or investigator) is aware of therapy being administered. In a double-blind study, neither investigators nor patients are aware of treatment assignments.

Types of Blinding

Type of Blinding	Definition
Single-blind	Either subjects or investigators are unaware of assignment of subjects to active or control groups
Double-blind	Both subjects and investigators are unaware of assignment of subjects to active or control groups
Triple-blind	Both subjects and investigators are unaware of assignment of subjects to active or control groups; another group involved with interpretation of data is also unaware of subject assignment.

Data Collection

Accuracy of measurements taken at study initiation may differ from those obtained towards study conclusion. Validation of data collection forms and instruments must also be undertaken. Accuracy of computer data entry should be determined periodically by comparing a portion of patient records to computer printouts.

Compliance

Subject compliance may also influence results and should be evaluated. There are many disadvantages to commonly used methods of compliance monitoring such as pill counts and urine or serum drug concentrations, but more accurate methods such as use of computerized prescription vials often are not feasible because of their expense. Monitoring of compliance is particularly important in studies where subjects receive medications on an outpatient basis and are responsible for self-administration of the study drugs. If study results indicate that a treatment is ineffective, but compliance for the study drug was low, lack of therapeutic benefit may be due to poor compliance of the study subjects rather than lack of efficacy of the drug therapy.

Statistical Analysis

Errors in statistical analysis of data are commonly encountered and invalidate study conclusion. Statistical tests are based on the study design and the type of data represented by outcome variable used for study endpoints. There are four types of data- nominal, ordinal, interval, and ratio. Nominal data are categorical (e.g. male/female, complete response/partial response/treatment failure), Ordinal data reflect a ranking (e.g., 1+/2+edema, $^{1/6}$ to $^{6/6}$, heart murmurs), Interval data have measurable equal distance between data points, but no absolute zero (e.g., temperature in degrees Fahrenheit), Ratio data are similar to interval data except an absolute zero point is present (e.g., serum drug concentrations, temperature in degrees Kelvin). Each type of data builds on the last, with nominal data being the weakest and interval/ratio data the strongest. Categories for nominal data should be specified a priori to avoid data dredging for statistically significant results at the conclusion of study.

Types of Data

Type of Data	Definition	Examples
Nominal	Categorical data	Yes/No; male/female; response/no Response/partial response
Ordinal	Data reflects ranking	Visual analog scales; Likert scales
Interval	Data with measurable equal distances between points but no absolute zero	Temperature in degrees Fahrenheit
Ration	Data with measurable equal distances between points and an absolute zero	Temperature in degree Kelvin; serum drug concentrations

Statistical tests are either one-sided or two-sided (also referred to as one-tailed or two-tailed). A one-sided test is used when the direction of the relationship between outcome variables is known (i.e., the variables can only vary in one direction from their original value). A two-sided test is used when the direction is unknown. For example, consider a drug being investigated for the treatment of asthma. If it is known that the drug will improve pulmonary function tests (PFTs), a one-sided test can be used; however, if the drug may either improve or worsen PFTs, a two-sided test would be used. A two-sided test requires a stronger relationship to achieve statistical significance than a one-sided test and is therefore often considered the preferred method. Whether one-sided or two-sided tests are used for study analysis should be specified a priori.

(e) *Results*

Data

Data should be presented in a clear and understandable format. Authors should indicate in the article how original data can be obtained, if desired. Confidence intervals and / or p values should be provided for any statistical analysis performed on the data. Efficacy results should be described in sufficient detail for readers to perform their own analysis of the data, if desired. Information on adverse effects should include severity of the event, how it was managed, and whether it was believed to be drug related. Variables that may have affected the prognosis in the control and treatment groups should be identified. If conduct of the study deviated from the protocol, reasons for the discrepancy should be provided (i.e., investigator error, patient noncompliance, laboratory error). Data should be presented as actual numbers, rather than percentage changes alone.

Type I and Type II Errors

A type I error occurs when the investigators accept the research hypothesis when it is incorrect (e.g., a false-positive result). The probability of a type I error is equal to alpha or the level of significance and by convention is usually set at .05. When a statistically significant difference is found between treatment groups at a significance level of .05 (e.g. $p<.05$), there is a 1 in 20 probability that it was a chance finding and does not indicate a true difference between treatment and control groups. For example, consider that the study comparing drug A and drug B in the treatment of acute otitis media with effusion showed that drug A was statistically better than drug B in achieving bacteriological cure at a significance level of .05%. For this study, there is a 95% probability that these results represent a "true" difference between efficacy for drugs A and B and a 5% probability that the results are a chance finding or false-positive result. Type I error is rarely discussed by the investigators, but should be considercd by readers. Study results are never 100% accurate; there is always the possibility that the results are a chance finding that would not be replicated if the study were repeated.

Type II errors (e.g., false-negative result) can occur whenever investigators conclude that two treatments are equally efficacious or equally safe. Type II errors are usually the result of chance or inadequate sample size.

Table 9.1 Type I and Type II Errors

Statistical Results of Study	Reality in population	
	No Difference	**Difference**
Null hypothesis rejected	Type 1 error Probability = alpha False positive	Correct results
Null hypothesis accepted	Correct results	Types II error Probability = beta False negative

Study Validity

Studies should be analyzed in terms of two types of validity – internal and external. Internal validity refers to the extent to which the study results reflect what actually happened in the study (e.g., are the results consequent to the drug under investigation or are they the result of another confounding factor?). Such confounding factors can include events that develop between initial and final measurements, changes that occur in subjects during the course of the study, accuracy of instruments and the investigators taking measurements, selection of subjects in a nonrandomized manner, and drop-outs and deaths that occur during the study resulting in elimination of important data points.

External validity is the degree to which the study results can be applied to patients routinely encountered in clinical practice (e.g., are the conditions of the study replicable or do factors such as concomitant medication use and presence of additional disease states in study subjects make it impossible to generalize results?). If study conditions are not similar to those routinely encountered clinical situations, the results may not be applicable to patient care.

(f) ***Conclusions***

The conclusion/discussion section allows authors to provide an interpretation of their data and how it relates to clinical practice. Study conclusions should be consistent with results and related to the initial study question. Results should be compared to a systematic review of all previously published data.

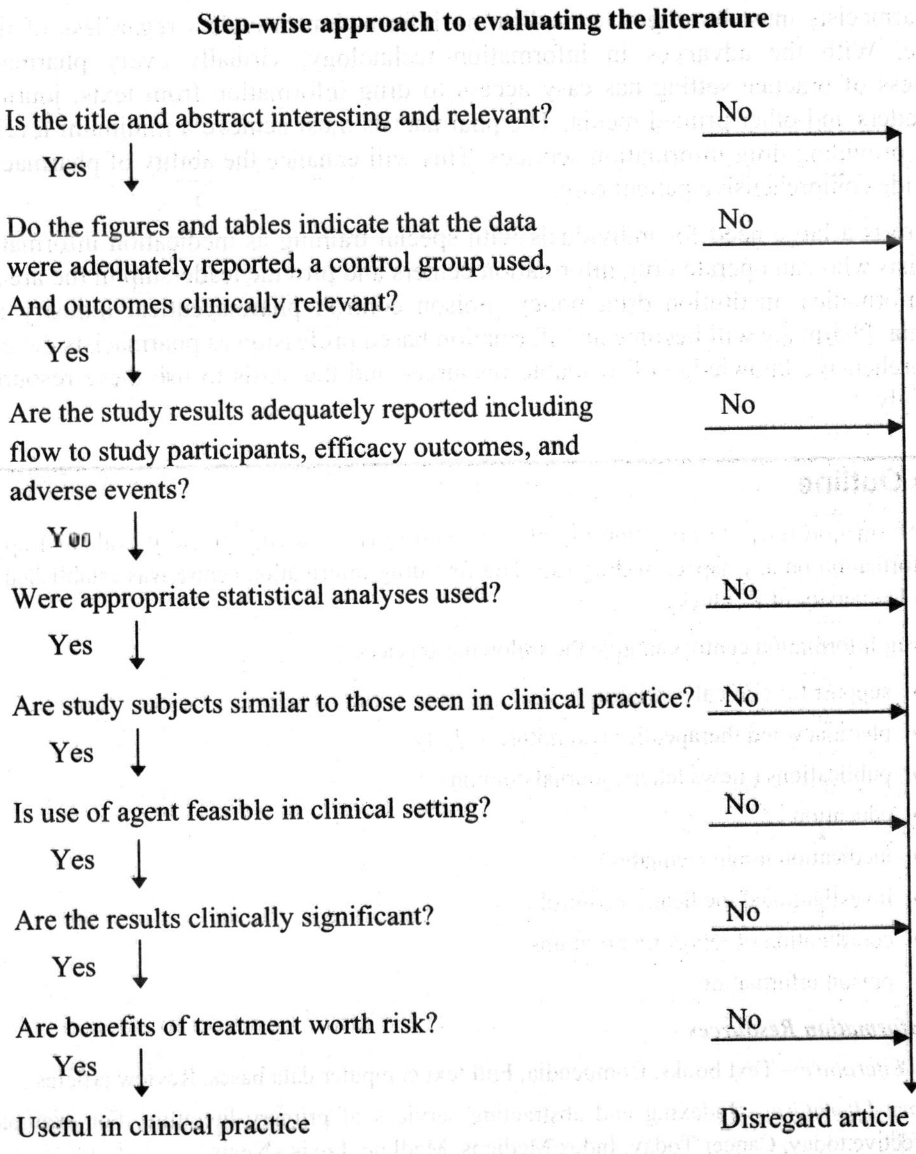

Fig. 9.1 Schematic representation for the step wise approach to evaluating the literature

Conclusion

All Pharmacists must be effective medication information providers regardless of their practice. With the advances in information technology, virtually every pharmacist regardless of practice setting has easy access to drug information from texts, journals, news letters and other printed media. The pharmacists must achieve a minimum level of skill in providing drug information services. This will enhance the ability of pharmacists to provide comprehensive patient care.

There is a large need for individuals with special training as medication information specialists who can operate drug information centers and provide leadership in the area of drug informatics, institution drug policy, poison control, pharmaceutical industry and academia. Pharmacy will become an information based profession as pharmacists develop a comprehensive knowledge of available resources and the skills to use these resources effectively.

Study Outline

Drug Information refers to provision of unbiased well referenced and critically evaluated up to date information on any aspect of drug use. The first drug information centre was established in 1962 in University of Kentucky.

A Drug Information centre can give the following services

- support for clinical services
- pharmacy and therapeutics committee activity
- publications (news letters, journal column)
- education
- medication usage evaluation
- investigational medication control
- coordination of reporting programs
- poison information

Drug Information Resources

Tertiary Literature – Text books, Compendia, Full text computer data bases, Review articles

Secondary Literature – Indexing and abstracting services of primary literature. For example, Anti-infective today, Cancer Today, Index Medicus, Medline, Lexis –Nexis

Primary Literature – Research studies published in biomedical journals

A pharmacist working in a Drug Information Centre should adopt a step wise systematic approach in formulating response to drug information queries.

Drug Information presentations can be through pharmacy news letters, formal lectures or verbal presentations.

Factors to be considered when formulating response

Several factors to be considered while formulating a response like,

- patient specific factors
- disease specific factors
- medication specific factors

The steps involved in formulating a response are

- securing demographics of requestor
- obtain background information
- determine and categorize ultimate question
- develop strategy and conduct research
- perform evaluation, analysis and synthesis
- formulate and provide response
- conduct follow up and documentation

Finally the drug information should be evaluated before being presented.

Drug Information Response Form*

Section 1 - General Information

1. **Pharmacist:** ______________________________
2. **Date:** ______
3. **Initial information request (i.e., the initial question received):**
4. **Actual information needed/requested:**
5. **Category of request:**

   ☐ Patient Specific (complete section 2)

   ☐ Non-patient specific drug information requests (do not complete section 2)

   ☐ Academic or educational information requests (do not complete section 2)

6. **Type of information requested** (choose only one)

___Adverse drug event	___Formulary issue	___Pharmaceutics (stability, etc.)
___Alternative agent (e.g. herbal)	___Foreign drug identification	___Pharmacokinetics
___Availability of drug	___General information	___Pregnancy/lactation
___Dosage and administration	___Identification of product	___Therapeutics
___Drug interaction	___Investigational drug	___Toxicology
		___Other ____________

7. **Method received:**

   ____ telephone

   ____ rounds

   ____ hand written

   ____ email

   ____ other

8. **Requestor information:**

   (a) Name: ____________________________________

   (b) Affiliation/practice site name: ______________________________

   (c) Telephone #: _______________________________

   (d) Mobile #: ______________

   (e) E-mail address: _____________________________

   (f) Fax #: ________________

   (g) Background and practice site:

________House staff physician	______Hospital
________Attending physician	______Ambulatory care clinic
________Nurse	______Community/retail
________Patient	______Managed care organization
________Family/Caregiver	Long-term care facility
________Other background	______Other practice site

Section 2 - Patient Data (if request related to specific patient)

1. **Age:** ___
2. **Sex:** ___M ___F
3. **Weight (kg):** _____
4. **Height (cm):** _____
5. **Ethnicity:**

   ___White

   ___Black

   ___Hispanic

   ___American Indian

   ___Asian

   ___Foreign

   ___Other (unknown)

6. **List allergies/ADEs/intolerances:**
7. **Pertinent medical history:**

8. **Current problems/diagnosis:**

9. **Organ function:**
   (a) Renal (ClCr):
   (b) Hepatic:
   (c) Cardiac:

10. **Medication history** (medication, dose, dosage forms, route of administration, frequency, duration):

11. **Pertinent laboratory values, other diagnostic test information:**

12. **Other pertinent information:**

Section 3 - Actual Question and Response

1. **Drug information response:**

2. **Response provided to:** ________________________________

3. **Method response was provided:**

   Face-to-face_____ Phone_____ Fax_____ Email_____ Mail_____ Other_____

4. **Approximate time to answer question (minutes):**

   ___< 5 ___6-15 ___16-30 ___31-60 ___61-119 ___120-239 ___ ≥ 240

5. **Were copies of references provided to requestor?** ___Yes ___No

6. **References:**

   List the sources and references (indicate primary or tertiary) used to formulate your response.

A minimum of two primary references must be cited. Note that drug information handbooks (print or electronic), PDA drug information programs, and class notes ARE NOT considered appropriate sources for the Drug Information Response. Electronic tertiary sources such as MICROMEDEX® may be used.

*(Adapted from Website of College of Pharmacy, University of Arizona. www.pharmacy.arizona.edu)

Drug Interactions

With the development of many new and potent therapeutically effective drugs considerable advances are made in the treatment of many diseases. However, equally significant and serious drug related problems are arising with these potent therapeutic agents.

Many drug related problems develop unexpectedly and are difficult to predict, whereas some are related to known pharmacologic actions of the drugs and can be reasonably anticipated. However, as drug therapy becomes more complex and many patients are treated with multiple drugs during the same period, the ability to predict the magnitude and seriousness of a specific action of any given drug is reduced. These situations point to a need not only for maintenance of complete and current medication records for patients, but also for closer monitoring and supervision of drug therapy. This will be useful to detect and prevent the problems at an early stage. The pharmacist is in a unique position to meet these needs and ample opportunities exist for involvement in and contribution to provision of drug therapy that is rationale, efficacious, economical and safe.

Increasing number of drug related problems are caused by drug interactions. We can define a drug interaction as a situation in which the effects of one drug are altered by prior or concurrent administration of another drug. Typically, interaction between drugs comes to mind (drug-drug interaction). However, the concept of drug interaction can be extended to the following situations:

- food or certain dietary items influence the activity of a drug (drug-food interactions)
- Environmental chemicals or smoking influences the activity of a drug
- A drug causes alterations of diagnostic laboratory test results (drug-lab test interactions)

We will be discussing the above topics in chapters 10, 11 and 12 respectively.

CHAPTER 10

Drug-Drug Interactions

Objectives

After reading this chapter, the student should be able to:

- Define the term drug interaction and differentiate it from incompatibility.
- Explain the different categories of drug interactions and understand their mechanisms.
- Understand the role of genetics, G-6-PD deficiency and p-glycoprotein in drug interactions.

10.1 Introduction

Definition: The term drug interaction has been defined as the phenomenon which occurs when the action of one drug is modified by the prior or concurrent administration of another (or the same) drug. Drug interactions may arise either from alteration of the absorption, distribution, biotransformation or excretion of one drug by another, or from combination of their actions or effects. The definition states "by the administration" this differentiates drug interaction from drug incompatibility. Although drug incompatibility may encompass the subject of interaction, the term incompatibility is ordinarily used for interactions which occur *in vitro*.

This is a fairly restrictive definition, describing a drug-drug interaction. Practical use of the term has enlarged the scope so much that the drug interaction literature considers the alteration of net effect of one substance (be it drug, chemical, food stuff, physiological substance or environmental agent) by another substance. Further, alteration of laboratory test results by ingested drugs is popularly considered in the drug interaction literature when, in fact, this may involve anything from an increase or decrease of an endogenous substance to simple interference with colour production.

As indicated in the definition, concurrent administration of two drugs is not necessary for an interaction to occur. For example, the prolonged effect of the monoamino oxidase inhibitors, the irreversible cholinesterase inhibitors or reserpine, each of which may have residual effects for sometime after the drug is discontinued. In some instances, chronic administration of one drug (e.g., meprobamate, glutethimide) may alter its own metabolism and hence its effectiveness. In other cases, a drug may have a different effect upon another substance depending on whether the drug is given acutely or chronically.

Before proceeding further we must define what we mean by the term "drug". A widely acceptable definition is "any biologically active substance". This encompasses not only synthetic or naturally occurring chemical products but also hormones, neurohormones and substances administered for diagnostic as well as for therapeutic purposes.

The terms used to describe the combined effects of drugs are often ambiguous. The words which we commonly hear like synergism, potentiation etc., are used, the exact meanings of which are not clear. Some of these terms are defined as per the classical pharmacology text books.

- *Homergic* – Two drugs produce the same overt effect.
  - *Summation:* If the combined effects are equal to the sum of their individual effect.
  - *Additive:* If the combined effects are equal to those expected for drugs acting by the same mechanisms.
  - *Synergism:* Has various meanings and is best avoided for homergic drugs.
- *Heterergic*: Only one of a pair of drug produces an effect.
  - *Synergism:* Combined effects of heterergic drugs that are greater than those of the active component alone (e.g., narcotic analgesic and chlorpromazine)
  - *Potentiation:* Often a synonym for synergism, should be avoided.
  - *Antagonism:* Combined effects of heterergic drugs that are less than that of the active component alone.
    - *Chemical Antagonism*: Interaction of an agonist and an antagonist to form an inactive complex (e.g., EDTA and lead, protamine sulfate and heparin sodium)
    - *Competitive antagonism*: Antagonist acts reversibly at the same receptor site as the agonist (e.g., atropine and acetylcholine). Drugs capable of

combining with receptors and initiating drug action are said to possess both affinity and efficacy (or intrinsic activity) and are termed agonists; those that react with receptors but lack efficacy are termed competitive antagonists. Agonists that produce a smaller maximal effect than other agonists acting on the same receptor are said to have intermediate efficacy and are termed partial agonists.

- *Non-Equilibrium Antagonism*: Agonist and antagonist act at different receptor sites.
- *Physiological or Functional Antagonism*: Antagonism between drugs having overtly opposite effects (e.g., histamine and epinephrine)

Using Drug Interaction Information

Generally, drug interactions are avoided, due to the possibility of poor or unexpected outcomes. However, drug interactions have been deliberately used, such as co-administering probenecid with penicillin prior to mass production of penicillin. Because penicillin was difficult to manufacture, it was worthwhile to find a way to reduce the amount required. Probenecid retards the excretion of penicillin, so a dose of penicillin persists longer when taken with it, and it allowed patients to take less penicillin over a course of therapy.

The information on drug interactions if used appropriately can be of immense help to the pharmacist in preventing several drug related problems and even can turn these problems into useful situations. Several factors should be kept in mind while studying the information on drug interactions, like

- *Interacting drugs can usually be used together:* Many a times two drugs which interact can be used together if certain precautions like closer monitoring of therapy, dosage adjustments to compensate for the altered response are taken. At times the use of one drug is contraindicated while the other is being given and in such situations the physician / pharmacist should look for alternatives.

- *Interacting drugs can be beneficial:* Sometimes a second drug interacts beneficially and is prescribed deliberately to modify the effects of the other drug. This information can be utilized either to enhance the effectiveness or to reduce the adverse effects of the primary drug. A contemporary example of a drug interaction used as an advantage is the co-administration of carbidopa with levodopa (available as Carbidopa/levodopa). Levodopa is used in the management of Parkinson's disease and must reach the brain in an un-metabolized state to be beneficial. When given by itself, levodopa is metabolized in the peripheral tissues outside the brain, which decreases the effectiveness of the drug and increases the risk of adverse effects. However, since carbidopa inhibits the peripheral metabolism of levodopa, the co-administration of carbidopa with levodopa allows more levodopa to reach the brain un-metabolized and also reduces the risk of side effects.

- *Patient variables:* A number of factors will influence the response to a drug either favorably or unfavorably. Patient related factors like age, genetic makeup, disease state, renal function, hepatic function, smoking, diet, alcohol, environmental factors etc., can influence drug interactions or adverse drug effects to some extent or other. Knowledge about these factors can be significant use to the physician / pharmacist to detect or prevent the drug interactions or adverse drug reactions

Reasons for drug interactions

Several reasons are cited for the increased number of drug interactions like,

- *Potency of the drug:* With advances in medical science very potent drugs are being synthesized and are available to physicians and patients. When multiple potent drugs are used together the chances of drug interaction occurring are increased several fold.
- *Patient visiting several physicians:* Patients with more than one problem normally visits different physicians. The physicians due to their busy schedule are not in a position to take the medication history of the patient and due to this they may prescribe certain medications which may have interactions with the drugs which the patient might be using already. To avoid such kind of drug related problems it is advisable that the patient visit a single pharmacy for all his medication needs so the pharmacist can properly counsel.
- *Patient noncompliance*: Due to various reasons the patient may not take the drugs as prescribed and as per the directions, which may lead to drug overdose or underdose. Some times they may take excessive medication and this may cause drug interactions.

10.2 Drug Interactions - Categories

Drug interactions can be broadly divided into 3 categories based on the severity: type A, type B, and type C.

Type A: Type A drug interactions are those that produce adverse outcomes in most patients. These interactions are usually easy for the pharmacist to handle. Very few drug interactions cause adverse outcomes in almost everybody who takes the combination and so type A interactions are relatively rare.

One example of a type A drug interaction is carbamazepine and clarithromycin. Patients stabilized on carbamazepine who are started on a CYP3A4 inhibitor such as clarithromycin are very likely to manifest symptoms of carbamazepine toxicity (e.g., nausea, vomiting, dizziness, drowsiness, headache, diplopia, and confusion).

Type B: Type B drug interactions are those that produce adverse outcomes in a minority of patients, and for which the risk factors are largely unknown. Type B drug interactions are the most common type. It is typical for drug interactions to cause adverse outcomes in only a small percentage of people who take the combination. Unfortunately, often little is known about the factors that predispose to the adverse outcome, so it is not possible to determine a priori which patients will manifest an adverse consequence.

For example, some patients on warfarin who receive a CYP2C9 inhibitor, such as trimethoprim-sulfamethoxazole for 10 days, will have a bleeding episode, but it is very difficult to tell with any degree of certainty which patients are at greater risk of bleeding. Depending on the potential severity of the adverse outcome, type B interactions may require action on the part of the pharmacist.

Type C: Type C drug interactions are those that produce adverse outcomes in a minority of patients, but enough is known about risk factors so that patients at higher risk can be identified. For a few drug–drug interactions, we know at least some of the risk factors, and can apply this information to identifying patients who may be predisposed to adverse outcomes. Although this is not the largest group of drug interactions, it is growing as we learn more about the characteristics of patients who manifest the adverse outcomes due to drug interactions. With advances in pharmacogenetics and other fields, most of the type B drug interactions may eventually be moved to the type C group.

A good example of a type C drug interaction would be the concurrent use of potassium-sparing diuretics such as amiloride, spironolactone, or triamterene in combination with angiotensin-converting enzyme (ACE) inhibitors. This interaction probably results in more drug interaction alerts to the pharmacist than any other drug interaction. It is clear that some patients do develop serious, even fatal, hyperkalemia when given this combination. Yet, it is also clear that the drug interaction alert is overridden, and the drug combination is dispensed by many pharmacists without adverse outcomes in the patients.

10.3 Drug Interaction Mechanisms

Drug interactions may occur as a result of one or more of the following mechanisms:

- A direct effect of one drug upon another
- By modification of the intestinal absorption
- By affecting the transport of a drug or substance across cell membranes
- By altering the distribution of a drug in the various body compartments
- By modification of a drug action at its receptor site
- By altering the binding of a drug to inactive binding sites
- By acceleration or retardation of the metabolism of a drug

- By affecting the rate of excretion
- By modification of the sensitivity of the receptor site

These mechanisms may be termed as "pharmacodynamic" actions.

Pharmacologic or pharmacokinetic actions would include the apparent enhancement or antagonism of drug's effect via a second drug acting on the same or a related physiologic system and producing either a similar or an opposite pharmacologic effect.

In essence, a drug interaction may occur when a substance either alters the ability of a drug to reach its receptor site in its usual manner and concentration, or alters the body's response to the drug.

Pharmacodynamic Drug Interactions

Pharmacodynamics is the study of the biochemical and physiological effects of drugs and their mechanisms of action. Pharmacodynamics deals with the absorption, distribution, biotransformation and excretion of drugs. These factors coupled with dosage, determine the concentration of a drug at its sites of action and, hence, both intensity and the time course of its effects. Substances which alter the pharmacodynamics of a drug would then alter its actions and effect on the body.

- ***Absorption***

  Passage of drugs across cell membranes is essential in the pharmacodynamics of a drug. It is believed that the cell or plasma membrane consists of a biomolecular lipoid sheet containing minute water-filled pores. The membranes are approximately 100 Angstrom units thick; the pores vary from 4 to 40 Angstrom units. The lipoid membrane is readily penetrated by lipid-soluble substances, and the aqueous pores allow rapid penetration of small water-soluble substances.

  Alteration of pH

  Most drugs are weak acids or bases, and are present in solution as both ionized and unionized species. The non-ionized portion is usually lipid and can readily diffuse across the cell membrane. In contrast, the ionized fraction is often unable to penetrate the lipoid membrane because of its low lipid solubility, or to traverse the membrane pores because of its size.

  Changes in acid-base balance may have a profound influence on the absorption of drugs and thus their action.

  For example, in the stomach a weak acid (e.g., salicylic acid, barbiturates) is almost entirely un-ionized and therefore diffuses freely across the gastric mucosal cells into the capillary blood. Weak bases are highly ionized in gastric juice and therefore are absorbed by diffusion through the stomach wall in negligible amount. Antacid therapy is expected to delay or partially prevent absorption of certain acidic drugs.

Similar principles occur in intestinal absorption, but here hydrogen ion gradients between the intestinal lumen and the capillary blood are much less extreme.

For example, weak bases, such as morphine, quinine, ephedrine and tolazoline are predominantly ionized at the *p*H of gastric juice, thus are poorly absorbed through the gastric mucosa. Sudden external changes of acid-base balance will then alter the concentration of drugs within the cell, and hence their activity.

Phenobarbital (a weak acid) owes its sedative action to the intracellular fraction. Breathing carbon dioxide decreases the concentration of phenobarbital in the plasma, increasing the concentration in the cell and hence increasing the potency of the drug. Ingestion of large doses of sodium bicarbonate, on the other hand, increases the alkalinity of the plasma, increasing the concentration of the phenobarbital therein, and reducing its potency. Conversely, mecamylamine's ganglionic blocking activity is a function of its plasma level. Being a base, carbon dioxide inhalation increases its concentration in the plasma, increasing its hypotensive effect. Thus, to predict accurately the effect that a change in the acid-base balance may have on the activity of a drug, one must know whether its activity is an intracellular or extracellular phenomenon, whether it is a weak acid or a weak base, and its response to change in acid-base balance.

Finally, changes in urinary pH may have a profound influence on the excretion of weak acids and bases.

Effect on Transport Systems

While the absorption of many drugs is a passive phenomena, governed by the physicochemical laws of diffusion, specialized active transport processes appear to be responsible for the rapid cellular transfer of certain foreign organic ions and polar molecules, as well as many natural substrates such as sugars, amino acids and pyrimidines.

Active transport processes differ from passive processes in that they exhibit selectivity, saturability and requirement for energy. Specialized active transport is generally thought to be mediated by carriers, membrane components that form a complex with the substance to be transported. The complex is presumed to be formed on one side of the membrane and diffuse to the other side where the substance is released, after which the carrier returns to the original surface to repeat the process. If the process transports a substance against an electrochemical gradient (uphill transport) and is blocked by metabolic inhibitors, it is called active transport; ions such as Na^+, K^+, amino acids, certain strong organic acids and bases, and ionized forms of weak electrolytes are transported across the renal tubule, choroids plexus and liver cells in this manner.

Carrier transport that shows selectivity, saturability and blockade by metabolic inhibitors, but in which the substance does not move against a concentration gradient is called *facilitated diffusion.* Glucose, pyrimidines and some of their anti-metabolites are transported by this process. Transport is facilitated by attachment to a carrier and is more rapid than simple diffusion.

Complex Formation

Drugs may form inactive or insoluble complexes with other drugs or foods in the intestinal tract. For example, the activity of penicillin G is diminished when administered with food, although this might be primarily an acid-instability problem. Tetracycline forms complexes with di- and tri- valent cations; such complexes inhibit or prevent the absorption of the drug from the gut. The use of milk with tetracycline has been disputed, but the inactive complex of tetracycline with aluminum has been well documented.

Miscellaneous Aspects

Drugs which affect the circulation to the site of absorption may affect drug absorption.

For example, the vasoconstrictor effect of epinephrine has been used for years in combination with local anesthetics. By slowing the absorption with local anesthetics the epinephrine prolongs the activity of the anesthetic and decreases its systemic toxicity. Taking drugs with meals may decrease gastric irritability but often delays absorption. Similarly, administration of drugs along with antacids or oils will delay gastric emptying and hence may affect absorption and rapidity of action.

Two drugs may be combined to form a precipitate which, when administered, will delay absorption and prolong blood level. The use of procaine penicillin G or of protamine zinc insulin adequately illustrates this point. Drugs may also be administered in oil (e.g., estrone in oil) for the same purpose. Conversely, one drug may be administered with another to enhance the latter's absorption.

For example, Hyaluronidase is added to large volume infusions delivered by hypodermoclysis. By breaking down hyaluronic acid, the infusion fluid spreads over a larger area, decreasing the swelling and pain of injection as well as increasing the rate of absorption. Although not commercially available, dimethyl sulfoxide serves as an effective carrier for drugs applied topically but not for systemic effect.

- ***Distribution***

Displacement of drug from storage tissue component

Pharmacodynamics, the study of the biochemical and physiological effects of drugs and their mechanisms of action, deals with the absorption, distribution, biotransformation and excretion of drugs. The distribution of drugs is via the plasma and body fluids, which transports then to sites of action, excretion and metabolism. Drug action depends upon absorption of the drug by an active receptor; the drug on the receptor is in equilibrium with the drug in the plasma. Hence, the response to a drug is determined in part by the concentration of unbound drug in the plasma which, in turn, is dependent upon a number of factors, not the least of which is the amount of bound drug.

Binding of a drug may be to plasma proteins, to connective tissue, to fat, in transcellular areas or even within cells. These may serve as reservoirs, since the pharmacologically inactive stored drug is in equilibrium with the free drug in the plasma and is released as the drug is metabolized, accumulated in other tissues or excreted. As a result of binding, effective plasma levels of the drug are maintained for a longer period of time and its pharmacological effects are correspondingly prolonged. However, to obtain therapeutically effective levels initially, adequate priming doses must be given to saturate the binding sites.

One drug may affect the action of another by altering its concentration at receptor sites. It may act directly by displacing the other drug from its specific site of action or, one drug may act indirectly by displacing the second drug from proteins in plasma or tissues, thereby increasing its concentration at specific receptors. In such a case, the biological activity of the first drug may be enhanced.

The binding of a single drug to plasma protein is not fully understood. Most therapeutic agents, however, are extensively bound to tissue or plasma proteins. Such binding is occasionally termed "sites of loss"; however, the drug is not really "lost", but held in reserve. Binding may be beneficial in that it may result in a diminished incidence of side effects and a prolonged duration of action.

A number of acidic drugs are attached to only one or two sites on the albumin molecule; for these drugs, the protein has a limited carrying capacity. Many of these acidic drugs appear to compete for the same limited number of protein binding sites. Hence, one acidic drug may be displaced by another, thereby increasing the concentration of the unbound (displaced) drug. As specific examples, highly bound acidic agents such as phenylbutazone, oxyphenbutazone, ethylbiscoumacetate, dicumarol, sulfinpyrazole and salicylic acid are able to displace the long-lasting, albumin-bound sulfonamides from plasma proteins. Since these sulfonamides are not rapidly metabolized or excreted, the displaced molecules diffuse from plasma into tissues with resultant enhanced antibacterial activity. By the same mechanism, phenylbutazone increases the antibacterial activity of acidic antibiotics such as penicillin.

Displacement of a drug can be dangerous if it is bound so extensively to plasma proteins that the unbound moiety is only a small fraction of the total. Displacement of only a small proportion of the drug from protein may then double or triple its unbound concentration at the target site. Thus a highly bound sulfonamide, such as sulfaphenazole, can induce hypoglycemic coma by displacing tolbutamide from protein. Similar results have been elicited by phenylbutazone and salicylates.

Other potentially hazardous drugs are anticoagulants of the coumarin type, which are highly bound to plasma albumin. A number of cases have been reported in which phenylbutazone, or oxyphenbutazone, has caused profound bleeding in patients being treated with warfarin. Likewise, methotrexate is bound in part to plasma albumin and is displaced by a number of drugs, including sulfonamides and salicylic acid. Since methotrexate is often used therapeutically in doses that are nearly toxic, the clinical implications are obvious. The fact that barbiturates, probenecid and coumarin do not displace sulfonamides from binding sites suggests that these acids are bound at sites different from those which take up tolbutamide, sulfonamides, phenylbutazone analogues, coumarin and salicylates.

Drugs can also be displaced from proteins in organ tissues. A particularly dramatic example of this occurs in the treatment of malaria. When primaquine is given to patients previously treated with quinacrine, the primaquine is displaced from organ tissues and its plasma concentration is increased five to ten fold.

Premature babies have relatively low quantities of albumin and the acidic binding sites are readily saturated with bilirubin. In such babies, sulfonamides can produce toxic effects by displacing bilirubin from the albumin, resulting in kernicterus. Because of this phenomenon, it is recognized that neonates should not be given sulfonamides, salicylates or other agents that can displace bilirubin from albumin.

Various hormones such as thyroxine, corticosteroids and perhaps, insulin are transported in plasma by specific proteins. An observation that rheumatic patients who developed obstructive jaundice became free of rheumatic effects suggested that bilirubin displaced corticosteroids from their protein binding sites. Further investigations with phenylbutazone derivatives demonstrated that only those analogues which displaced corticosteroid from transcortin have antirheumatic effects. A similar mechanism is proposed for the antirheumatic effects of salicylate, flufenamic acid and indomethacin. Likewise, it has been postulated that the primary action of the sulfonylurea drugs in diabetes is the freeing of endogenous insulin from protein-bound complexes in the pancreatic beta cells, the plasma and the tissues.

Tyramine causes norepinephrine to be released from its storage granules, producing sympathomimetic effects. On the other hand certain anti-adrenergic drugs (such as reserpine) inhibit binding of norepinephrine at the sympathetic nerve endings or else decrease the synthesis of this important neurohormone (e.g., α-methyldopa), producing a decrease in sympathetic activity.

Modification of Drug Action at Receptor Site

The cell component directly involved in the action of a drug is usually termed its receptive substance or, simply, its receptor. The chemical groups that participate in drug-receptor combination and the adjacent portions of the receptor that favour or hinder access of the drug to these active groups are known as receptor sites. Other drug-cell interactions that do not initiate drug action (such as binding of drugs to plasma or to enzymes concerned with biotransformation and transport of drugs) are said to involve secondary receptors, silent receptors, sites of loss, storage sites or drug acceptors. As stated previously, such drugs are not lost but held in reserve.

Receptor groups, like the active centers of enzymes, are thought to be carboxyl, amino, sulfhydryl, phosphate and similar reactive groups spatially oriented in a pattern complementary to that of the drugs with which they react. There are a number of theories to explain how a drug interacts with the receptor and produces its effect; however, none of the theories is completely satisfactory.

Receptors are best categorized on the basis of the effects, or lack of effects, of representative agonists and antagonists (e.g., muscarinic or nicotinic receptors, or alpha or beta-adrenergic receptors).

Some drugs act only on certain cells, tissues or organs and thereby exert localized effects. Other drugs act in or on most cells of the body, hence produce generalized effects. Some drugs act extracellularly; others at the cell surface; and still others, intracellularly. Certain drugs act directly on effector cells, others influence effector cells indirectly. For the most part, the actual biochemical and biophysical mechanisms of action of drugs are not known.

In biochemical terminology, a drug would be considered a substrate, and the substrate would react with an enzyme in a reversible reaction to form an enzyme substrate (enzyme-drug) complex, a transition state (the active site on the enzyme is the receptor). This enzyme substrate complex now breaks down to form a product (response). The *intrinsic activity* or ability to initiate a drug action, is a measure of the tendency of the enzyme-substrate (enzyme-drug) complex to form (produce) a product (response). A competitive inhibitor would also react with the enzyme forming a complex which is not active. This, then, means that some of the enzyme is tied up and unavailable to the drug. The degree to which the inhibitor blocks the enzyme depends on the concentration of the inhibitor and its affinity for the enzyme. "Partial agonists" would lie somewhere between the inhibitor and the substrate, with a high affinity for the enzyme but the product (or response) is very poor.

Two important concepts then enter into the picture of drug interaction at the receptor site, the affinity of the drug for the receptor and the intrinsic activity or effectiveness of the drug-receptor complex. In interactions, a drug may have a biphasic action if it has a high affinity for the receptor, but the complex so formed has a low intrinsic activity. In small doses, such a drug may inhibit the action of the original drug or neurohormone, but in high doses weakly mimic it.

Competitive inhibition occurs when the antagonist acts reversibly at the same receptor site as the agonist. Atropine, for example, is an inert substance, but is widely taken up by the receptor at the parasympathetic nerve ending. Consequently, acetylcholine is crowded out and prevented from discharging its normal function. Sufficiently high doses of acetylcholine would eventually displace some of the atropine and produce a cholinergic effect.

If a receptor antagonist acts irreversibly, the antagonism is termed non-equilibrium. The non-equilibrium antagonism often cited is that of the anticholinesterase agents which produce their effect by destroying pseudocholinesterase (isofluorophate, demecarium bromide). Some of the insecticides act in this manner. Serious consequences have been reported in persons who use cholinergic drugs and who were exposed to such insecticides.

Partial agonists usually have a high affinity for the receptor but a low intrinsic activity. The antidotal effects of nalorphine and levorphan to the respiratory depressant effect of the narcotic analgesics are based on this mechanism.

Non-competitive antagonism occurs when the agonist and antagonist act at different receptor sites. One such interaction might be illustrated by the effect atropine has on the ganglionic stimulating effect of small doses of nicotine. In this case, atropine would be acting at the post-ganglionic ending.

- ***Biotransformation***

Many drugs are lipid-soluble, weak electrolytes. To facilitate excretion or detoxification, many are transformed into more polar compounds. While this biotransformation usually results in inactivation of the drug, occasionally a drug may be converted from an inactive moiety to an active one (prontosil to sulfanilamide), or transformed into an active metabolite (acetohexamide to hydroxyhexamine). Biotransformation may be a non-synthetic reaction (such as oxidation, reduction or hydrolysis), or a synthetic reaction, also called conjugation. The latter involves coupling between the drug and an endogenous substrate.

Biotransformation of drugs occurs mainly in the liver, although some also takes place in plasma, kidney and other tissues. Oxidative enzymes (such as those which dehydrogenate alcohols) and reducing enzymes (which cause nitro reduction of chloramphenicol) are found primarily in the liver microsomes. Esterases involved in the hydrolysis of procaine, meperidine, acetylcholine, etc., are located in the plasma, liver microsomes and many other tissues. Conjugating enzymes occur mainly in the liver but also in other tissues.

Those enzyme systems concerned in the biotransformation of many drugs appear to be located in the hepatic endoplasmic reticulum. The microsomal enzymes catalyze many of the non-synthetic and synthetic biotransformations described above. The activity of these drug-metabolizing enzymes in liver microsomes as well as the structure and amount of smooth-surfaced endoplasmic reticulum (the microsomal part believed to possess the drug-metabolizing enzymes) are influenced markedly by the administration of various drugs and hormones, and by age, sex, strain, temperature, nutritional status and pathological state of the individual.

Stimulation of Drug Metabolism

Prior treatment of individuals with certain drugs increases their ability to metabolize both the administered drug as well as other related and unrelated drugs. Chronic administration of one drug can then reduce the pharmacological activity of another drug by stimulating its metabolic inactivation. This effect is produced by increasing the amount of drug metabolizing enzymes in the liver microsomes, sometimes referred to as *enzyme induction.* The increased activity of the microsomal enzymes is probably due to enhanced enzyme synthesis. Drug metabolism can be stimulated by various types of drugs including hypnotics, analgesics, tranquilizers, antihistamines, oral antidiabetics or uricosuric agents.

There are numerous examples of enzyme induction by clinically available drugs. Phenobarbital stimulates the enzymes which inactivate the muscle relaxant zoxazolamine, the hypnotic hexobarbital, the anticoagulants such as bishydroxycoumarin and warfarin, the anticonvulsant diphenylhydantoin, the antifungal antibiotic griseofulvin and the analgesic aminopyrine. Not only drugs, but substances present in the environment stimulate drug-metabolizing enzymes in liver microsomes. Insecticides, such as chlordane and DDT, acting via this mechanism, shorten the duration of action of hexobarbital and phenylbutazone.

Inhibition of Drug Metabolism

Examples are known where drugs can inhibit the metabolic detoxification of other drugs and thus cause an increase in their duration and intensity of pharmacological action. The first compound described that accomplished this interference was SKF 525A. Others include iproniazid, nialamide, chloramphenicol, aminosalicyclic acid and narcotics (meperidine, morphine sulfate). The exact mode of action of the inhibitors is not known; apparently the inhibition may be noncompetitive with one set of enzymes and competitive antagonism with other enzymes.

Oxyphenbutazone has been shown to potentiate the anticoagulant action of warfarin by its ability to inhibit the metabolizing enzymes. Further studies demonstrated that oxyphenbutazone metabolism could be slowed by administration of the anabolic steroid, methandrostenolone. Probably the most familiar example of enzyme inhibition is that of the monoamine oxidase (MAO) inhibitors. The unusual sensitivity to subsequent doses of sympathomimetic amines is well documented. These drugs, however, may inhibit enzymes which act on many compounds with amino groups. Hence, the MAO inhibitors may potentiate the action of large number of drugs.

Some drugs may exhibit a biphasic mechanism, depending on whether they are given acutely or chronically. Chlorcyclizine, phenylbutazone and glutethimide all have produced a biphasic response in animals. An acute dose of these drugs markedly inhibits certain enzymes, producing, for example, a prolongation of the hypnotic action of hexobarbital. On the other hand, chronic administration accelerated the activity of the enzymes, with enhanced metabolism of hexobarbital and reduction of its hypnotic action.

Cytochrome P 450

Enzymes responsible for drug metabolism often belong to a family of enzymes called CYP450 enzymes. These enzymes enable the oxidative metabolism of drugs and endogenous substances, such as prostaglandins and steroids. Most of this metabolic activity takes place in the liver or in the wall of the small intestine. Although more than 30 different families of enzymes have been identified, only 3 families, CYP1, CYP2, and CYP3, are responsible for the metabolism of most drugs. Subfamilies within each family are designated by a capital letter and individual enzymes are named with a final Arabic number. Thus the individual enzymes CYP2C9 and CYP2C19 both belong to the CYP2 family and the CYP2C subfamily. Other common drug metabolizing enzymes include CYP1A2, CYP2D6, and CYP3A4. Table 10.1 lists 5 enzymes and the common drugs that are metabolized by them. A drug that is metabolized by an enzyme is said to be a substrate for that enzyme. Table 10.1 presents a list of drugs that can inhibit or induce the activity of the enzyme.

Theoretically, any two drugs that are metabolized by the same enzyme could produce a drug interaction. The two drugs could compete for the same enzyme, and one drug might be metabolized while the other drug metabolism is reduced. In some drugs, this effect can be demonstrated in vitro but not in vivo. When two drugs compete for the same metabolizing enzyme, it is known as competitive enzyme inhibition. Whether this leads to a significant reduction in the metabolism of one of the drugs depends on the concentrations of the drugs and their affinities for the enzyme receptor binding site. Fortunately, because the liver and the intestinal wall contain a large quantity of enzymes relative to the amount of drug to be metabolized, the administration of two drugs having the same metabolic pathway rarely results in a measurable change in the metabolism of either drug. For an interaction to occur, one of the substrates must partially saturate the enzyme so that the ability of the enzyme to metabolize the other drug is impaired.

Table 10.1 Selected Cytochrome P450 Substrates, Inhibitors, and Inducers

Isozyme	Substrate	Inhibitors	Inducers
CYP1A2	Acetaminophen,Caffeine, Clozapine,Amitriptyline, Tacrine, Theophylline	Cimetidine,Ciprofloxacin, Diltiazem,Enoxacin,Fluvoxamine, Tacrine	Barbiturates, Cigarettes, Rifampin
CYP2CP	Fluvastatin,Ibuprofen, Glipizide,Losartan, Mephenytoin,Phenytoin, Rosiglitazone,Tolbutamide, Warfarin	Amiodarone,Cimetidine, Fluconazole,Isoniazid, Metronidazole, Sulfamethoxazole	Barbiturates, Phenytoin, Rifampin
CYP2C 19	Diazepam,Citalopram, Esomeprazole,Lansoprazole, Omeprazole,Pantoprazole, Sertraline	Esomeprazole,Fluconazole, Fluoxetine,Fluvoxamine, Omeprazole	Barbiturates, Phenytoin, Rifampin
CYP2D6	Amitriptyline,Codeine, Desipramine,Dextromethorphan Flecainide,Haloperidol, Imipramine,Metoprolol, Nortriptyline,Peroxetine, Propafenone,Propranolol, Thioridazine, Timolol	Amiodarone,Fluoxetine, Haloperidol,Paroxetine, Propafenone,Propoxyphene, Quinidine,Terbinafine, Thioridazine	Rifampin (weak)
CYP3A4	Amiodarone,Alprazolam, Buspirone,Cisapride, Cyclosporine,Diltiazem, Erythromycin,Felodipine, Indinavir,Lovastatin, Midazolam,Nifedipine, Pimozide,Pioglitazone, Quinidine,Sertraline, Sildenafil, Simvastatin, TAO, R-warfarin, Tacrolimus,Triazolam, Verapamil, Zolpidem	Clarithromycin,Cyclosporine, Erythromycin,Flucanozole, Grape fruit-juice,Indinavir, Itraconazole,Ketoconazole, Miconazole, TAO, Ritonavir, Verapamil	Barbiturates, Carbamazepine, Griseofulvin, Nevirapine, Phenytoin, Rifampin, St,Johns wort

- **Alteration of Excretion**

The kidney is the most important organ for drug excretion. Drugs may be eliminated from the body either unchanged or as metabolites. Generally, the more polar compounds are excreted unchanged; the less polar, lipid-soluble drugs, however, are not readily eliminated until they are metabolized to more polar, less lipid-soluble compounds. In the kidney, most of the drug molecules filtered at the glomerulus returns to the blood stream by diffusing across the lipid-like membrane of the tubular cells. More polar compounds cannot penetrate the membrane; consequently, they are readily excreted in the urine.

Excretion of drugs in the urine involves three processes: *passive glomerular filtration, active tubular secretion and passive tubular reabsorption.* In the proximal and distal tubules, the non-ionized forms of weak acids and bases undergo reabsorption or excretion by passive diffusion. The diffusion is potentially bidirectional. The direction of diffusion depends upon the concentrations of the drug and the pH on the two sides of the tubular cells.

Changes in Urinary pH

Changes in urinary pH induced by ingestion of ammonium chloride, sodium bicarbonate, carbonic anhydrase inhibitors, etc, may have a profound influence on the excretion of weak acids and bases. In general, an acidic or basic drug may be expected to show the phenomenon of pH-dependent excretion if the un-ionized fraction is lipid-soluble and if the pKa is within a favorable range of 7.5-10.5 for weak bases, and 3.0-7.5 for weak acids. Weak acids are excreted at a higher clearance in highly alkaline urine, and weak bases in acidic urine. Drugs which are known to show the phenomenon of pH-dependent excretion include the weak acids salicylic acid, phenobarbital, nitrofurantoin, nalidixic acid and some sulfonamides. The weak bases include quinacrine, chloroquine, procaine, mecamylamine, meperidine, levorphanol, quinine, amphetamine, imipramine and amitryptyline.

Drugs which alter the pH of the tubular urine can markedly affect the excretion of other drugs. Examples include the hastened excretion of streptomycin and the reduced excretion rate of mecamylamine in alkaline urine, and the enhanced effectiveness of the mercurial diuretics in acidic urine.

Direct Effect on Kidney

A number of drug interactions may be attributed to a direct effect on the kidney. Penicillin is both filtered at the glomerulus and excreted through the tubules. The mechanism for excretion of penicillin can be clogged by administration of para aminohippuric acid (PAH, a substance which seeks the same transport system). The blood level of penicillin can be prolonged by the administration of probenecid, which inhibits the penicillin-transport mechanism. Hypochloremia results in a diminished diuresis in response to administration of mercurial diuretics.

Complex Reactions

Seemingly unrelated drug interactions may have their origin in an effect on the kidney. The hypokalemia produced by the thiazide diuretics has wide spread implications. Increased potency of skeletal muscle relaxants and toxicity to digitalis has both been produced by this very mechanism. The use of diuretics to enhance the excretion of toxins is one of the recognized mechanisms of treating drug poisoning.

10.4 Genetics – Drug Interactions

The amount of enzyme found in patients is quite variable and depends on a number of factors, including genetics. For the enzymes CYP2C9, CYP2C19, and CYP2D6, there are patients who have very little active enzyme due to the presence of a genetic defect. These genetic defects result in a change in the structure of the protein making up the CYP enzyme. The defective enzyme is unable to facilitate the oxidation of drugs, and a loss of enzyme activity and drug metabolism is the result. For the enzyme CYP2C19, patients can be classified as either fast or *extensive metabolizers (EMs) or slow or poor metabolizers (PMs)*. The majority of all populations studied are EMs for CYP2C19, but the percentage of the population that is PMs varies based on ethnic origin. For example, 3% of Caucasians are CYP2C19 PMs, and about 20% of Asians carry the defective gene. About 8% to 10% of Caucasians are PMs for CYP2D6, and about 3% are PMs for CYP2C9.

Genetic differences in drug metabolism can influence drug interactions in several ways. First, inhibition of drug metabolism was greater in patients with more rapid baseline metabolism. Diazepam is partially metabolized by CYP2C19. Due to higher incidence of CYP2C19 PMs in diseased patients, the clearance of diazepam is lower in Chinese than Caucasians.

Metoprolol is primarily metabolized by CYP2D6. When quinidine, a potent inhibitor of CYP2D6, was co administered, only patients who were EMs for CYP2D6 had a reduction in their metoprolol metabolism. No effect of quinidine on metoprolol pharmacokinetics was noted in the CYP2D6 PMs. This demonstrates a second effect of genetics on drug interactions. Patients who are PMs are protected from most drug interactions caused by enzyme inhibitors (or inducers) of the enzyme they lack. Simply stated, *an inhibitor cannot inhibit an enzyme that is not present due to a genetic deficiency.*

In some instances, being a PM may increase the risk of an adverse outcome during a drug interaction. Some antidepressants, such as amitriptyline and imipramine, are metabolized by more than one enzyme, including CYP2C19, CYP2D6, and CYP3A4. Imipramine will normally use all three pathways for its metabolism. If the patient is a PM for CYP2C19, the metabolism of imipramine will be shifted to the CYP2D6 and CYP3A4 pathways. Should that patient be administered a CYP3A4 inhibitor, the remaining CYP2D6 pathway may not be able to compensate, and the patient would likely have an interaction of greater magnitude than a patient receiving a CYP3A4 inhibitor who was an EM for CYP2C19.

Glucose -6-Phosphate Dehydrogenase (G-6-PD) Deficiency - G-6-PD Deficiency is most common inherited enzyme deficiency affecting red blood cells. G-6-PD is a critical antioxidant, a deficiency can predispose to oxidation and subsequent hemolysis of the red blood cell.

Common oxidants that should be avoided in G-6-PD deficiency patients are - sulfonamides, furantoins, chloramphenicol, large doses of ascorbic acid, dapsone(>200mg/day), chloroquine, methylene blue, nalidixic acid, penicillamine, primaquine, quinidine, quinine.

The degree of hemolysis induced by a drug may be accentuated by the presence of additional factors (infection or disease state etc). The severity of the reaction is dependent on the type of G-6-PD deficiency [(Mediterranean deficiency-Caucasian (most severe)]; Blacks (usually mild to moderate). The sex of the patient is also important; males are at greater risk based on severity compared to females.

G-6-PD deficiency is not an absolute contraindication to the use of oxidizing agents. Decisions should be based on a risk vs. benefit analysis (consider severity of disease; sex of patient; availability of other agents; type of deficiency). If therapy is initiated, the patient should be monitored closely for adverse effects. Patients with G-6-PD deficiency will exhibit signs within 1-3 days of initiation of treatment. Symptoms may include abdominal or back pain in severe cases. The urine of the patient will darken in color.

10.5 P-glycoprotein-Drug Interactions

P-glycoproteins are part of a larger family of efflux transporters found in the gut, gonads, kidneys, biliary system, brain and other organs. They appear to have developed as a mechanism to protect the body from harmful substances. Using ATP as an energy source, they transport certain hydrophobic substances in the following directions:

- into the gut
- out of the brain
- into urine
- into bile
- out of the gonads
- out of other organs

PGPs play a large role in the distribution and elimination of many clinically important therapeutic substances. Prescription and OTC drugs, foods and substances made by the body may be inhibitors and/or inducers of these transporters. Some drugs like cyclosporine are both substrates and inhibitors of PGP, other drugs like nifedipine are inhibitors only and some drugs like digoxin are substrates only.

Since PGPs block absorption in the gut, they should be considered part of the "first-pass effect". In fact, they can "set up" or act as "gatekeepers" for later P450 Cytochrome actions. If one drug is a substrate of both PGP and CYP3A4 (both found in close proximity in the intestinal wall), and a second drug is added that is an inhibitor of both PGP and CYP 3A4 (e.g., ketoconazole, erythromycin, mibefradil), then the first drug will be allowed in increased amounts. Since CYP3A4 is inhibited, levels of unmetabolized drug will enter the blood. The effect of PGP blockade is to "open the gates" so that the later actions of CYP3A4 inhibition will be increased.

P-Glycoprotein, is a 170 kDa membrane-bound protein which has been implicated as a primary cause of multidrug-resistance in tumors. An understanding of the physiological regulation of these transporters is key to designing strategies for the improvement of therapeutic efficacy of drugs which are their substrates. PGP activity is controlled by a variety of endogenous and environmental stimuli which evoke stress responses including cytotoxic agents, heat shock, irradiation, genotoxic stress, inflammation, inflammatory mediators, cytokines and growth factors.

Another example is loperamide and quinidine. Loperamide is an opiate antidiarrheal that is normally kept out of the brain by the blood brain barrier due to transport away from the brain by PGP. When given with quinidine which inhibits PGP, more loperamide can enter the brain and cause respiratory depression.

10.6 Drug Interaction – Arrhythmias (Torsades)

Torsades de Pointes (TdP) is a ventricular tachycardia that can be asymptomatic, and it produces syncope or dizziness, and rarely is a cause of sudden death. TdP occurs when the ventricle repolarizes too slowly and then prematurely depolarizes, initiating an arrhythmia. Drugs that slow potassium efflux from the ventricular cells can lead to delayed ventricular repolarization. Slow repolarization of the ventricle can be seen as a prolongation of the QT interval on the electrocardiogram. Several antiarrhythmic drugs (e.g., amiodarone, procainamide, quinidine, dofetilide, and sotalol) prolong ventricular repolarization by inhibiting potassium efflux at therapeutic plasma concentrations. The incidence of TdP with these drugs has been estimated at <5 per 1000 patients. Other drugs that are not considered to be antiarrhythmic agents may also delay potassium efflux and slow repolarization. Drugs such as phenothiazines, some antibiotics, and tricyclic antidepressants have been noted to affect repolarization, particularly at elevated or toxic plasma concentrations. Table 10.3 lists commonly used drugs that have been reported to prolong repolarization, either at therapeutic concentrations or at elevated levels. The exact risk of TdP with these agents is not known, but it is believed to be very low, perhaps approaching 1 per 100,000.

Table 10.2 Selected P-Glycoprotein Substrates, Inhibitors, and Inducers

Substrate	Inhibitor	Inducer
Amprenavir	Amiodarone	Phenobarbital
Cyclosporine	Clarithromycin	Rifampin
Digoxin	Cyclosporine	St. John's wort
Doxorubicin	Diltiazem	
Etoposide	Erythromycin	
Fentanyl	Felodipine	
Fexofenadine	Itraconazole	
Indinavir	Ketoconazole	
Loperamide	Nicardipine	
Morphine	Quinidine	
Mycophenolate	Ritonavir	
Nelfinavir	Tamoxifen	
Quinidine	Testosterone	
Rifampin	Verapamil	
Ritonavir		
Saquinavir		
Sirolimus		
Tacrolimus		
Verapamil		
Vinblastine		
Vincristine		

(Adapted from Hansten P, Horn J. The Top 100 Drug Interactions: A Guide to Patient Management. Edmonds, WA: H &H Publications; 2002: 425-743-1908. Available at: www.hanstenandhorn.com.)

The potential for interacting drugs to produce sufficient delay in repolarization to initiate an arrhythmia is very difficult to discern. Interactions between drugs that can prolong repolarization can be pharmacodynamic, pharmacokinetic, or both. Management of potential interactions between these drugs depends on which drugs are combined and how they interact.

Potential interacting combinations to avoid

The combination of two drugs known to prolong the QT interval at therapeutic concentrations (e.g., antiarrhythmic drugs in column A Table 10.3) would produce a pharmacodynamic interaction that should probably be avoided because the risk of torsades is likely to be markedly increased. The coadministration of an antiarrhythmic drug (column A) and a drug that can increase the QT interval at elevated concentrations (column B) should be avoided if there is also a pharmacokinetic interaction between the two drugs. For example, quinidine prolongs repolarization at therapeutic concentrations and is an inhibitor of CYP2D6. If it is administered with thioridazine, it will elevate the concentration of thioridazine, perhaps to levels sufficient to produce a significant increase in the QT interval. This type of a dual mechanism interaction (both drugs can prolong repolarization plus quinidine increases the concentration of thioridazine) may result in the development of an arrhythmia.

Potential interacting combinations are to be used only when the benefit outweighs the risk. The coadministration of a drug that prolongs repolarization at therapeutic concentrations (column A) and one that may do it at elevated concentrations (column B), without a pharmacokinetic interaction, represents a risk for TdP that should be carefully considered. If a patient taking procainamide is prescribed haloperidol, the patient's electrocardiogram should be carefully monitored for QT prolongation. Because this is a pharmacodynamic interaction, the risk of developing an arrhythmia is somewhat increased somewhat but may be acceptable, particularly at lower doses of haloperidol. If two drugs that can prolong repolarization at elevated concentrations and have a pharmacokinetic interaction are combined (dual interaction mechanism), the risk of excessive prolongation may be increased. This type of interaction mechanism is the basis for the widely described interaction between cisapride and erythromycin. Erythromycin-induced inhibition of cisapride metabolism leads to an elevation of cisapride concentration. The patient's risk of TdP increases with the elevation of cisapride concentrations and the presence of a second drug (erythromycin) that may also affect the ventricle. If two drugs from column B are administered concomitantly, there appears to be only a small risk of arrhythmia, provided that they do not have a pharmacokinetic interaction and both drugs are at therapeutic concentrations. Most of the drugs in column B increase the QT interval by less than 5%.

Table 10.3 Common Drugs Reported to Prolong Ventricular Repolarization (QT Interval)

A. Drugs that prolong the QT interval at therapeutic concentrations	B. Drugs that may produce prolongation of the QT interval at elevated concentrations
Amiodarone	Amitriptyline
Disopyramide	Bepridil
Dofetilide	Chlorpromazine Cisapride
Ibutilide	Clarithromycin
Procainamide	Clomipramine
Propafenone	Clozapine
Quinidine	Desipramine
Sotalol	Droperidol
	Erythromycin
	Gatifloxacin
	Haloperidol
	Levofloxacin
	Mesoridazine
	Moxifloxacin
	Pimozide
	Thioridazine
	Ziprasidone

(Adapted from Hansten P, Horn J. The Top 100 Drug Interactions: A Guide to Patient Management. Edmonds, WA: H&H Publications; 2002: 425-743-1908. Available at: www.hanstenandhorn.com).

10.7 Some Important Drug Interactions with Over-the-Counter Medications

Aspirin can modify the effectiveness of arthritis medications, strong prescription steroids and diuretics. Combining aspirin with diabetic medications can drop blood sugars to dangerous levels. Aspirin can also cause toxicity when taken with glaucoma and anticonvulsant (anti-seizure) drugs and cause bleeding episodes when combined with a blood thinner, like warfarin.

Acetaminophen can also cause interaction complications when overused. Heavy drinkers who take acetaminophen for hangover relief risk liver damage. Taking high doses of acetaminophen with Coumadin can cause bleeding episodes.

Antacids taken with antibiotics, heart and blood pressure or thyroid medications can decrease drug absorption up to 90 percent.

Over-the-counter antihistamines - should be avoided with antianxiety or antidepressant medications.

Oral contraceptives are less effective when taken with barbiturates, antibiotics, anti-fungal or tuberculosis drugs.

Table 10.4 Important Drug-drug Interactions*

Sl.No	Drug combination	Impact	Mechanism of action	Prevention	Management
1	Warfarin – NSAIDs (NSAIDs does not include COX-2 inhibitors) (Diclofenac,piroxicam, flurbiprofen, ibuprofen, indomethacin, ketoprofen, ketorolac, mefenamic acid, meloxicam,nabumetone,naproxen tramadol etc.,)	Serious gastrointestinal bleeding	NSAIDs increase gastric irritation and erosion of protective lining of stomach	Avoid concomitant use of an NSAID with warfarin. Consider acetaminophen for antipyretic effect and COX-2 inhibitors for anti-inflammatory effects.	Prothrombin time and INR to be monitored every week. Signs and symptoms of an active bleed should be monitored.
2	Warfarin – Sulfa Drugs (Sulfamethoxazole-trimethoprim)	Increased effects of warfarin, with potential for bleeding.	Mechanism unknown; Warfarin's activity is prolonged due to a decreased production of vitamin K by intestinal flora affected by antibiotic administration.	Avoid concomitant use of a sulfa drug with warfarin, particularly sulfamethoxazole-trimethoprim. Identify microbial pathogen prior to initiation of antibiotic therapy. Reduce warfarin dose by 50% if use of sulfa drug is imperative.	Monitor prothrombin time and INR every week. Signs and symptoms of active bleed should be monitored daily.
3	Warfarin-Macrolides (azithromycin, clarithromycin, dirithromycin, erythromycin base, erythromycin ethyl succinate, erythromycin stearate, troleandomycin)	Increased effects of warfarin, with potential for bleeding.	Erythromycin inhibits the metabolism and subsequent clearance of warfarin from the body. The activity of warfarin may also be prolonged due to alterations in the intestinal flora and its production of vitamin K.	Interaction is highly probable. Avoid concomitant use of a macrolides with warfarin. Switch to an alternative antibiotic.	If use of macrolide is imperative, monitor INR every other day and adjust warfarin dosing as necessary. Signs and symptoms of active bleed should be monitored daily.

Table 10.4 *Contd...*

Sl.No	Drug combination	Impact	Mechanism of action	Prevention	Management
4	Warfarin- Quinolones (alatrofloxacin, ciprofloxacin, enoxacin, gatifloxacin, levofloxacin, lomefloxacin, moxifloxacin, norfloxacin, ofloxacin, sparfloxacin, trovafloxacin)	Increased effects of warfarin, with potential for bleeding.	Exact mechanism is not known. Reduction of intestinal flora responsible for vitamin K production by antibiotics is probable with decreased metabolism and clearance of warfarin	Identify the microbial pathogen prior to antibiotic therapy. Metabolism of warfarin delayed particularly with enoxacin, ciprofloxacin, norfloxacin and ofloxacin. Select newer quinolones that have not demonstrated significant impairment of warfarin metabolism.	Prothrombin time and INR should be monitored regularly. If ciprofloxacin use is imperative, monitor INR every other day. Monitor signs and symptoms of active bleed daily.
5	Warfarin- Phenytoin	Increased effects of warfarin and / or phenytoin	Mechanism unknown. One theory suggests a genetic basis involving liver metabolism of warfarin and phenytoin.	Obtain baseline phenytoin levels prior to initiation of warfarin. Monitor INR during co-administration. Target INR should be towards the lower end of the therapeutic range.	Prothrombin time, INR and phenytoin levels should be monitored. Signs and symptoms of active bleed should be monitored daily.
6	ACE inhibitors – Potassium supplements (benazepril,captopril, enalapril, fosinopril, ramipril, lisinopril quinapril, trandolapril)	Elevated serum potassium	Inhibition of ACE results in decreased aldosterone production and potentially decreased potassium excretion.	Draw potassium level prior to initiation of ACE-inhibitor in a patient.	Potassium levels greater than 5 should be monitored carefully due to risk of severe hyperkalemia and EKG changes. Watch renal function (BUN, SCr) also. Adjust potassium supplementation if levels increase.

Table 4 *Contd...*

Sl.No	Drug combination	Impact	Mechanism of action	Prevention	Management
7	ACE Inhibitors – Spironolactone	Elevated serum potassium levels	Unknown, possibly an additive effect.	Draw potassium level prior to initiation of spironolactone in a patient.	Potassium levels greater than 5 should be monitored carefully due to risk of severe hyperkalemia and EKG changes. Watch renal function (BUN, SCr) also. Avoid potassium supplements.
8	Digoxin – Amiodarone	Digoxin toxicity	Mechanism unknown. Amiodarone may decrease the clearance of digoxin, resulting in proloned digoxin activity.	Obtain digoxin level prior to initiation of amiodarone therapy. Then decrease dose of digoxin by 50% and monitor digoxin levels once weekly for several weeks.	Maintain digoxin level between 1-2. Monitor for signs and symptoms of digoxin toxicity.
9	Digoxin – Verapamil	Digoxin toxicity	Synergistic effect of slowing impulse conduction and muscle contractility leading to bradycardia and possible heart block.	Monitor heart rate and EKG-PR interval. Evaluate selection of verapamil and digoxin.	Monitor heart rate and EKG-PR interval. Monitor for signs and symptoms of digoxin toxicity.
10	Theophylline – Quinolones (alatrofloxacin, ciprofloxacin, enoxacin, gatifloxacin, levofloxacin, lomefloxacin, moxifloxacin,norfloxacin, ofloxacin, sparfloxacin, trovafloxacin)	Theophylline toxicity	Inhibition of hepatic metabolism of theophylline by the quinolones	Obtain theophylline level prior to initiation of a quinolone. The quinolones, enoxacin, and ciprofloxacin reduce theophylline clearance by 30-84%. Consider switching to gatifloxacin, levofloxacin, moxifloxacin, or trovafloxacin.	Monitor theophylline levels. Maintain level within targeted range of 5-15mcg/ml;

(*Adapted from www.rphworld.com – "Top ten dangerous drug interactions").

Conclusion

There is a lot of literature available on the internet about drug-drug interactions and there are certain clinical situations where it is not possible to completely avoid a particular interaction. It is important to understand the clinical significance of potentially interacting drug combinations. Most interacting drug combinations can be administered concurrently if the patient is monitored appropriately and corresponding adjustments are made in the drug dose, dosing interval or route of administration. The clinical pharmacist can play a crucial role because of his knowledge, skills and expertise in predicting a particular interaction. This is possible only when the clinical pharmacist has thorough and in-depth knowledge of drug interactions and keeps himself updated with the latest available information on drug interactions.

Study Outline

Drug interaction is a situation in which a substance affects the activity of a drug i.e., the effects are increased or decreased or produces a new effect.

Interaction can be of the following types

Drug – drug interactions

Drug – food interactions

Drug – herb interactions

Drug – lab tests interactions

Some terms used in describing drug interactions are –

Homergic – two drugs produce the same overt effect

- Summation
- Additive
- Synergism

Heterergic – only one of a pair of drug produces an effect

- Synergism
- Potentiation
- Antagonism
    - Chemical
    - Competitive
    - Non-equilibrium
    - Physiological

Drug Interactions – categories (based on severity)

Type A – resulting in adverse outcomes in most patients.

Type B – Produce adverse outcomes in minority of patients and for which risk factors are largely unknown.

Type C – produce adverse outcomes in minority of patients but enough is known about risk factors so that situation can be avoided.

Drug Interaction Mechanisms

- a direct effect of one compound upon another
- by modification of intestinal absorption
- by affecting transport of such substances/ drugs across cell membrane
- by altering drug distribution in various body compartments
- by modification of drugs action at receptor site
- by altering the binding of a drug to inactive binding sites
- by acceleration or retardation of the metabolism of drug
- by affecting rate of excretion
- by modification of sensitivity of receptor site

Pharmacodynamic drug interactions

Substances which alter pharmacodynamics of a drug would then alter its actions and effect on the body.

- Absorption – can be affected by alteration of pH, complex formation
- Distribution – displacement of drug storage tissue compartment
  - modification of drug action at receptor site
- Biotransformation – stimulation of drug metabolism
  - inhibition of drug metabolism
- Excretion – alteration in urinary pH
  - direct effect on kidneys

Genetics

Genetic differences in drug metabolism influence drug interactions in several ways

E.g., G-6-PD deficiency is genetic and causes hemolysis of RBC resulting in hemolytic anemia when antioxidants like sulfonamides, chloramphenicol, chloroquine are administered.

CHAPTER 11

Drug – Food / Herb Interactions

Objectives

After reading this chapter, the student should be able to:

- Understand the term drug-food interactions and their nature.
- Explain the mechanism of drug-food interactions
- Discuss various pharmacologically active substances present in food products
- Discuss the role of grape fruit juice, alcohol and herbs in drug interactions

11.1 Introduction

Herbs and foods may interact with medications we normally take resulting in serious adverse reactions. Food-drug interactions are often overlooked resulting in unforeseen complications. These interactions commonly occur during multiple medications for chronic medical conditions. Physiological changes affect drug absorption, distribution, metabolism and excretion as well as its action. This variability in drug action may be further enhanced by interaction with foods. Individuals on multiple medications are usually prone to these effects. In addition, endocrine dysfunction, restrictive diets and alcoholism in many patients may further complicate these interactions.

Interactions of drugs and dietary components have been primarily directed toward reports of drug induced malabsorption phenomena or drug effects on nutritional status.

Foods are known to contain a variety of pharmacologically active substances, some of which are capable of producing severe toxicity and even death. Some drugs interfere with the body's ability to absorb nutrients. Similarly, some herbs and foods can lessen or increase the impact of a drug. Apart from the naturally occurring pharmacologically active substances in food, lots of chemicals and pharmaceuticals are used in the food processing industry due to our changing dietary pattern that can interact with the drugs causing severe drug-food interactions.

Pharmacologically active substances present in foods can be categorized in the following manner:

- *Foods of Plant and Animal Origin*: In this class one can cite the presence of 5-hydroxytryptamine in pineapples and bananas, 3,4-dihydroxyphenylalanine (DOPA) in broad beans, oxalates in spinach, rhubarb and celery, and various metals such as selenium, potassium, calcium, magnesium and sodium in grains and other foods. Also the presence of tyramine in various cheeses and chicken livers as well as fatty acids and lipids in meats has been noted.
- *Foods of Marine Origin*: Neurotoxins have been found in species of poisonous fish and paralytic toxins in polluted shellfish. Pesticide and heavy metal residues also have been detected in several species of edible fish.
- *Food Additives and Contaminants*: Increasing quantities of intended food additives such as preservatives, antioxidants, sequestrants, surface active agents, stabilizers and thickeners, bleaching and maturing agents, buffers, food colors, nonnutritive and special dietary sweeteners, flavors, and so forth are used in food processing technology to enhance the taste, structure or storage life of food. Examples of naturally occurring contaminants are the potent mycotoxins and bacterial toxins which result from fungal or bacterial contamination of foods. Man-made contaminants include antibiotics, pesticides, radio nuclides, metals, and processing degradation products.
- *Water, Soft Drinks and Alcoholic Beverages:* These dietary constituents may contain various metals, xanthines, histamines, alcohol and congeners.

Examples

- Alcohol is a drug that interacts with almost every medication, especially antidepressants and other drugs
- Theophylline, a medication administered to treat asthma, contains xanthines, which are also found in tea, coffee, chocolate, and other sources of caffeine. Consuming large amounts of these substances while taking theophylline increases the risk of drug toxicity that affect the brain and nervous system.
- Certain vitamins and minerals too have an impact on medications. Large amounts of broccoli, spinach, and other green leafy vegetables high in vitamin

K, which promotes the formation of blood clots, can counteract the effects of heparin, warfarin, and other drugs given to prevent clotting.

- Dietary fiber also affects drug absorption. Pectin and other soluble fibers slow down the absorption of acetaminophen, a popular painkiller. Bran and other insoluble fibers have a similar effect on digoxin, a major heart medication.

11.2 The Nature of Drug-Food Interactions

There are two major areas of concern with regard to drug effects and food:

- Some drugs are capable of impairing the absorption and utilization of nutrients and
- Certain foods or patterns of dietary consumption may alter drug absorption and response.

There are numerous examples of the first phenomenon, which in some instances may result in markedly altered nutritional states. With the exception of anti-infective agents, most of those drugs implicated in the impairment of absorption and utilization of nutrients are used for long-term treatment and hence are more prone to induce malabsorption syndromes.

The absorption characteristics of drugs and foods are strikingly dissimilar. The absorption of most drugs is governed to a large extent by

- Relative lipid solubility (the more lipid-soluble the greater the extent of absorption)
- Rate of dissociation (characterized by pKa)
- pH of the medium
- Particle size or molecular size and
- Physical form (crystal state, etc).

Transport across gastric or intestinal mucosa is mostly by passive non-ionic diffusion rather than active transport. (Exceptions are digitalis glycosides and pyrimidine compounds which are believed to be actively transported). Weak acids (those with a pKa less than 2) are as a rule absorbed in the stomach, while weak bases (those with a pKa less than 8) are usually absorbed in the upper intestine. Digestive enzymes or competitive inhibition are not thought to be factors in drug absorption.

The absorption of food, unlike the absorption of drugs, is largely dependent on gastrointestinal secretions, pH and enzyme activity. Transport mechanisms are not limited to passive diffusion, and lipid solubility is only of significance in lipid absorption.

Various dietary constituents also have been shown to alter clinical laboratory test values. Bananas, pineapples, coffee, chocolate, tea and vanilla may alter results of vanilmandelic acid, catecholamine and 5-hydroxyindole acetic acid determinations, while carrots may interfere with serum bilirubin determination. Dietary restriction of these substances for at least twenty-four hours prior to the respective test is therefore advisable.

11.3 Mechanism of Drug-Food Interactions

Food-drug interactions can be either pharmacodynamic or pharmacokinetic. Both of these pharmacologic properties can be enhanced or antagonized by food.

(A) ***Effects of drugs on nutrient and electrolyte absorption and utilization***

There are numerous citations of drug-induced impairment of nutrient and electrolyte absorption and utilization in man. They can be classified accordingly:

- *Drugs affecting gastric and / or intestinal motility:* Mineral oil has been shown to decrease the absorption of carotenes, vitamins A, D, E, and K. Chronic use of certain cathartics such as podophyllin, jalop and colocynth may cause calcium and potassium loss, and steatorrhea, while oxphenisatin, bisacodyl and phenophthalein are capable of inhibiting intestinal uptake of glucose. It also has been suggested that chronic and excessive antacid use can lead to thiamine deficiency, presumably because of alkaline destruction of thiamine within the bowel lumen. Orally administered calcium carbonate and mannitol have been implicated in causing steatorrhea by possible intraluminal fat binding and direct injury to absorptive mucosal cells. In addition, certain ganglionic blocking agents and anticholinergic substances may be capable of inhibiting the absorption of some nutrients by their action on the autonomic system of the gastrointestinal tract. Examples of such drugs are methantheline, propantheline and mecamylamine.

- *Hypocholesterolemic agents:* The hypocholesterolemic agents like neomycin, clofibrate and cholestyramine resin, while being relatively effective hypocholesterolemic agents, have been associated with a variety of malabsorption phenomena including vitamin B_{12}, d-xylose, carotene, and medium chain triglyceride, and electrolyte, iron and sugar absorption.

- *Surfactants:* Stool softening agents are capable of affecting fat dispersion and permeability of the lipoprotein membrane of mucosal cells with resultant changes in the absorption of a number of nutritional factors.

- *Anti-Infective agents:* Cycloserine, para-aminosalicylic acid, neomycin, erythromycin, sulfonamides, broad spectrum antibiotics such as tetracyclines, penicillins, isoniazid, chloramphenicol and others have been implicated in decreased folic acid utilization, vitamin B_{12} malabsorption, decreased bacterial synthesis of vitamin K, impaired absorption of calcium and magnesium, pyridoxine inactivation and impaired amino acid transfer in protein synthesis.

- *Cytotoxic drugs:* Methotrexate, aminopterin and other folic acid antagonists are inhibitors of folic acid, interfere with vitamin B_{12} and d-xylose absorption and are responsible for nonspecific changes in the jejunal mucosa. Colchicine, a specific therapeutic tool in the management of acute episodes of gout, is also associated with vitamin B_{12}, carotene, fat, lactose and electrolyte and d-xylose malabsorption.

- *Anticonvulsant drugs:* Diphenylhydantoin, primidone and phenobarbital have been specifically indicated for their role in the impairment and utilization of folic acid, vitamin B_{12} and d-xylose.

- *Alcohol:* The effects of alcohol on nutritional status are well known with malabsorption of folic acid, vitamin B_{12} and increased excretion of magnesium. Transient hypomagnesemia has been observed in alcoholic patients undergoing convulsive seizures during acute withdrawal phases.

- *Diuretics:* Most diuretics with the exception of triamterene and spironolactone are capable of precipitating dangerous episodes of hypokalemia through excessive renal clearance of potassium. Some diuretics such as the thiazides also have been reported to be diabetogenic.

- *Oral Contraceptives:* Some oral contraceptives have been implicated in impaired folic acid absorption and utilization.

(i) *Drug Effects on Taste and Appetite*

There have been reports of decreased taste acuity and unpleasant or altered taste sensation associated with griseofulvin, D-penicillamine, clofibrate, lincomycin, oxyphedrin and some tranquilizers. It should be noted that these reports are not associated exclusively with concomitant ingestion of foods, but appear to be systemically mediated. Exact mechanisms explaining these effects remain obscure at this time.

Any unpleasant tasting drugs, on the other hand, such as chloral hydrate, paraldehyde, vitamin B complex, uncoated penicillin preparations as well as suspensions, and a host of other drugs may precipitate transient states of altered taste sensation or aftertastes when foods are administered concomitantly or shortly after ingestion of such drugs. The long-term use of many of the psychotropic agents such as the phenothiazines, benzodiazepines and tricyclic antidepressants also has been associated with substantial weight gain in some patients. Such effects appear to be secondary to altered mental status and resultant appetite improvement.

(ii) *Effects of Food Upon Drug Absorption and Response*

Four possible means in which drug-food interaction phenomena might theoretically occur include:

- The effect of food upon drug absorption.
- Dietary constituents may alter drug metabolism (i.e., through enzyme induction or inhibition, etc.)
- Foods may possibly alter the rate of excretion of certain drugs (i.e., excessive acidification or alkalinization of urine).
- Pharmacologically active substances present in foods may alter the response of a concomitantly administered drug (i.e., monoamine oxidase inhibitors and tyramine-containing foods with resultant increases in pressor responses).

Antibiotic and Sulfonamide Drugs

Antibiotic and sulfonamide drugs have received more attention than any other group of therapeutic agents with regard to impairment of absorption by foods. Food has been shown to reduce the absorption of tetracycline, dimethylchlortetracycline, chlortetracylcline and methacycline. Penicillin G, penicillin V, nafcillin, oxacillin, ampicillin, erythromycin base, erythromycin propionate, erythromycin stearate, triacetyloleandomycin and lincomycin absorption have also been reportedly delayed by concomitant administration with food.

Griseofulvin levels have been found to be markedly increased after ingestion of a high fat content meal. This could be a significant problem in patients receiving anticoagulant therapy, as there have been several case reports of decreased prothrombin time when griseofulvin and warfarin were administered concurrently.

Tetrachloroethylene is often used to treat hookworm infestations. Patients should be cautioned against excessive fat intake when taking this anthelmintic in order to avoid systemic absorption and possible central nervous system toxicity.

(iii) *Drug Administration and Food Ingestion*

There are many drugs whose absorption may be apparently delayed or impaired by concomitant administration of foods. There are a number of drugs which are intrinsically irritating to gastric mucosa and should therefore be taken immediately before, with or immediately after meals, or with food or milk. This list is quite extensive but the more popular drugs are indomethacin, steroids, metronidazole, iron salts, aminophylline, potassium supplements, reserpine and many others. The following drugs should be taken on an empty stomach, preferably one hour before meals or three hours after meals: ampicillin, cloxacillin, erythromycin base, lincomycin, penicillin G potassium, pentaerythritol tetranitrate and penicillamine.

Drugs are often mixed with various juices and beverages in an attempt to mask their unpleasant taste or assist in oral administration in patients having difficulty swallowing oral solid dosage forms. This is very often the case in pediatric or geriatric patient populations. The practice of extemporaneously mixing drugs with various juices and beverages may precipitate problems with regard to acid labile substances whose absorption might be impaired in the stomach through decreased gastric pH or in vitro inactivation in acidic media. Most beverages and juices as seen in Tables 11.1 and 11.2 are quite acidic. Whole milk, by contrast, has an approximate pH range of 6.4 – 6.8. In light of the relative acidity of most beverages other than milk, acid labile antibiotics such as ampicillin, erythromycin base, and penicillin G potassium should not be mixed and allowed to stand for any length of time in the beverages represented

Table 11.1 pH Range of selected commercially available canned Juice and other beverages

Canned Juices	Approximate pH range
Cherry	3.4 – 3.6
Grape	3.5 – 4.5
Lemon	2.2 – 2.6
Lime	2.2 – 2.4
Pineapple	3.4 – 3.7
Tomato	3.9 – 4.4
Other beverages	
Milk (cow's)	6.4 – 6.8
Milk (evaporated)	5.9 – 6.3
Beers	4.0 – 5.0
Wines	2.3 – 3.8

Table 11.2 Approximate pH of carbonated beverages

Beverage	**pH**
Club soda	4.7
Cherry soda	3.0
Cola	2.4
Grape	3.0
Lemon	2.9
Lemon-lime	3.1
Orange	3.2
Raspberry	3.1
Beet Root	4.0

(B) *Dietary Constituents and Drug Metabolism*

There are numerous literature citations of apparent enzyme induction as well enzyme inhibition caused by drugs and their resultant impact on rates of drug metabolism; however, reports of diet-induced changes in human drug metabolism have been limited to food contaminants. Pesticide residues such as DDT (cholorophenothane), lindane (gamma benzene hexachloride), aldrin and dieldrin can be found in all levels of the food chain in varying concentrations. These residual concentrations are a function of such factors as the nature of the pest control treatment used in seed preparation, spraying and sprinkling, weathering, climate and soil conditions. Untreated plants may also absorb pesticides from the soil. Organo-chlorine insecticides are stored for prolonged periods in the body fat and livers of man and animals after having been absorbed from contaminated food. Although acute toxicity from such accumulation has not been observed in man thus far, residuals of certain pesticides (e.g., DDT, aldrin and dieldrin) have been shown to induce microsomal enzymes.

Alcohol has been shown to stimulate a microsomal enzyme system responsible for the metabolism of the oral hypoglycemic agent, tolbutamide. Resultant two fold reductions in the half-life of this drug have been observed in chronic alcoholic patients. This may well explain the relatively high failure rate in treating diabetics in this population.

(C) *Alteration in Urinary Excretion*

Changes in urinary pH have been shown to markedly influence the activity of some drugs by altering their respective rates of excretion. Such alterations in rates of excretion are functions of pH influence on the ionization of weak acids and weak bases. A drug in its nondissociated form, for example, will more readily diffuse from the urine back into the blood. The action of acidic drugs will be prolonged in acid urine because there is larger proportion of the drug in its undissociated form in acid urine than in alkaline urine where it would exist primarily as an ionized salt. The opposite phenomenon will occur for a basic drug such as amphetamine or quinidine.

Although it is generally thought that extreme shifts in urinary pH (i.e., well below 5 and above 8) are difficult to achieve through changes in dietary patterns alone, increased urinary acidification or alkalinization has been observed with concomitant ingestion of acid-or alkaline-ash diets and urinary acidifying or alkalinizing drugs (i.e., ammonium chloride and carbonic anhydrase inhibitors, respectively). Extreme shifts in urinary pH can have important clinical significance.

11.4 Pharmacologically Active Substances Present in Foods

Table 11.3 Tyramine-Containing Foods and MAO Inhibitors

Meat	Vegetable
Meat, fish fowl, shellfish	Corn and lentils
Eggs	
Cheese (all types)	
Peanut butter	
Fat	**Fruit**
Bacon	Plums
Nuts	
Peanuts, walnuts	
Bread	**Dessert**
Breads (all types),	Cakes and cookies, plain
Crackers	
Macaroni, Noodles	

Table 11.4 Potentially Basic or Alkaline -Ash Foods

Milk, Cream and Buttermilk
Nuts
Almonds, chestnuts, coconut
Vegetable - All types (except corn and lentils)
Fruits - All types (except cranberries, prunes, plums)

Pharmacologically active substances present in some foods have been shown to alter the response of a concomitantly administered drug. This type of interaction has been observed with the concomitant administration of monoamine oxidase inhibitors (e.g., pargyline, phenelzine, nialamide, tranylcypromine and isocarboxazid) and the ingestion of foods containing large amounts of tyramine and other biologically active amines. Several deaths were initially reported from this interaction as a result of exaggerated pressor responses and subsequent hypertensive crisis with intracranial bleeding. The hypertensive syndrome observed in this drug/food interaction has been described clinically similar to that seen in pheochromocytoma. Headache usually heralds the onset of the syndrome, with fever frequently accompanying the hypertensive episode. Most of the attacks have occurred between a half-hour and two hours after patients have eaten the cheese. Monoamine oxidase inhibition appears to modify and intensify the effects of endogenous biogenic amines as well as the precursors of biogenic amines (i.e. DOPA and 5-hydroxytrytophan). Evidence accumulated thus far, also indicates that the indirectly acting sympathomimetic amines such as amphetamine and tyramine are more potentiated than the direct acting amines such as nor epinephrine and epinephrine. Amphetamine and tyramine have been shown to act peripherally, primarily by releasing the stores of catecholamines in nerve endings. With monoamine oxidase inhibition, the levels of catecholamines are raised significantly, thereby producing profound potentiation of effects such as pressor actions.

Tyramine-containing foods (notably cheeses) and beverages have been the major offenders in this interaction, although DOPA (3, 4-dihyroxyphenylalanine) containing substances also have been implicated. It is imperative that patients receiving MAO inhibitors be appropriately counseled to avoid those foods which contain unusually high amounts of tyramine.

Other Foods

Licorice when ingested in excessive amounts has caused hypokalemic myopathy and myoglobinuria. This is thought to be due to an active principle, the 18-beta isomer of glycyrrhetinic acid, which has mineral corticoid, antidiuretic and anti-inflammatory activity. In addition to hypokalemia, excessive licorice ingestion has been associated with salt and water retention, hypertension, paresthesias, and alkalosis. Although this substance is only found in the foot of the *Glycyrrhiza* species, the natural extract of this plant is still used in some candy manufacturing as a licorice flavor.

Monosodium L-Glutamate

This widely used food additive monosodium L-glutamate has definitely been implicated as the causative agent in the "Chinese restaurant syndrome" in certain predisposed individuals. This syndrome is characterized by headaches, burning sensation of the extremities, facial pressure, and chest pain which may mimic the pain of angina. The pharmacological effects appear to be dose related. However, there is a considerable variation in oral threshold doses among individuals.

Goiterogenic Foods

Cabbage, cauliflower, turnips have been known to possess goiterogenic activity as a result of their thio-oxazolidine content. Under normal circumstances, however, there is usually enough iodine in the normal diet to counteract any such effect.

11.5 Drug – Food Interactions

- ***Grapefruit Juice***

  Grapefruit juice is a potent inhibitor of the intestinal cytochrome P-450 3A4 system (specifically: CYP3A4 - mediated drug metabolism) which is responsible for the first-pass metabolism of many medications. This interaction can lead to increases in bioavailability and corresponding increases in serum drug levels. Here are a few examples of adverse effects that are possible when the following medications are taken concurrently with grapefruit.

  - Excessive sedation: benzodiazepines
  - Increased risk of rhabdomyolyis: HMG-CoA reductase inhibitors (statins), (some exceptions exist)
  - Symptomatic hypotension: dihydropyridine calcium antagonists (some exceptions exist)
  - QT interval prolongation: astemizole, cisapride, pimozide, terfenadine. Drug interactions may be most apparent when patients are stabilized on the affected drug and the CYP3A4 inhibitor is then added to the regimen.

  There may be some pharmacological advantages to this interaction. If the interaction is taken into account during the initialization of drug therapy it is possible to decrease drug dosages. This concept can be applied to cyclosporine therapy. If a patient regularly consumes grapefruit, lower dosages of cyclosporine will be required, which will lead to lower drug costs.

  Grapefruit juice is not the only inhibitor of this enzyme system. Other drugs which have a similar effect include: clarithromycin, erythromycin, itraconazole, ketoconazole, nefazodone, and ritonavir.

  Many drugs interact with grapefruit (juice, segments, extract and certain related citrus fruits, e.g. Seville oranges, pummelos, and some exotic orange varieties). Several components in grapefruit called furanocoumarins (two of the most common are bergamottin and 6'7'-dihydroxybergamottin) irreversibly inhibit cytochrome P450 3A4 isoenzymes (3A4) in the intestinal wall, decreasing the pre-systemic metabolism of affected drugs taken up to 72 hours after grapefruit consumption. Intestinal 3A4 activity can remain inhibited during this time, as the body produces more enzymes. Greater amounts of 3A4-metabolized drugs can then enter the systemic circulation. The resulting increase in drug levels can lead to an increase in therapeutic effect, adverse effects and/or toxicity. Interactions are most pronounced for drugs that normally undergo a large amount of pre-systemic metabolism (low oral bioavailability). Grapefruit weakly inhibits intestinal cell wall p-glycoprotein (p-GP), an efflux pump in enterocytes that actively secretes some absorbed drugs back into the gut lumen. Not all 3A4-metabolized drugs are p-GP substrates. Organic anion transporting polypeptide (OATP) is another transporter system affected by grapefruit. Drugs handled by OATP may have decreased absorption when taken with grapefruit, possibly leading to loss of efficacy.

Medications that should be avoided with grapefruit

Amiodarone, astemizole, atorvastatin, budesonide, buspirone, cerivastatin, cilostazol, cisapride, colchicines, eletriptan, etoposide, halofantrine, lovastatin, mifepristone, pimozide, qinidine, sildenafil, simvastatin, sirolimus, terfenadine, ziprasidone.

Medications that should be used with caution

Albendazole, alfentanil, alfuzosin, almotriptan, aprepitant, aripiprazole, bupropion, carbamazepine, cinacalcet, clomipramine, cyclosporine, delavirdine, dextromethorphan, diazepam, dofetilide, efavirenz, erythromycin, eszopiclone, felodipine, fexofenadine, fluvoxamine, gefitinib, imatinib mesylate, indinavir, itraconazole, losartan, methadone, methylprednisolone, midazolam, montelukast, nicardipine, nifedipine, nimodipine, nisoldipine, oxybutynin, propafenone, quetiapine, fumarate, quinine, saquinavir, sertraline, solifenacin, tacrolimus, tamoxifen, tamsulosin, tolterodine, triazolam, trazodone.

Medications with no significant interaction with grapefruit

Acebutolol, alprazolam, amlodipine, amprenavir, caffeine, carvedilol, clarithromycin, clozapine, digoxin, diltiazem, eplerenone, ethinyl estradiol, fentanyl, haloperidol, lansoprazole, levothyroxine, omeprazole, phenytoin, pravastatin, prednisone, scopolamine, estradiol, telithromycin, theophylline, verapamil, warfarin.

Medications considered safe for use with grapefruit

*C*etirizine, desloratadine, fluvastatin, loratadine, praziquantel, rosuvastatin

- ***Orange juice***

  Orange juice shouldn't be consumed with antacids containing aluminum. The juice increases the absorption of the aluminum. Orange Juice and milk should be avoided when taking antibiotics. The juice's acidity decreases the effectiveness of antibiotics, as doe's milk.

- **Milk** doesn't mix with laxatives containing bisacodyl.
- Large amounts of **oatmeal** and other high-fiber cereals should not be eaten when taking digoxin. The fiber can interfere with the absorption of the drug.
- **Leafy green vegetables**, high in vitamin K, should not be taken in great quantities while taking warfarin. These vegetables could totally negate the affects of the drug and cause blood clotting.
- **Caffeinated beverages** and asthma drugs taken together can cause excessive excitability.
- **Grilled meat** can lead to problems for those on asthma medications containing theophylline. The chemical compounds formed when meat is grilled somehow prevent this type of medication from working effectively, increasing the possibility of an unmanageable asthma attack.
- Regularly consuming **a diet high in fat** while taking anti-inflammatory and arthritis medications can cause kidney damage and can leave the patient feeling drowsy and sedated.
- **Alcoholic beverages** tend to increase the depressive effects of medications such as benzodiazepines, antihistamines, antidepressants, antipsychotics, muscle relaxants, narcotics, or any drug with sedative actions.
- **Black licorice** with **digoxin** (which contains the ingredient glycyrrhizin) can produce irregular heart rhythms and cardiac arrest; licorice and diuretics will produce dangerously low potassium levels, putting a patient at risk for numbing weakness, muscle pain and even paralysis. Licorice can also interact with blood pressure medication or any calcium channel blockers.
- **Aged cheese** (brie, parmesan, cheddar and Roquefort), fava beans, sauerkraut, Italian green beans, some beers, red wine, pepperoni and overly ripe avocados should be avoided by people taking MAO antidepressants. The interaction can cause a potentially fatal rise in blood pressure.

Table 11.5 Some prominent Drug - Food Interactions*

Drugs	Effects and Precautions
	Antibiotics
Cephalosporins, Penicillin	Take on an empty stomach to speed absorption of the drugs.
Erythromycin	Don't take with fruit juice or wine, which decrease the drug's effectiveness.
Sulfa drugs	Increase the risk of Vitamin B-12 deficiency
Tetracycline	Diary products reduce the drug's effectiveness. Lowers Vitamin C absorption
	Anticonvulsants
Dilantin, Phenobarbital	Increase the risk of anemia and nerve problems due to deficiency of folate and other B vitamins.

Table 5 *Contd...*

Drugs	Effects and Precautions
Antidepressants	
Fluoxetine	Reduce appetite and can lead to excessive weight loss
Lithium	A low-salt diet increases the risk of lithium toxicity; excessive salt reduces the drug's efficacy
MAO Inhibitors	Foods high in tyramine (aged cheeses, processed meats, legumes, wine, and beer, among others) can bring on a hypertensive crisis.
Tricyclics	Many foods, especially legumes, meat, fish, and foods high in Vitamin C, reduce absorption of the drugs.
Antihypertensives, Heart Medications	
ACE inhibitors	Take on an empty stomach to improve the absorption of the drugs.
Alpha blockers	Take with liquid or food to avoid excessive drop in blood pressure.
Antiarrhythmic drugs	Avoid caffeine, which increases the risk of irregular heartbeat.
Beta blockers	Take on an empty stomach; food, especially meat, increases the drug's effects and can cause dizziness and low blood pressure.
Digitalis	Avoid taking with milk and high fiber foods, which reduce absorption, increases potassium loss.
Diuretics	Increase the risk of potassium deficiency.
Potassium sparing diuretics	Don't take diuretics with potassium supplements or salt substitutes, which can cause potassium overload.
Thiazide diuretics	Increase the reaction to MSG.
Asthma Drugs	
Pseudoephedrine	Avoid caffeine, which increase feelings of anxiety and nervousness.
Theophylline	Charbroiled foods and high protein diet reduce absorption. Caffeine increases the risk of drug toxicity.
Cholesterol Lowering Drugs	
Cholestyramine	Increases the excretion of folate and vitamins A, D, E, and K.
Gemfibrozil	Avoid fatty foods, which decrease the drug's efficacy in lowering cholesterol.
Heartburn and Ulcer Medications	
Antacids	Interfere with the absorption of many minerals; for maximum benefit, take medication one hour after eating.
Cimetidine, Famotidine, Sucralfate	Avoid high protein foods, caffeine, and other items that increase stomach acidity.
Hormone Preparations	
Oral contraceptives	Salty foods increase fluid retention. Drugs reduce the absorption of folate, vitamin B-6, and other nutrients; increase intake of foods high in these nutrients to avoid deficiencies.

Table 5 *Contd...*

Drugs	Effects and Precautions
Hormone Preparations	
Steroids	Salty foods increase fluid retention. Increase intake of foods high in calcium, vitamin K, potassium, and protein to avoid deficiencies.
Thyroid drugs	Iodine-rich foods lower the drug's efficacy.
Laxatives	
Mineral Oils	Overuse can cause a deficiency of vitamins A, D, E, and K.
Painkillers	
Aspirin and stronger non-steroidal anti-inflammatory drugs	Always take with food to lower the risk of gastrointestinal irritation; avoid taking with alcohol, which increases the risk of bleeding. Frequent use of these drugs lowers the absorption of folate and vitamin C.
Codeine	Increase fiber and water intake to avoid constipation.
Sleeping Pills, Tranquilizers	
Benzodiazepines	Never take with alcohol. Caffeine increases anxiety and reduce drug's effectiveness
*(Adapted from www.foodmedinteractions.com)	

11.6 Drug – Alcohol Interactions

Taking certain drugs with alcohol can cause very harmful effects. Certain drugs belonging to the categories of antianxiety, antiepileptic, antidiabetic, antihistamines, antianginal, antihypertensives, hypercholesterolemic drugs, analgesics etc., can cause some reactions when used with alcohol. Sometimes they cause serious and fatal reactions which can be life threatening. Certain medications like pain killers, cold and cough remedies, anti allergy drugs contain more than one ingredient that can react with alcohol. Some cough syrups and laxatives, and some vitamin tonics may contain very high concentration of alcohol even to the extent of 10%.

Women in general have a higher risk for problems than men when she consumes alcohol. The alcohol concentration reaches higher level than in men, even when both are drinking the same amount. This is because female bodies generally have less water than male bodies. As alcohol mixes with body water, a given amount of alcohol is more concentrated in a female body than in male. As a result females are more susceptible to alcohol related damage of organs such as liver. Older people are at particularly high risk for harmful alcohol-medication interactions. Aging slows the body's ability to break down alcohol, so alcohol remains in a person's system longer. Alcohol and medicines can interact harmfully even when they are not taken at the same time.

Table 11.6 Commonly used medicines (Prescription and OTC) that interact with alcohol*

Symptoms / Disorders	Medication taken	Some possible reactions with alcohol
Allergies / Cold / Flu	Loratadine, Fexofenadine, Diphenhydramine, Desloratadine, Brompheniramine, Chlorpheniramine, Cetirizine,	Drowsiness, dizziness; increased risk for over dose.
Angina, Coronary Heart Disease	Isosorbide, Nitroglycerin	Rapid heart beat, sudden changes in blood pressure, dizziness, fainting
Anxiety and Epilepsy	Lorazepam, Clonazepam, Chlordiazepoxide, Paroxetine, Diazepam, Alprazolam	Drowsiness, dizziness; increased risk for over dose; slowed or difficulty breathing; impaired motor control; unusual behaviour and memory problems.
Arthritis	Celecoxib, Naproxen, Diclofenac	Ulcers, stomach bleeding, liver problems
Blood clots	Warfarin	Occasional drinking may lead to internal bleeding; heavier drinking also may cause bleeding or may have the opposite effect, resulting in blood clots, strokes, or heart attacks.
Cough	Dextromethorphan, Guaifenesin Codeine	Drowsiness, dizziness; increased risk for overdose.
Depression	Clomipramine, Citalopram, Trazodone, Venlafaxine, Amitryptiline, Escitalopram, Fluvoxamine, Desipramine, Paroxetine, Fluoxetine, Nefazodone, Bupropion, Sertraline	Drowsiness, dizziness; increased risk for over dose; increased feelings of depression or hopelessness in adolescents (suicide)
Diabetes	Metformin, Glyburide, Tolbutamide	Abnormally low blood sugar levels, flushing reaction (nausea, vomiting, headache, rapid heart beat, sudden changes in blood pressure)
Enlarged prostrate	Doxazosin, Terazosin, Tamsulosin, Prazosin	Dizziness, light headedness, fainting
Heartburn, indigestion, sour stomach	Nizatidine, Metoclopramide, Ranitidine	Rapid heartbeat, sudden changes in blood pressure (metoclopramide); increased alcohol effect.
High blood pressure	Quinapril, Hydrochlorthiazide, Doxazosin, Clonidine, Losartan, Terazosin, Benzapril, Prazosin, Enalapril	Dizziness, fainting, drowsiness,; heart problems such as changes in the heart's regular heartbeat (arrhythmia)

Table 11.6 *Contd...*

Symptoms / Disorders	Medication taken	Some possible reactions with alcohol
High Cholesterol	Lovastatin, Rosuvastatin, Niacin, Atorvastatin, Pravastatin, Simvastatin, Ezetimibe	Liver damage (all medications); increased flushing and itching (niacin); increased stomach bleeding (pravastatin + aspirin).
Infections	Nitrofurantoin, Metronidazole, Griseofulvin, Ketoconazole, Isoniazid, Cycloserine, Tinidazole	Fast heartbeat, sudden changes in blood pressure; stomach pain, upset stomach, vomiting, headache, or flushing or redness of the face; liver damage (isoniazid, ketoconazole)
Muscle pain	Cyclobenzaprine, Carisoprodol	Drowsiness, dizziness; increase risk of seizures; increased risk for over dose; slowed or difficulty breathing; impaired motor control; unusual behaviour; memory problems.
Nausea, motion sickness	Meclizine, Hydroxyzine, Dimenhydrinate, Promethazine	Drowsiness, dizziness; increased risk for overdose.
Pain, fever, inflammation	Ibuprofen, Naproxen, Aspirin, Acetaminophen,	Stomach upset, bleeding and ulcers; liver damage (acetaminophen); rapid heartbeat.
Seizures	Phenytoin, Clonazepam, Phenobarbital	Drowsiness, dizziness; increased risk of seizures.
Severe pain from injury, post surgical care, oral surgery, migraines	Propoxyphene, Meperidine, Oxycodone, Hydrocodone	Drowsiness, dizziness; increased risk for over dose; slowed or difficulty breathing; impaired motor control; unusual behaviour; memory problems.
Sleep problems	Zolpidem, Eszopiclone, Estazolam, Temazepam, Diphenhydramine, Doxylamine	Drowsiness, sleepiness, dizziness; slowed or difficulty breathing; impaired motor control; unusual behaviour; memory problems
***Adapted from (www.nlm.nih.gov)**		

11.7 Drug – Herb Interactions

Most drug interactions involving herbal products are not well documented. For example, many herbal products are reported to increase the bleeding risk in patients receiving warfarin, but very few of them could be considered well documented.

Herbal products may not contain what is indicated on the label. Some herbal products simply do not contain the product that is stated, while others are adulterated with other medications, some of which could produce serious toxicity. So, even if a patient has taken one herbal product with prescription medications without mishap, switching to a different brand of the same herbal product may produce an adverse drug interaction. In addition, because of the lack of regulatory requirements on the accuracy of labeled amount of herb products, large variations in content within products are known to occur. Even if a patient buys the same brand of herbal products, the amount consumed may vary from lot to lot.

St John's wort is an enzyme inducer and may reduce drug effect. St John's wort is one of the few herbals for which there is credible and extensive information on drug interactions. St John's wort is a well-documented inducer of CYP3A4 and tends to reduce the serum concentrations and effect of a variety of CYP3A4 substrates. Given that CYP3A4 is estimated to be involved in the metabolism of about half of all drugs that patients take, the potential for St John's wort drug interactions is substantial. Already, numerous examples of reduced drug effects have been documented with concurrent use of St John's wort with cyclosporine, indinavir, irinotecan, nifedipine, simvastatin, tricyclic antidepressants, and warfarin.

The decision to use herbal products in patients on prescription medications should be based on estimated benefit vs. risk. With the exception of St John's wort, little is known about the risk of using herbal products with prescription medications. There may be a few cases, such as reports of bleeding in patients on warfarin who take ginkgo biloba. Since there are no controls in such cases, however, it is not possible to be sure that the patient would not have had the bleeding episode in the absence of ginkgo. So, the risk of adding ginkgo is not known. Yet, the benefit is also unknown; indeed, there is little credible clinical information to suggest that ginkgo improves mental functioning.

Therefore, when considering whether a patient on warfarin should take ginkgo, one is left with an unknown risk of bleeding and an unknown benefit on mental functioning. Given the unknown (and questionable) benefit, however, one's tolerance for risk should be quite low. So, even though it is not clear whether ginkgo can be dangerous in patients on warfarin, most people should probably not be inclined to take the risk.

Some Prominent Drug-Herb Interactions

The following are the examples of known interaction between popular herbs and drugs.

Hawthorn, touted as effective in reducing angina attacks by lowering blood pressure and cholesterol levels, should never be taken with Lanoxin (digoxin), the medication prescribed for most heart ailments. The mix can lower heart rate too much, causing blood to pool, bringing possible heart failure.

Ginseng, according to research, can increase blood pressure, making it dangerous for those trying to keep their blood pressure under control. Ginseng, garlic or supplements containing ginger, when taken with the blood-thinning drug, Coumadin, can cause bleeding episodes. Warfarin is a very powerful drug that leaves little room for error, and patients taking it should never take any medication or otherwise before consulting a qualified health professional. In rare cases, ginseng may overstimulate resulting in insomnia. Consuming caffeine with ginseng increases the risk of overstimulation and gastrointestinal upset. Long tern use of ginseng may cause menstrual abnormalities and breast tenderness in some women. Ginseng is not recommended for pregnant or lactating women.

Garlic capsules combined with diabetes medication can cause a dangerous decrease in blood sugars. Some people who are sensitive to garlic may experience heartburn and flatulence. Garlic has anti-clotting properties.

Goldenseal is used for coughs, stomach upsets, menstrual problems and even arthritis. However, the plant's active ingredient will raise blood pressure, complicating treatment for those taking antihypertensive medications, especially beta-blockers. For patients taking medication to control diabetes or kidney disease, this herb can cause dangerous electrolyte imbalance. High amount of consumption can lead to gastrointestinal distress and possible nervous system effects. Not recommended for pregnant or lactating women.

Feverfew, believed to be the natural remedy for migraine headaches, should never be taken with Imitrex or other migraine medications. It can result in the patient's heart rate and blood pressure to reach dangerous levels.

Guarana, an alternative remedy being used as a stimulant and diet aid, contains 3-5 % more caffeine than a cup of coffee. So, any medicine that should not be taken with any drink containing caffeine, should not take guarana. It may cause insomnia, trembling, anxiety, palpitations, urinary frequency, and hyperactivity. Avoid during pregnancy and lactation period. Long term use of Guarana may lead to decreased fertility, cardiovascular disease, and several forms of cancer.

Kava, an herb that has antianxiety, pain relieving, muscle relaxing and anticonvulsant effects, should not be taken together with substances that also act on the central nervous system, such as alcohol, barbiturates, anti depressants, and antipsychotic drugs.

St. John's Wort is a popular herb used for the treatment of mild depression.The active ingredient of St. John's Wort is hypericin. Hypericin is believed to exert a similar influence on the brain as the monoamine oxidase (MAO) inhibitors such as the one in major antidepressants. Mixing MAO inhibitors with foods high in tyramine, an amino acid, produces one of the most dramatic and dangerous food-drug interactions. Symptoms, which can occur within minutes of ingesting such foods while taking an MAO inhibitor, include rapid rise in blood pressure, a severe headache, and perhaps collapse and even death. Foods high in tyramine include aged cheese, chicken liver, Chianti (and certain other red wines), yeast extracts, bologna (and other processed meats), dried or pickled fish, legumes, soy sauce, ale, and beer.

Some patients report that St. Johns Wort caused excessive stimulation and sometimes dizziness, agitation and confusion when taken with other antidepressants. It also caused their blood pressure to shoot up.

White Willow, an herb traditionally used for fever, headache, pain, and rheumatic complaints may lead to gastrointestinal irritation, if used for a long time. It exhibits similar reactions as aspirin (aspirin is derived from white willow). Long term use may lead to stomach ulcers.

Turnips contain two goitrogenic substances, progoitrin and gluconasturtin, which can interfere with the thyroid glands ability to make its hormones. Although moderate consumption of goitrogens is not a hazard for healthy people, they can promote development of a goiter (an enlarged thyroid) in persons with thyroid disease.

Tomato contains small quantities of a toxic substance known as solanine that may trigger headaches in susceptible people. They are also a relatively common cause of allergies. An unidentified substance in tomatoes and tomato-based products can cause acid reflux, leading to indigestion and heartburn. Individuals who often have digestive upsets should try eliminating tomatoes for 2 to 3 weeks to see if there is any improvement.

Strawberries, Raspberries, Spinach, and Rhubarb These contain oxalic acid, which can aggravate kidney and bladder stones in susceptible people, and reduce body's ability to absorb iron and calcium.

Raspberries contain a natural salicylate that can cause an allergic reaction in aspirin sensitive people.

The **seeds from fruits such as Apple, apricot, and Quinces** contain amygdalin, a compound that turns into Hydrogen Cyanide in the stomach. Eating large amount of seeds can result in cyanide poisoning.

Potatoes with a green tint to the skin will taste bitter and may contain solanine, a toxic substance that can cause diarrhea, cramps, and fatigue.

Plums, Peaches, Apricots, and Cherries may produce allergic reaction in individuals with confirmed allergies to apricots, almonds, peaches, and cherries. People who are allergic to aspirin may also encounter problems after they have eaten plums or peaches as they contain salicylates. The pits of plums, peaches and apricots contain a compound called amygdalin. When consumed in large amounts, amygdalin breaks down into hydrogen cyanide, a poison.

Very high doses of **horseradish** can cause vomiting or excessive sweating. Avoid if you have hypothyroidism.

Turmeric should be avoided by persons with symptoms from gallstones.

Table 11.7 Drug – Herb Interaction Chart*

Herb (botanical name)	Interaction/Side effects (SE)
Agrimony	warfarin ↓ INR → herb may be a coagulant **SE**: photo dermatitis
Alfalfa (Medicago sativa)	cholesterol meds → herb may further ↓ lipid levels cyclosporin/steroids → herb immuno-stimulating hypoglycemic meds → herb may cause further hypoglycemia warfarin ↑↓ INR → herb may contain warfarin constituents or ↓ effect because of Vitamin K content in herb **SE**: rare pancytopenia & worsening of lupus **CI**: Lupus
Aloe (Aloe vera)	digoxin & thiazide ↑ cardiac toxicity → due to electrolyte imbalance Not recommended with breastfeeding. **SE**: contact dermatitis
Angelica	Warfarin ↑ **INR** → herb may contain warfarin constituents Not recommended with breastfeeding. **SE**: photo dermatitis
Anise (Aniseed)	MAOI's → herb may ↑ risk of hypertensive crisis warfarin ↑ INR → herb may contain warfarin constituents
Aristolochia	amiodarone, anabolic steroids, ketoconazole, methotrexate → herb may have additive **hepatotoxicity** effect **SE**: **nephrotoxic**
Arnica (Wolf bane)	warfarin ↑ INR → herb may contain warfarin constituents
Asafoetida	Warfarin ↑ INR → herb may contain warfarin constituents- in vivo
Ayurvedic syrup	phenytoin → herb **may** ↓ **phenytoin levels** as well as ↓ efficacy **SE**: heavy metal poisoning from contamination
Betel nut (Areca catechu)	Antipsychotics → herb may ↑ **extrapyramidal SE** (strong cholinergic effects); **asthmatics** → inadequate control of asthma
Black cohosh (Cimicifuga racemosa) **Remifemin 20 mg bid**	Hormones → herb may have estrogen-like effect. Dose: 40-80mg/day. iron → herb contains tannic acids which may ↓ iron absorption warfarin ↑ INR → herb may contain **salicylates SE**: For menopausal symptoms → may cause mild GI effects & ↓ BP
Bladderwrack (Fucus, Kelp)	warfarin ↑ INR → herb may have anticoagulant action levothyroxine → herb is a source of iodine → caused **hyperthyroidism**
Bogbean	Warfarin ↑ INR → herb may have hemolytic activity
Borage	antipsychotics/anticonvulsants/TCA's → herb may ↑ **seizures** amiodarone, anabolic steroids, ketoconazole; methotrexate → herb may have additive **hepatotoxicity** effect. Generally **unsafe**

Table 11.7 *Contd...*

Herb (botanical name)	Interaction/Side effects (SE)
Broom	Antihypertensive meds → herb may ↑ BP by itself
Calamus	Sedatives → herb may potentiate sedation. Generally **unsafe**
Capsicum (Chili peppers)	MAOI's → herb ↑ risk of hypertensive crisis SE: dermatitis, GI upset. **ACE inhibitor** → may ↑ **cough**; **theophylline** → may ↑ absorption
Cascara (Rhamnus purshiana)	Various meds →↓ absorption since going quicker via GI system Digoxin/thiazides/steroids → herb may potentiate **hypokalemia**
Cassia	warfarin ↑ INR → herb may inhibit platelet aggregation
Celery (seed/extract)	warfarin ↑ INR → herb may contain warfarin constituents sedatives → herb may potentiate sedation. Herb →? diuretic action.
Cereus	MAOI's/SSRI's/TCA's → herb may↑ risk of serotonin syndrome
Chamomile (Natricaria reutita) (German/Roman)	warfarin ↑ INR → herb may contain warfarin constituents iron → herb contains tannic acids which may ↓ iron absorption **sedatives** → herb may potentiate sedation
Chaparral (Larrea tridentata)	amiodarone, anabolic steroids, ketoconazole, methotrexate → herb may have additive **hepatotoxicity** effect. Generally **unsafe**
Chinese herb mixture	Rare: heavy metal exposure due to **contamination**
Chondroitin 1200mg/day	warfarin↑ **INR** → herb may increase bleeding & chondroitin sulfate is a component of the antithrombotic danaparoid **SE**: GI. Poor **oral** absorption ~<10%, IM form in other countries.
Chromium picolinate	nephrotoxic drugs → herb may↑ cause renal failure & rhabdomyolysis hypoglycemic → herb may cause hypoglycemia
Clove	warfarin ↑ INR → herb contains eugenol –a platelet inhibitor
Coltsfoot (Tussilago farfar)	amiodarone, anabolic steroids, ketoconazole, methotrexate → herb may have additive **hepatotoxicity** effect. Not received with breastfeeding
Comfrey (Symphytum species)	amiodarone, anabolic steroids, ketoconazole, methotrexate → herb may have additive **hepatotoxicity** effect. Generally **unsafe**
Co-enzyme Q10 (Ubiquinone)	betablockers, phenothiazines, TCA's, doxorubicin → herb may ↓ cardiac side effects from these medications cardiac & antihypertensives → may improve effect of cardiac meds HMG-Co A & hypoglycemic → may ↓ natural levels of **Q10** in body warfarin ↓ INR → herb may decrease effect of warfarin
Couchgrass	diuretics → herb may↑ potassium loss; lithium → herb may alter level. sedatives → herb may potentiate sedation

Table 11.7 *Contd...*

Herb (botanical name)	Interaction/Side effects (SE)
Dandelion	diuretics & lithium → herb may ↑ diuretic effect & ↑ lithium toxicity warfarin ↓ INR →↓ effect due to Vitamin K content in the herb
Danshen	Warfarin ↑ **INR** → **clinical bleed** due to acetylsalvianolic acid
Dehydroepiandrosterone DHEA	Warfarin ↑ INR → herb may have fibrinolytic potential. triazolam level can ↑ due to DHEA. Banned by the NBA.
Devil's Claw (Harpagophytum procumbens)	heart & blood pressure meds → herb may interfere (↑↓) with BP hypoglycemics → herb may cause **hypo/hyperglycemia** **warfarin → purpura** **SE:** headache, ringing ears, ↓ appetite, ↓ taste
Dong Quai (Angelica sinensis)	heart meds → herb has **quinidine** like activity warfarin↑ **INR** → herb contain warfarin constituent-**Case reports** Not recommended with breastfeeding. **SE**: photosensitive
Echinacea Ⓟ **Purple Coneflower E. purpurea, pallida & angustifolia**	amiodarone, anabolic steroids, ketoconazole, methotrexate → herb may have additive **hepatotoxicity** if used for > 8 weeks **corticosteroids/cyclosporine** → avoid combination glycemic control → herb may cause hypo/hyperglycemia warfarin ↑ INR → herb in vitro ↑ INR → by ↓ warfarin metabolism **SE**: Often used for 2 weeks for an acute infection but can cause allergic reaction, tiredness, somnolence, dizziness, headache & GI upset. **CI**: HIV, TB, transplant pts, RA, MS, lupus → herb immunostimulant
Elecampane	sedatives → herb may potentiate sedation
Ephedra Ⓟ **(Ma huang) Herbal Ecstasy Ephedrine/ Pseudoephedrine (Ban in olympics) ?~1% ephedrine. Tea~15-30mg ephedrine/cup.**	Anticonvulsants → herb may cause **seizures** caffeine,decongestants, stimulants → herb may ↑ nervousness & tremor **heart & blood pressure** meds → herb may ↑ heart rate & BP hypoglycemics → herb may cause hypo/**hyper**glycemia **SE**: Used in many weight loss or energy products but **over 800 reports** of nervousness, insomnia, irritability, psychosis, headache, dizziness, seizures, stroke, premature ventricular contraction, hypertension, **myocardial infarction & death** FDA maximum: 8mg/dose & 24mg/day for no more than a week. Not recommended with breastfeeding. **NOT considered SAFE**
Evening Primrose oil (Oenothera biennis)	**anaesthetics/antipsychotics**/anticonvulsants → herb↑ **seizures SE**: For menopause but can cause nausea, headache & soft stools
Fenugreek	warfarin↑ INR → herb may contain warfarin constituents
Feverfew Tanacet 125mg daily (Tanacetum parthenium)	iron → herb contains tannic acids which may ↓ iron absorption **NSAIDS/STEROIDS** → may ↓ the therapeutic **effect** of feverfew warfarin ↑ INR → herb in vitro ? inhibit binding of platelets Recommend 0.2% but most products contain <0.1% parthenolide **SE**: Often used for migraine headaches but can cause gastric discomfort, oral ulcers, lip & tongue swelling & rebound headache when herb stopped. Not recommended with breastfeeding.

Table 11.7 *Contd...*

Herb (botanical name)	Interaction/Side effects (SE)
Flaxseed	warfarin ↑ INR → herb may ↑ bleeding time **(Linum usitatissimum)**
Garlic Ⓟ (Allium sativum) Active agents: allicin & ajoene Need high doses to work. Only short 3hr half life & acid labile → enteric coated better	antihypertensive meds → this herb may ↓ BP thus caution advised aspirin/warfarin ↑ **INR** → ajoene, a product of allicin breakdown is believed to be responsible for **reversible** inhibition of platelet aggregation- clinical bleeding has occurred (**Case reports**) hypoglycemic → herb may cause hypoglycemia; **saquinavir** →↓ level **SE**: Often used for hypertension & high **cholesterol** but can cause burning sensation, nausea, heartburn, menorrhagia, diaphoresis, lightheadedness, **odor**iferous skin & breath & contact dermatitis.
Germander (Teucrium chamaedrys)	amiodarone, anabolic steroids, ketoconazole, methotrexate → herb may have additive **hepatotoxicity** effect Generally considered **unsafe- 30 cases of acute liver failure**.
Ginger (Zingiber officinale)	heart & antihypertensives → herb may ↑ or ↓ effect with these meds hypoglycemics → herb may cause hypoglycemia warfarin ↑ **INR** → herb may inhibit platelet aggregation (in vitro) **SE**: Used for antiemetic but cause heart burn & allergic reactions.
Ginkgo biloba Ⓟ (Maidenhair Tree) ~40mg po tid ac	acetaminophen & ergotamine/caffeine → subarachnoid **hemorrhage** & subdural hematoma anticonvulsant/TCA/trazodone → may ↓ seizure threshold → ↑ seizures **aspirin/clopidogrel/dipyridamole/ticlopidine/ warfarin** ↑ **INR** → ginkolide B may inhibit platelet activating factor by displacement from its receptor binding sites (**Case reports**) thiazides → with herb may lead to hypertension (1 case) **SE**: Often used to help circulation & cognition but may cause **headache**, dizziness, restlessness, nausea, vomiting, diarrhea & dermal sensitivity.
Ginseng, Eleuthero or Siberian Eleutherococcus senticosus)	digoxin → herb **may↑ digoxin** serum level (? Maybe assay interference with level or from contaminated P. sepium) heart & blood pressure meds → herb may change BP/ ↑ heart rate warfarin↑ INR → herb ? ↓ platelet aggregation & contain coumarin. Not recommended with breastfeeding.
Ginseng, Ⓟ American (Panax quinquefolius) Korean/Asian (Panax ginseng) Only 25% of ginseng products actually contained ginseng in a recent study, plus **85% did not contain ginseng in a 1990 survey.**	alcohol → may↑ alcohol clearance from the body corticosteroids → herb may affect steroid concentrations heart & blood pressure meds → herb has negative chronotropic & inotropic activity, as well as possible ↓ **blood pressure estrogens/corticosteroids** → herb may have possible additive effects (reported mastalgia & postmenopausal bleeding) **furosemide** → case report of diminishing furosemide effect hypoglycemics → herb may have additive **hypoglycemic** effect **MAOI's** → may inhibit reuptake of various neurotransmitters & ↑ tremor/**mania** thus contraindicated mood stabilizers → herb may **induce mania** oral contraceptives → herb may interfere in effectiveness of sex hormone treatment **sedatives** → herb may potentiate/antagonize sedative side effects warfarin ↑↓ **INR** → herb may cause reduction of blood coagulation or ↓ **INR** (**Case reports**) **SE**: in general for ALL species: nervousness, excitation, diarrhea, insomnia, inability to concentrate, headache, hypertension, epistaxis, allergies & skin eruptions. Not recommended with breastfeeding

Table 11.7 *Contd...*

Herb (botanical name)	Interaction/Side effects (SE)
Glucosamine ~500mg po tid	hypoglycemics/insulin → ? herb may ↑ glucose or insulin resistance. Well absorbed ~90%. Inj avail other countries. Some efficacy Arch Int Med Jul 03 **SE**: For osteoarthritis but may cause GI side effects such as diarrhea.
Goldenseal (Hydrastis canadensis)	heart & antihypertensives → herb can alter heart & blood pressure heparin → herb can oppose the action of heparin sedatives → herb may ↑ sedation. **Expensive & often adulterated.**
Gotu kola	sedatives → herb may ↑ sedation statins → lipids herb may ↑
Green tea	iron → herb contains tannic acids which may ↓ iron absorption warfarin ↓ **INR** → herb may contain ↑ vitamin K content (in vitro). Contains 10-80mg caffeine/cup. **Lithium** level ↑ if stop caffeine is stopped.
Guar gum (Cyamopsis tetragonolobus)	digoxin & penicillin V → slows absorption in the stomach glyburide, iron & **metformin** →↓ absorption with some formulations **SE**: rare gastric obstruction. May ↓ cholesterol levels.
Hawthorn (Crataegus monogyna)	**digoxin & antihypertensives** → herb may interfere with these meds MAOI's → may contain tyramine thus ↑ risk of hypertensive crisis
Hops	**sedatives** → herbs may ↑ sedation; herb has estrogen like chemicals
Horse chestnut	aspirin & warfarin ↑ INR → herb may contain warfarin constituents **SE**: irritant to stomach & hypoglycemia **(Aesculus hippocastanum)**
Horseradish	warfarin ↑ INR → peroxidase stimulates arachidonic acid metabolites
Indian snakeroot	antihypertensives & digoxin → herb can ↑ effect antidepressants → can ↓ effect (reserpine found in herb)
Jamaican Dogwood	sedatives → herb may potentiate sedative SE
Karela (Bitter melon)	hypoglycemic → herb may affect blood glucose levels
Kava kava Ⓟ (Piper methysticum) -a social drink in South Pacific	alcohol/antipsychotics/sedatives → herb may ↑ **sedation** alprazolam /benzodiazepines → has led to additive depression (Case report of ↑ lethargy/?coma with alprazolam) antiparkinsonian meds → herb may exacerbate Parkinson's–case report **SE**: Often used for anxiolytic but causes headache, dizziness, GI discomfort & local numbess after oral ingestion; **dry scaly skin** & discoloration **(yellow)**, leukopenia, **thrombocytopenia**, photosensitivity & eye redness with long term use or high dosages. Reports of **hepatotoxicity FDA Mar/02**.Not recomm. with breastfeeding
Kelp	Levothyroxine → herb source of iodine → caused hyperthyroidism
Kombucha	amiodarone, anabolic steroids, ketoconazole, methotrexate → herb may have additive **hepatotoxicity** effect. Source of **anthrax** outbreak.
Kyushin	digoxin → herb may interfere with dynamics/ monitoring

Table 11.7 *Contd...*

Herb (botanical name)	Interaction/Side effects (SE)
Life root (Senecio aureus)	amiodarone, anabolic steroids, ketoconazole, methotrexate → herb may have additive **hepatotoxicity** effect. Generally **unsafe**
Licorice (Glcyrrhiza glabra) **High dose is >50 grams/day** **Most licorice in the USA contains anise oil rather than licorice.**	antihypertensives/digoxin/loop diuretics/spironolactone/thiazides → herb may cause **hypokalemia**, plus **sodium & fluid retention** which can ↑ blood pressure (ie. Pseudoaldosteronism) corticosteroids → herb **may↑ oral & topical steroid** effects digoxin → herb may interfere with pharmacodynamically/monitoring hypoglycemic → herb may cause ↓ glucose tolerance thus caution oral contraceptive → may lead to hypertension, edema & ↓ potassium warfarin ↑ INR → herb may inhibit platelet activity **SE**: lethargy, headache & electrolyte imbalances. Not recommended with breastfeeding. Generally **unsafe**
Meadowsweet	warfarin ↑ INR → herb may contain salicylate constituents
Melilot (Sweet clover)	warfarin ↑ INR → herb may contain warfarin constituents
Milk thistle (Silybum marianum)	hypoglycemics → herb may have additive hypoglycemic effect **SE**: Gastric pain, diarrhea, vomiting & allergic reactions. In Europe available IV to "detoxify the liver". Oral ~25% absorbed.
Mistletow	warfarin ↓ INR → herb may contain lectins → ↓ agglutination
Nettle	iron → herb contains tannic acids which may ↓ iron absorption sedatives → herb may potentiate sedation warfarin ↓ INR → herb may contain Vitamin K
Papain/Papaya	warfarin ↑ INR → may ↑ INR **(Carica papaya) SE:** gastritis
Parsley	Antihypertensives → herb has sympathomimetics → watch for ↑ BP **MAOI's** → herb ↑ risk of hypertensive crisis. Herb may contain Vit K
Passionflower	MAOI's/SSRI's/TCA's → herb may ↑ risk of **serotonin syndrome** **sedative** → herb ↑ sedation; warfarin ↑ INR → may contain coumarins
Pennyroyal (Mentha puleguim)	amiodarone, anabolic steroids, ketoconazole, methotrexate → herb may have additive **hepatotoxicity** effect (? Treat → acetylcysteine)
Plantain (Black psyllium)	carbamazepine/digoxin/iron/lithium/warfarin →↓ absorption by herb digoxin → herb may interfere with absorption/dynamics/monitoring
Pleurisy root	MAOI's → herb ↑ risk of hypertensive crisis
Poplar	warfarin ↑ INR → herb may contain salicylate constituents
Prickly Ash	warfarin ↑ INR → herb may contain warfarin constituents
Psyllium (P.ovata)	carbamazepine/digoxin/iron/lithium/warfarin → herb ↓ absorption
Quassia	warfarin ↑ INR → herb may contain warfarin constituents

Table 11.7 *Contd...*

Herb (botanical name)	Interaction/Side effects (SE)
Red Clover (Promensil)	oral contraceptive → herb may ↓ effect. Made cheetah's sterile. warfarin INR → herb may contain warfarin. **SE**: rash
Royal jelly	asthma medications → herb may cause bronchospasm Expensive source of "B" vitamins. Food for queen bee.
Sage	Sedatives → herb may potentiate sedation
Saiboku-to Asian herb mixture	corticosteroids → herb may ↑ prednisolone levels Same herbs → **sho-saiko-to**, Poria cocos, Mangolia officinalis & Perillae frutescens
Sassafras	**SE**: sedation. Generally considered **unsafe (S. albidum)**
Sauropus androgynus	amiodarone, anabolic steroids, ketoconazole & methotrexate → herb may potentiate **hepatotoxicity**
Saw palmetto (Serenoa repens) Sabal fruit May cause false negative PSA test	**estrogen/contraceptives/hormone** → herb may have antiandrogen & estrogenic activity iron → herb contains tannic acids which can ↓ iron absorption **SE**: Often used for benign **prostatic hyperplasia** but causes **headache,** GI discomfort (nausea, abdonimal pain, constipation & diarrhea) & rare hormonal actions (breast tenderness, loss of libido & venous thrombosis). Efficacy: ≤ Proscar but likely < than ∝ 1 blockers
Scullcap	amiodarone, anabolic steroids, ketoconazole, methotrexate → herb may have additive **hepatotoxicity** effect (? due to adulterants) **sedatives** → herb may potentiate sedation
Senna (Cassia senna)	digoxin/thiazides/steroids → herb may potentiate hypokalemia various meds →↓ absorption → going quicker via GI system
Shanka pushpi	phenytoin → herb **may** ↓ **phenytoin levels** as well as ↓ efficacy **(Ayurvedic mixed herb syrup)**
Shepherds Purse	MAOI's → may contain tyramine thus ↑ risk of hypertensive crisis sedatives → herb may potentiate sedation
Sho-saiko-to	prednisolone →↓ levels for prednisolone **(Asian herb mixture)**
St. John's Ⓟ Wort (Hypericum perforatum) ~300mg po tid -not for major depressionJAMA APR 01 & 02 **Active agents:** **0.3% hypericin & hyperforin (Used commonly –esp. in Germany)** Only **2/54 products** contained within 10% of the labeled amount. CJC Pharmacol 2003	antihypertensive meds → this herb may ↑ BP thus caution advised barbiturates → herb may ↓ barbiturate induced sleeping time **cyclosporin/digoxin/fexofenadine/indinavir/midazolam/nevirapine/omeprazole/oral contraceptives/sumatriptan/theophylline/warfarin** → herb may **↓ levels** of these drugs via ↑ metabolism (P450 3A4 inducer) iron → herb contains tannic acids which can ↓ iron absorption **MAOI's/SSRI's/TCA's** → herb may ↑ risk of **serotonin syndrome (6 case reports-tremor, delirium...)** by ↑ serotonin levels plus since MAOI action → restriction tyramine food is wise. **narcotics** → may prolong narcotic induced sleeping time piroxicam/tetracyclines → can ↑ photosensitize reaction sedatives → herb may potentiate **sedation SE**: Often for mild to moderate depression but may cause allergic reactions, headache, dizziness, restlessness, fatigue, dry mouth, nausea, vomiting, constipation, dreams, hair loss & **photosensitivity & possible uterotonic activity.** Possible **cataract link** thus rec to wear wrap around sunglasses. Hold for 2 weeks before any surgery.

Table 11.7 *Contd...*

Herb (botanical name)	Interaction/Side effects (SE)
Tamarind	aspirin →↑ bioavailability of aspirin **(Tamarindus indica)**
Tonka Bean	Warfarin ↑ INR → herb may contain warfarin constituents
Umbelliferae	Warfarin ↑ INR → herb may contain dicumoral constituents
Herb (botanical name)	**Interaction/Side effects (SE)**
Uzara root	**Digoxin** → herb may have additive effects or interfere with monitoring
Valerian Ⓟ **(Valeriana officinalis)**	sedatives → herb may potentiate **sedation** Possible acute hepatitis reported (? Due to adulterants). **SE**: Often used for sedative & anxiolytic action but may cause headache, excitability, ataxia & gastric complaints. (Case report of withdrawal syndrome involving **cardiac abnormalities & delirium**)
Verbena (Vervain)	MAOI's → herb ↑ risk of hypertensive crisis
Vitamin E	warfarin ↑ INR → herb may ↓ platelet aggregation. In **sunflower seeds**.
Wild Carrot	sedatives → herb may potentiate sedation
Wild Lettuce	sedatives → herb may potentiate sedation
Willow/Wintergreen	**Warfarin ↑ INR** → herb may contain **salicylate constituents**
Woodruff	warfarin ↑ INR → herb may contain warfarin constituents
Yarrow	warfarin ↓ INR → herb may be a coagulant in vivo
Yohimbe (Pausinystalia yohimbe)	clonidine & antihypertensives → herb may ↑ BP since is α 2 blocker **TCA antidepressants** → herb may ↑ **risk of hypertension SE:** nervousness, tremor, headache, dizzy, flushing & nausea
Xaio chai hu tang	Corticosteroids → herb may ↓ **blood level of prednisolone**

*(Adapted from www.$R_x$files.ca)

Conclusion

Although it is apparent that relationships between diet and drug therapy are not as common or as frequent as drug-drug interactions, the pharmacist should be constantly aware of their potential contribution to therapeutic failures and adverse effects in the clinical setting. Same can be said of drug-herb and drug-alcohol interactions. It is the knowledge and the expertise of the clinical pharmacist which can avoid such interactions because drugs may be absolutely necessary in certain situations but the interacting food and herbs can be withheld or substituted with another food and herb which does not interact, for that period of time during which drug is being administered. A constant vigil of the clinical literature as well as a balanced perspective of judgement will indeed facilitate the appropriate application of drug-food relationships in therapeutics.

Study Outline

Drug – food interactions

Two major areas of concern

- some drugs are capable of impairing absorption and utilization of nutrients
- some foods or patterns of dietary consumptions may alter drug absorption and response

Mechanisms of Drug food interactions

- Drugs affect nutrient and electrolyte absorption and utilization

  e.g., hypercholesterolemic agents, surfactants, anticonvulsants, alcohol, cytotoxic drugs, certain antimicrobial agents, diuretics, oral contraceptives

- Drugs affect taste and appetite

  e.g., griseofulvin, d-penicillamine, clofibrate

- Effect of foods upon drug absorption and response

  e.g., reduced absorption of tetracycline, penicillin etc., in presence of food

- Drug administration and food ingestion

  Drugs like Indomethacin, metronidazole, iron salts, reserpine which are highly irritant to gastrointestinal tract mucosa should be taken with food or milk. Drugs whose absorption is delayed in presence of food should be taken on empty stomach (ampicillin, lincomycin etc.,)

- Drug interactions with grape fruit juice, orange juice, caffeinated beverages and green leafy vegetables are well documented

Drug – herb interactions

Not well documented but some well known interactions are as follows:

Hawthorn should never be taken with digoxin

Ginseng, garlic taken with coumadin can cause bleeding

Ginseng can increase blood pressure which is dangerous in hypertensive patients

Garlic capsules combined with diabetes can cause dangerous decrease in blood sugar levels.

Drug - alcohol interactions

Well documented

CHAPTER 12

Drug – Lab Interactions

Objectives

After reading this chapter, the student should be able to:

- Understand the effects of drugs on laboratory tests
- Explain various mechanisms involved in drug-lab interactions
- Discuss some prominent drug-lab interactions

12.1 Introduction

Laboratory tests are important tools in the diagnosis of disease; they also serve as useful parameters for monitoring the course of a patient's progress throughout his hospital stay. Monitoring the effects of drugs on patients has become a responsibility of many pharmacists. With this responsibility comes the necessity for an understanding of laboratory tests, their relationship to a variety of disorders and to drugs being administered to patients. This later consideration is important since many drugs can affect test results with the possibility of producing an erroneous diagnosis.

In general, diagnostic tests are attempts to measure the level or the presence or absence of chemical constituents in the body. Disease states can alter these levels from normal or from levels obtained in patients without some disease state. Laboratory 'normals', which in most instances are ranges of values, are obtained by measuring a specific chemical in a group of individuals considered to be healthy. Statistical calculations are used to obtain means, standard deviations and boundaries of normality. Since testing procedures may vary from one laboratory to another, normal or ranges of normality may also vary. It becomes important then to know the specific procedure used by a given laboratory and the normals associated with that procedure.

12.2 Effects of Drugs on Laboratory Tests

Mechanisms by which drugs affect laboratory tests can be considered from either of two viewpoints. Knowledge of the specific mechanism responsible for a particular drug-induced laboratory test modification is essential for assessing the clinical significance of the effect and recommending appropriate action, if any, to be taken. However, a consideration of such particular mechanisms for each reported drug-laboratory test modification is beyond the scope of this chapter. Mechanisms can, however, be categorized into two types and it is these types which will be considered with reference to specific modification mechanism by way of examples.

As discussed above, clinical laboratory tests are basically an attempt to measure the level (or presence or absence) of some chemical constituent of the body. Drugs, being chemicals with biologic (or pharmacologic) activity, can alter such measurements. A drug, or a metabolite, present in a sample obtained for analysis may be active or interfere with the procedure used in the laboratory. Modification of this type is termed *chemical interference* and causes a false test result (false positive and false negative). If the circumstances warrant, a way of circumventing the interference may be sought or the drug discontinued and the test repeated.

On the other hand, a drug may, through a biologic effect, alter the level of a constituent to be analyzed. A sample subsequently obtained may contain increased or decreased levels of the substance. Such modification produces a true result (true positive or true negative). The alteration may be due to a *pharmacological* effect of the drug, an *adverse reaction* or an *allergic response.* The common feature is that the test result reported from the laboratory is correct and represents the actual level in that patient. However, the effect is drug-induced rather than disease-related. This is not to imply that the result may then be ignored. Consideration of the mechanism by which the drug produces the abnormal result and its clinical significance may draw attention to an adverse or allergic reaction which might otherwise go undetected for a period of time. A caution common to the use of many drugs is the monitoring of renal, hepatic and/or hemolytic function with common laboratory tests.

Chemical Interference

Chemical interference represents a self-limiting type of drug-induced laboratory test modification. If the interference is marked, it will usually be detected by the laboratory technician as the result will be grossly beyond the usual abnormal range and the report returned as interfering substance rather than a specific result. For example, such reports are common when, through oversight, measurement of protein-bound iodine (PBI) is attempted a day or two after the administration of iodine containing radiopaque media.

When less obvious interference is present, the fact that tests are generally run as groups or batteries prevents a false test result from leading to misdiagnosis. As discussed above, diagnosis of a specific disease is generally based on a pattern of abnormal results rather than a single value. When the modification of a test result is due to chemical interference, the effect is usually specific for one test in the battery. For example, erythromycin estolate causes a false elevation in glutamic-oxalacetic transaminase (SGOT). However, other tests for hepatic disease or cardiac damage will be normal if disease is not present. If, in a set of tests run as an organ or system battery, a single value does not fit the pattern established by the other results and the patient's clinical picture, it is usually not pursued.

If more than one test related to a particular organ or system is falsely abnormal, the pattern may point to a drug effect. For example, in the presence of thyroid disease, PBI and T-3 uptake results deviate from normal in the same direction. Iodine contamination, however, causes an *elevated* PBI and a decrease in T-3 uptake. Thus, a drug effect is readily recognized.

When a falsely abnormal result is obtained on a screening test, the battery of tests associated with that organ or system may be ordered in the belief that disease is present. Essentially normal results will be obtained with the exception of the screening test which is generally repeated as part of the group. However, even if the clinician is aware of a drug effect, it would be advisable to perform at least one of the other tests, if not the battery, to ensure that the abnormal result is due solely to drug interference, particularly if there was an initial suspicion of disease in the organ or system associated with that test.

When accurate evaluation is necessary, there are several alternatives. Choosing the most appropriate is contingent on an understanding of the specific mechanism responsible for the modification.

It may be possible to measure the same substance using an alternate analytical procedure not affected by the drug. Obviously, knowledge of the chemistry of the procedure and the way in which the drug interferes is necessary.

Many substances can be measured by more than one technique. If the analytical or biochemical bases are different, one procedure may be used when chemical interference occurs with the other.

The ability to utilize alternate procedures may be limited by the equipment available in a given laboratory. Additionally, accuracy and reproducibility (usually with standards provided by another laboratory) and, in some instances, range of normal limits for a given procedure should be established independently in each laboratory. Even if this is not required, the necessity of running simultaneous controls or establishing a standard curve may represent more effort than the test is worth to the physician. However, if a laboratory is not able to offer a given procedure, a sample can usually be sent out for analysis by a commercial laboratory.

Where an alternate procedure is not available, consideration can be given to discontinuing the interfering drug and, if necessary, substituting other therapy.

If treatment can be interpreted, knowledge of the time required for clearance of the drug or its metabolites from the body is desirable. Thus, sufficient time between discontinuing the drug and obtaining the sample for analysis can be permitted to elapse.

The specific mechanism of the drug interference should also be considered, in addition to clearance time, when the clinical situation requires continued therapy with an alternate drug. Obviously, the drug substituted should produce the same therapeutic effect as the former. However, potential for causing the same interference must also be evaluated. A drug's ability to react or interfere with a given analytical procedure is usually related to its basic chemical structure or the presence of a functional group in the molecule.

Pharmacologic Effect

The use of the term, pharmacological effect, as a type of drug-induced modification of laboratory test results has several connotations. It implies explanation of the mechanism of the effect by the drug's currently known pharmacology, *i.e.,* consistent occurrence of the effect from patient to patient (magnitude of the effect being dependent on dose and patient variability) and that the result reported by the laboratory is the true value. The clinical significance of a drug induced alteration of the level of a substance in the body is related to the nature of the substance and its significance to the patient condition. The situation may only require edge that the effect is drug, rather than disease related. If necessary, taking an alternate approach to evaluating function of the organ or system in question can be considered. Third, the fact that the substance is present in abnormal quantities may, in itself, have adverse implications to the patient's condition, requiring substitution of a drug which does not have the pharmacological property responsible for producing the abnormal diagnostic test.

Adverse Reactions

The alteration of laboratory parameters as manifestations of adverse reactions is probably the most common type of drug-induced laboratory test modification. Diagnostically, however, importance must be given to recognition of possible relationships between drugs and the abnormal tests. The association, if established, is generally secondary in that the test results indicate the presence of drug-induced disease. Certainly a low hemoglobin and haematocrit will be found in anemia secondary to drugs. Drug-induced hepatotoxicity or renal damage will manifest in abnormal diagnostic tests as well as symptoms and physical signs.

Prospectively, judicious use of drugs often requires that appropriate laboratory tests be performed periodically to detect incipient adverse effects. Retrospectively, however, drug therapy is often overlooked as a possible etiology for the disease being evaluated and should certainly be considered when abnormal laboratory results, consistent with an adverse reaction to one of the patient's drugs, are obtained.

In evaluating such a possibility, assumptions based on simple one to one relationships should be avoided. Superficially, a drug may be incriminated. However, the mechanism of the specific abnormality known to be produced by the drug may be inconsistent with the clinical laboratory data regarding the patient's problem.

For example, lists of drugs having the potential for decreasing hemoglobin and/or haematocrit can be found in various references. But the drugs included may cause various anemias such as blood loss, marrow depression, folate deficiency (antagonism) or hemolysis. Furthermore, with blood loss, the route (gastrointestinal ulceration, haematuria) must be considered and with hemolytic anemias, the particular type (G-6-PD) deficiency.

Obviously, the details of the suspected drug effect must be consistent with the patient's clinical picture before a causal relationship can be assumed. In addition to mechanism, other available data in the literature (such as dose, rationale of therapy and predisposing factors) should be considered, if applicable.

The same reasoning also applies to the evaluation of possible abnormalities mediated by chemical interferences, pharmacologic effect or allergic response. In short, all available data should be considered before a decision is made.

Corrective action depends on the clinical significance of the adverse effect. If alternate therapy is indicated, a drug should be selected which has little, if any, potential for producing the same effect. If it has been elucidated, knowledge of the specific mechanism of the adverse reaction may be helpful. Comparison of this with the known effects of possible alternate drugs may provide a basis for selection. On the other hand, it may be necessary to rely on the fact that the reaction has not been reported for a particular drug. This assumption should be made cautiously and be based on an adequate review of the literature.

Allergy

Laboratory test modifications due to drug allergy could be considered as a sub-group of the adverse reaction type. However, the theoretical distinction of an antibody-mediated response has additional practical implications both diagnostically and therapeutically.

In some instances, it is possible to demonstrate antibodies to drug in vitro. Examples include several of both the hemolytic anemias characterized by a positive Coomb's reaction and the drug-induced thrombocytopenias. If available, such tests can be valuable in evaluating a drug as a possible etiology.

Other allergic reactions may be associated with an elevated eosinophil count. Eosinophilia usually occurs with phenothiazine-induced hepatitis.

Alternate therapy requires selection of an antigenically dissimilar substitute. In patients allergic to it, the substitute again may itself be capable of the same effect. However, this does not contraindicate its use for a given individual if it is unrelated chemically to the offending drug in that patient.

Caution is indicated in the use of pharmacologically different, but chemically similar drugs in a patient who has had such a response. Chemical relationships between drugs of different groups are often not considered. For example, Coomb's positive hemolytic anemia has been reported with the antibacterial sulfonamides, the sulfonamide diuretics and the sulfonylureas. Cross-sensitivity to these compounds may be exhibited by the same individual.

Table 12.1 Some Drug-Lab interactions.

Drug	Laboratory Test	Increase / Decrease
Acetaminophen	Alkaline phosphatase	Increase
	Bilirubin	Increase
	Glucose	Decrease
Acyclovir	Alkaline phosphatase	Increase
	Bilirubin	Increase
	Creatinine	Increase
Aluminum Antacids	Phosphorus	Decrease
Amiodarone	Alkaline phosphatase	Increase
	Bilirubin	Increase
	Prealbumin	Decrease
Amitriptylline	Alkaline phosphatase	Increase
Amphotericin B	Bilirubin	Increase
	BUN	Increase
	Creatinine	Increase
	Magnesium	Decrease
	Potassium	Decrease
Ampicillin	Sodium	Increase
Ascorbic acid	Bilirubin	Increase
	Urine sugar	(false +)
Atenolol	Glucose	Increase
Barium	Potassium	Decrease
Beta-2-agonists	Potassium	Decrease

Table 12.1 *Contd...*

Drug	Laboratory Test	Increase / Decrease
Beta-adrenergic blockers	Potassium	Increase
Bicarbonates	Chloride Potassium	Decrease Decrease
Calcium	Potassium Sodium	Increase Increase
Captopril	Potassium	Increase
Carbamazepine	Alkaline phosphatase Bilirubin	Increase Increase
Chlorambucil	Bilirubin	Increase
Chloramphenicol	Bilirubin BUN BUN	Increase Decrease Increase
Chlordiazepoxide	Bilirubin	Increase
Clofibrate	Sodium	Decrease
Chloroquine	Bilirubin	Increase
Chlorpromazine	Alkaline phosphatase Glucose	Increase Increase
Chlorpropamide	Sodium	Decrease
Cholestyramine	Cholesterol	Decrease
Cisplatinum	Potassium Magnesium	Decrease Decrease
Citrates	Calcium Magnesium	Decrease Decrease
Clonidine	Sodium	Increase
Cephalexin	Alkaline phosphatase Creatinine	Increase Increase
Corticosteroids	Calcium Chloride Chloride Glucose Phosphorus Potassium Sodium	Decrease Decrease Increase Increase Decrease Decrease Increase
Cyclophosphamide	Bilirubin Sodium	Increase Decrease
Cyclosporine	Potassium	Increase
Diethylstilbestrol	Bilirubin Calcium	Increase Increase
Digoxin	Potassium	Decrease
Diltiazem	Alkaline phosphatase Bilirubin Uric acid	Increase Increase Increase
Enalapril	Potassium	Increase
Erythromycin	Alkaline phosphatase Bilirubin	Increase Increase
Estrogens	Dexamethasone Suppression	(false +)

Table 12.1 Contd...

Drug	Laboratory Test	Increase / Decrease
Ethacrynic acid	Bicarbonate	Increase
	Calcium	Decrease
	Chloride	Decrease
	Magnesium	Decrease
	Potassium	Decrease
	Sodium	Decrease
Fat emulsion	Bilirubin	Decrease
Furosemide	BUN	Increase
	Calcium	Decrease
	Chloride	Decrease
	Glucose	Increase
	Magnesium	Decrease
	Potassium	Decrease
	Sodium	Decrease
Gentamicin	Magnesium	Decrease
	Potassium	Decrease
Glutamine	Phenytoin	Increase
Growth hormone	Total protein	Increase
	Phosphate	Increase
Heparin	Calcium	Decrease
	Potassium	Increase
	Sodium	Decrease
Hydrochlorothiazide	Bicarbonate	Increase
	Bilirubin	Increase
	Calcium	Increase
	Glucose	Increase
	Potassium	Decrease
Indomethacin	Alkaline phosphatase	Increase
	Bilirubin	Increase
	Glucose	Increase
	Urea nitrogen	Increase
	Potassium	Increase
Insulin	Total protein	Increase
	Potassium	Decrease
Isoniazid	Alkaline phosphatase	Increase
	Bilirubin	Increase
Laxatives	Magnesium	Decrease
	Potassium	Decrease
	Sodium	Decrease
Lithium	Magnesium	Increase
Magnesium hydroxide	Phosphorus	Decrease
Magnesium salts	Calcium	Increase
Mannitol	Sodium	Decrease
Meperidine	Glucose	Increase
Metformin	Bicarbonate	Decrease
	Iron	Decrease

Table 12.1 Contd...

Drug	Laboratory Test	Increase / Decrease
Methotrexate	Alkaline phosphatase Bilirubin	Increase Increase
Methyldopa	Bilirubin Chloride Sodium Urine ketone	Increase Increase Increase Increase
Metoclopramide	Potassium	Decrease
Metoprolol	Alkaline phosphatase	Increase
Metronidazole	Glucose	Decrease
Morphine	Urine volume	Decrease
Niacin	Alkaline phosphatase Bilirubin Glucose Uric acid	Increase Increase Increase Increase
Nitrofurantoin	Bicarbonate Creatinine	Decrease Increase
NSAIDS	Potassium	Increase
Oral contraceptives	Glucose Sodium Total protein	Increase Increase Decrease
Oxazepam	Bilirubin Glucose	Increase Increase
Oxytocin	Sodium	Decrease
Penicillin	Albumin Urine Glucose Potassium	Decrease Increase Decrease
Phenobarbital	Calcium Folate	Decrease Decrease
Phenothiazines	Bilirubin Phosphate	Increase Decrease
Phenytoin	Alkaline phosphatase Glucose Folate	Increase Increase Decrease
Phosphates	Calcium	Decrease
Probenecid	Bilirubin Urine protein	Increase Increase
Procainamide	Potassium	Increase
Propranolol	Glucose Glucose Triglycerides	Decrease Increase Increase
Quinidine	Bilirubin	Increase
Rifampin	Bilirubin Glucose	Increase Increase

Table 12.1 Contd...

Drug	Laboratory Test	Increase / Decrease
Risperidone	Glucose Potassium Sodium	Increase Decrease Decrease
Saline infusions	Chloride	Increase
Sildenafil	Alkaline phosphatase Glucose Sodium	Increase Increase Decrease
Spironolactone	Sodium Potassium	Decrease Increase
Succinylcholine	Potassium	Increase
Sucralfate	Phosphate	Decrease
Sulfonylureas	Alkaline phosphatase BUN Sodium	Increase Increase Decrease
Tetracycline	Glucose Phosphate Sodium	Decrease Increase Decrease Increase Increase
Theophylline	Bilirubin Glucose Potassium	Decrease Decrease Decrease
Thiazide diuretics	Calcium Bilirubin Chloride Glucose Magnesium Sodium	Increase Increase Decrease Increase Decrease Decrease
Thyroid preparations	Glucose	Increase
Tolbutamide	Alkaline phosphatase Cholesterol	Increase Decrease
Triamterene	Bicarbonate	Decrease
Valproic Acid	Alkaline phosphatase Bilirubin Sodium	Increase Increase Decrease Increase
Valsartan	Potassium	Increase
Vancomycin	BUN	Increase
Vasopressin	Sodium	Decrease
Verapamil	Urine sodium	Increase
Vincristine	Sodium	Decrease
Vitamin K	Bilirubin	Increase

BUN = blood urea nitrogen; ADH = antidiuretic hormone; G6PD = glucose-6-phosphate dehydrogenase; ISE = Ion sensitive electrode; NSAIDS = Non-steroidal anti-inflammatory drugs; EDTA = Ethylenediaminetetraacetic Acid.

Table 12.2 Drug – Urine Interactions (Urine discoloration).

Urine discoloration	
Cascara	Chloroquine
Ferrous salts/ iron dextran	Levodopa
Methocarbamol	Methyldopa
Metronidazole	Nitrates
Nitrofurantoin	Quinine
Senna	Sulfonamides
Yellow-brown	
Bismuth	Chloroquine
Cascara	Metronidazole
Nitrofurantoin	Primaquine
Senna	Sulfonamides
Blue or blue green	
Amitriptyline	Methylene blue
Triamterene	Methocarbamol
Orange/yellow	
Chlorzoxazone	Dihydroergotamine
Heparin	Phenazopyridine
Rifampin	Sulfasalazine
Warfarin	
Red / Pink	
Daunorubicin or Doxorubicin	Heparin
Ibuprofen	Methyldopa
Phenothiazines	Phenytoin
Phenylbutazone	Rifampin
Salicylates	Senna

Table 12.3 Drugs that might cause discoloration of feces.

Therapeutic Category	Color Imparted	Drug(s) Responsible
Analgesics (CNS)	Pink to red to black (resulting from internal bleeding)	Salicylates
Analgesics (urinary)	Orange-red	Phenazopyridine (Pyridium)
Antacids	Whitish discoloration	Iminum hydroxide preparation
Anthelmintic	Blue Red	Dithiazinine, Pyrvinium pamoate
Antibacterial agents	Black	Bismuth sodium triglycollamate
Anticoagulants	Pink to red to black (resulting from internal bleeding)	all anticoagulants
Antiprotozoal agents	Black	Bismuth glycolylarsanilate
Haematinic agents	Black	Iron preparations (e.g., ferrous sulfate

Conclusion

Drug-lab interactions are very important because they affect the diagnosis and prognosis of a disease. It is difficult to avoid such interactions and the best way out in such situations is that all the health professionals associated with the patient should have knowledge of such interactions. Working knowledge of the common diagnostic tests and their relationship to disease states is an important asset to the clinical pharmacy practitioner. The phenomena of drug induced modifications of test data are complex. The potentialities are legion. The magnitude of the problem with respect to the data creates an almost impossible task for the physician who is attempting to consider all possibilities which might account for test abnormalities. A pharmacist monitoring patient's therapy program is faced with this problem. Alternative methods of diagnosis should be taken up wherever possible and the interaction should be considered while reporting the diagnosis.

Avoiding an unpleasant situation for the patient lies in the hands of the alert and responsible clinical pharmacist.

Study Outline

Lab tests are important tools in the diagnosis of a disease. Diagnostic tests are attempts to measure the level or presence / absence of chemical constituents in the body.

Effect of drugs on lab tests can be divided into 2 types

Chemical interference - a drug /metabolite can interfere with the lab procedure and can cause false positive or false negative test result.

Pharmacologic interference – a drug / metabolite can alter the level of a constituent to be analyzed in the lab test causing a true positive or true negative result.

Here the pharmacist should use his knowledge of drug-lab test interactions to diagnose the condition of the patient.

The drug –lab tests interactions are well documented.

Medication Misadventures

The role of Pharmacists is very important in the medication use process. During the process of medication use, there is a large potential for unexpected adverse events, errors in prescribing, drug administration, idiosyncratic and allergic reactions and other adverse effects. All these events together can be termed as medication misadventures. Pharmacists can play a pivotal role in recognizing and preventing such events.

Medication misadventure is a very broad term, referring to any iatrogenic hazard or incident associated with medications. All adverse drug events (ADEs), adverse drug reactions (ADRs), and medication errors fall under the umbrella of medication misadventures. ADRs and medication errors are the most specific terms. *ADRs* refer to any unexpected, unintended, undesired, or excessive response to a medicine. A *medication error* is any preventable event that has the potential to lead to inappropriate medication use or patient harm.

We will be discussing the above topics in chapters 14 and 15 respectively.

Chapter 13

Medication Errors

Objectives

After reading this chapter the student should be able to:

- Understand and define the term medication errors
- Differentiate between a medication error and adverse drug event
- Classify and evaluate various types of medication errors
- Explain factors contributing to medication errors
- Plan strategies for error prevention

13.1 Introduction

Patients depend on health systems and health professionals to help them stay healthy. As a result, frequently patients receive drug therapy with the notion that these medications will help them lead a more healthy life. In fact, the initiation of drug therapy is the most common medical treatment received by patients. Virtually in all cases, patients and their health care providers understand that when medications are given, there are some known and some unknown risks. Many patients may experience expected side effects. However, patients also experience significant unexpected drug-related morbidity and mortality. Errors in medication use process, including errors in medication prescribing, dispensing, administering, and monitoring, are responsible for a significant number of drug-related deaths.

The fundamental criteria to be strictly implemented in treating any patient is the common adage as known to many health care practitioners is "First do no harm". It is the responsibility of all health professionals and health systems to maintain this adage and contribute to the minimization of medication errors. The medication use process is complex and involves multiple individuals representing several health professionals and some nonprofessionals. Communication and teamwork among the various professionals is a necessity. Society perceives pharmacists to be responsible for the safe and effective use of drugs. The pharmacy profession needs to take a prominent role in the maximization of safe medicine use as a core responsibility of pharmaceutical care.

The responsibility for preparation and administration of medications includes reporting and recording errors, omissions and incidents. Each person who prepares and administers medications is responsible for his or her actions.

Most institutions require incident reports or other special forms to protect the patient, the person who prepares and administers the medication, and the hospital. For legal reasons, detailed description and accuracy in such statements is essential. These forms, which must be completed immediately following the incident, provide for statements by the individual involved as well as the physician who is notified of the error or incident.

Misinterpretation and misunderstanding resulting from incorrect interpretation of the physician's order, the medication card, or the label on the container contribute to the greatest frequency of medication errors. Disruptions that interfere with concentration on the immediate task also increase the incidence of errors, as do overcrowded medication trays, inadequate lighting, telephone interruptions, physician's rounds, and patient requests. The important aspect is that the person who prepared and administered the medication must re-evaluate his or her actions to prevent similar occurrences. This is part of the judgment and decision-making process to determine whether other choice of action could have been overlooked, environmental factors could have been improved, and safe versus unsafe practices could have been identified and corrected.

Listings of look-alike and sound-alike drugs are published periodically in the pharmaceutical literature. Potential danger for error always exists in the interpretation of the correct drug name. Such lists can be of value in 1) stressing respect for drugs by the beginner as well as the experienced professional; 2) use as a teaching and working tool for all health team members in self-study, group-study, and divisional and departmental study; and 3) demonstrating the need for review of present systems of medication administration.

In service orientation and continuing education programs play an important role in the prevention of medication errors and incidents and the improvement of patient care. Pharmacy staff often conducts employee training programs on medication reviews and intravenous administration and additives. Seminars for the nursing staff on drug interactions, adverse effects, new drugs and dosages, and orientation to pharmacy policies and procedures are helpful. Instructions can be supplied to the medical and dental staff in the form of policies and procedures in prescription writing, ordering drugs, the formulary, investigational drugs, and special requests.

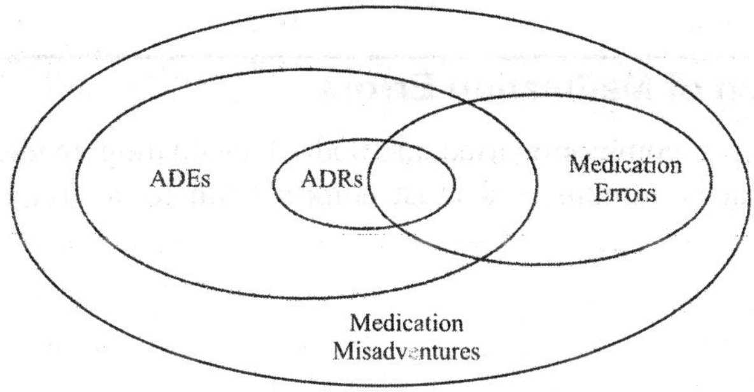

Fig. 13.1 Relationship among medication misadventures, adverse drug events, medication errors, and adverse drug reactions. Adapted from Am J Health-Syst Pharm 1998; 55:165-6.

13.2 Definition

In general terms, "an error is a failure to perform an intended action that was appropriate under the given circumstances". The National Coordinating Council for Medication Error Reporting and Prevention (NCC MERP) an organization composed of 19 national organizations including FDA and American Pharmaceutical Association (APhA) has developed a detailed definition of what constitutes a medication error.

Any preventable event that may cause or lead to inappropriate medication use or patient harm while the medication is in the control of health care professional, patient, or consumer. Such events may be related to professional practice, health care products, procedures, and systems, including prescribing; order communication; product labeling, packaging, and nomenclature; compounding; dispensing; distribution; administration; education; monitoring, and use.

Based on the above definition, medication errors also occur when a prescriber writes an incorrect dose on a prescription pad. Even if the prescriber is called by a dispensing pharmacist to clarify and change the order and the patient eventually receives an appropriately dosed medication, an error did occur in the process. An adverse outcome does not necessarily have to occur to classify an event as a medication error.

A medication error can also be broadly defined as a dose of medication that deviates from the physician's order as written in the patient's chart or from standard hospital policy and procedures. Except for errors of omission, the medication dose must actually reach the patient; i.e., a wrong dose that is detected and corrected before administration to the patient is not a medication error. Prescribing errors (e.g., therapeutically inappropriate drugs or doses) are excluded from this definition.

The precise definitions for medication errors may vary among institutions. The general principles will be similar, but there may be differences in what qualifies as a reportable error.

13.3 Evaluation of Medication Errors

The "five rights" is a commonly used method of evaluating medication errors. Each medication dose that is administered must comply with these five rights to be free of error:

- Right patient
- Right drug
- Right dose
- Right time
- Right route.

The five rights are a tool to assist health care professionals at every step in the medication use process to minimize the occurrence of errors. This method is not so precise though used very commonly. Every health care professional, when prescribing, or administering, should clarify that the five rights are in order before furthering the process of medication use. The five rights also provide an easy and understandable way to identify when medication errors occur.

13.4 Classification

Classification of medication errors helps to determine where errors are occurring and the severity of the errors, and assists with development of measures to improve the medication use process and minimize the occurrence of such errors.

Medication errors can be classified in a variety of ways. Some medication error reporting systems focus on the type of error. Other systems may be more interested in the outcome of the error.

The most common way to classify errors is to identify them by type. This classification focuses on whether an error was related to dispensing, administering, prescribing, or patient compliance. American Society for Hospital Pharmacists defines 11 categories of medication errors based on the type of error.

- *Prescribing error*: Prescribing errors are those errors which occur due to inappropriate drug selection, dose, dosage, form, or route of administration. Examples may include ordering duplicate therapies for a single indication, prescribing a dose that is too high or too low for a particular patient, writing a prescription illegibly, prescribing an inappropriate dosage interval, or ordering a drug to which the patient is allergic. Failing to monitor side effects and serum drug levels, prescribing an inappropriate medication for a particular indication, and inappropriate duration of therapy are the other types of prescribing errors.

- *Omission error:* An omission error occurs when a patient does not receive a scheduled dose of medication. This is considered to be the second most common error in the medication use process, next only to wrong time errors.
- *Wrong time error:* A wrong time error generally occurs when a dose is not administered in accordance with a predetermined administration interval. Every institution / hospital must establish a policy to indicate what exactly constitutes an error in this category.
- *Unauthorized drug error:* This type of error occurs when patients receive a drug that was not authorized by an appropriate prescriber. This might include giving the wrong patient a medication.
- *Improper dose error:* In this type of error, the dose given is inconsistent with what was prescribed, assuming the prescribed dose was appropriate. This type of error is different from that which occurs when a prescriber orders an inappropriate dose of a medication. If a prescriber orders an inappropriate dose, an "improper dose error" did not occur; however, a prescribing error did occur. This kind of error may occur when a dose is miscalculated or determined based on improper units or measured improperly.
- *Wrong dosage form error:* This error occurs when a patient receives a dosage form different from that prescribed, assuming the appropriate dosage form was originally ordered. This error is different from the type described in the prescribing error section.
- *Wrong drug preparation error:* When medications require some type of preparation, such as reconstitution, this type of error may occur. These kinds of errors may also occur in the compounding of various intravenous admixtures and other products.
- *Wrong administration technique:* These errors occur when a drug is given to a patient inappropriately. An example is when an intravenously administered agent is given at an excessive rate or when an agent meant for intramuscular administration is given intravenously.
- *Deteriorated drug error:* This error occurs when drugs are administered that has expired or has deteriorated prematurely due to improper storage conditions.
- *Monitoring error:* These errors occur when patients are not monitored appropriately either after receiving a drug or before they received a drug. For example, if a patient is placed on warfarin therapy and adequate blood tests are not performed to assess the patient's response, resulting in life-threatening hemorrhage, monitoring error has occurred. Further, in a community pharmacy, if

a pharmacist fails to review patient's medication history prior to dispensing a medication, resulting in a significant drug-drug interaction, a monitoring error has occurred.

- *Compliance error:* This type of error occurs when patients use medications inappropriately. Proper patient education and follow-up may play a significant role in minimizing this type of error. This type of error may be a direct result of insufficient patient counseling from a dispensing pharmacist, a prescribing physician, or both.

Table 13.1 Common sources of drug error and misuse.

Over dosage
• Taking more than the prescribed dose at any one administration.
• Taking more than the prescribed number of doses in any one day.
• Taking a dose, prescribed as needed, at a time other than when needed.
• Taking the same medication from two or more different bottles simultaneously.
Under dosage
• Taking less than the prescribed dose at any one administration.
• Omitting one or more doses.
• Discontinuing the drug before the prescribed time
• Omitting the dose of a medication, prescribed as needed, when it is needed.
Other Misuse
• Taking a dose at a different time if a time has been specified in the instructions.
• Taking a dose in a form other than that specified in the directions.
• Using the wrong route of administration.
• Taking medication that has been discontinued.
• Taking out-dated medication.
• Taking someone else's medication.
• Taking two or more medications that are therapeutically contraindicated.
• Failing to get the prescription filled.

13.5 Factors Contributing to Medication Errors

The factors responsible for Medication errors can be broadly categorized into,

- Performance lapses,
- Lack of knowledge, and

- Lack or failure of safety systems.

  Personal and environmental factors can contribute to the occurrence of medication errors. There are several factors specific to the professional involved and their working environment that may contribute to their committal of an error.

- *Excessive task demand:* Many dispensing pharmacists attribute their errors to this situation, complaining that their workload is so heavy and they are overloaded with tasks, making it difficult to work error free. Most pharmacists and experts in medication errors agree that work overload may be the most significant factor contributing to medication errors.
- *Personal characteristics:* Personal factors such as age, sensory deficits, or state of health may contribute to performance lapses. Personal levels of stress or fatigue may also have an impact. Someone who is bored at work may also be more error prone.
- *Extra-organizational factors*: Factors such as similar product names or packaging from pharmaceutical companies may have an extensive impact on the committal of errors with particular drugs.
- *Work environment*: Poor working conditions may influence the rate of error committal. Poor illumination and high noise levels have been shown to affect the dispensing error rate in pharmacies. Other factors in this category may include high ambient temperatures and frequent interruptions from the telephone or patients.
- *Intra-organizational factors:* In the era of managed care, there is a significant emphasis on the bottom line. Policies and procedures demanding high output or mandating long working hours may significantly affect cognition and the ability to prevent error occurrence.
- *Interpersonal factors:* Conflicts among co-workers or with patients may distract professionals from the tasks at hand and contribute to error committal. General interruptions from people may also fall into this category.

Other Factors

- *Lack of communication:* This factor may also fall under interpersonal factors listed above. Failure to communicate among fellow employees or among health care professionals has frequently been named as contributing to medication error. For example, an error may be more likely to occur if a pharmacist chooses not to clarify unclear physician orders. Poor physician handwriting and verbal orders are also significant factors.
- *Failure to comply with policy:* This is a common factor in dispensing and administering drugs. Non-compliance with policy has also been associated with drug administration errors. Often nurses develop specific personal routines for

administration of certain agents, which they perceive to be an improvement in the medication administration process, despite contrary policy.

- *Lack of knowledge:* This is a frequently cited factor in the committal of medication errors. Mistakes rather than slips are typically committed as a result of inadequate knowledge. Placing inexperienced recent graduates in positions where they cannot interact with more experienced practitioners may increase medication errors. Non specialists covering a service that is normally staffed by a specialist may also lead to errors. Nurses untrained in pharmacology may be more unlikely to recognize potential inconsistencies in disease state and medication usage and doses, resulting in the possibility of increased medication errors.
- *Lack of patient counseling:* Counseling of patients before dispensing of medication is the last safety check. Talking to the patient allows the pharmacist to correlate the medication and dose with the patient's conditions and helps the pharmacist to detect any errors that may have occurred in the medication use process. However, errors may occur not only from lack of counseling, but also from providing incorrect information during patient counseling. Providing incorrect information may also fall in the *lack of knowledge* category.

13.6 Medication Error Reporting

Institutional Reporting

Individual institutions must develop a reporting system specific to their institution, designed to meet their specific needs. There are at least four methods for collecting reports to medication errors. These methods may be used alone or in combination.

- *Anonymous self-reports:* In this system, anyone detecting or committing an error can report it without associating their name with the error. It is essentially risk free for the reporter and therefore it may increase the likelihood of having an error reported. Despite this theoretical advantage, there is still under reporting, particularly in cases that do not result in patient harm.
- *Incident reports:* This type of self-reporting system is the most commonly used. In this system, errors are highly underreported.
- *Critical-incident technique:* Although not really a reporting system, this technique uses observations and interviews of professionals involved in medication errors to analyze and identify weaknesses in the system. This method uses errors reported by other systems in an attempt to provide solutions to existing medication use problems.

- *Disguised observation:* Instead of relying on individuals to report errors, this method places an observer among health care professionals to watch for the occurrence of errors. The purpose of the observation is unknown to the professionals. Errors are then recorded and reported. This method is more reliable than self-reporting, but is time consuming and expensive.

13.7 Medication Error Prevention

The ultimate purpose for defining, classifying, analyzing, and reporting medication errors is to enable individuals and organizations to implement better systems that prevent medication errors. American Society of Health System Pharmacists has identified a multitude of risk factors associated with the occurrence of medication errors as outlined below.

- Work shift – more errors occur during the night shift.
- Inexperienced or inadequately trained staff.
- Medical services with special needs (e.g., pediatrics, oncology, etc).
- Higher number of medications per patient.
- Environmental factors such as high levels of noise, poor lighting, and frequent interruptions.
- High workload for staff.
- Poor communication among health care providers.
- Dosage form – more errors with injectable drugs.
- Drugs category – more errors with certain classes of drugs (e.g. antibiotics).
- Type of drug distribution systems – unit dose system is associated with fewer errors; high levels of floor stock are associated with increased errors.
- Improper drug storage.
- Calculations –increased errors with increased complexity and frequency of amount of calculations required.
- Poor handwriting.
- Verbal orders.
- Lack of effective policies and procedures.
- Poorly functioning oversight committees.

Practitioner Strategies

Individual health care practitioners play an integral role in the medication use process and must be familiar with factors that may contribute to medication errors. Although individuals are merely one part of a medication use system, each must take some responsibility for ensuring that their individual practices are consistent with the goal of reducing medication errors. Practitioners that recognize the potential for errors in various situations and implement personal practice habits to minimize errors can have a significant impact on error reduction. Individual Practitioners can do the following to minimize medication errors.

- *Patient communication:* Interaction with the patient may significantly reduce medication errors. A pharmacist who counsels patients before handing out the medication is more likely to catch a dispensing error. Similarly, nurses may minimize errors that reach a patient by asking the patient about allergies and describing the medication to the patient just prior to administration. Physicians may similarly contribute to better medication use by counseling a patient more thoroughly when writing the prescription. When the pharmacist also counsels, there will be reinforcement of the information. Also, if the directions are different from the pharmacist compared to the physician that may indicate that an error was committed somewhere in the medication use process.
- *Intra-professional communication:* In addition to communicating with patients, health care professionals need to improve communication among them. Illegible writing, extensive verbal medication orders, and a lone ranger approach to practice have no place in a health system devoted to reducing medication errors. When a medication order is unclear, it is a necessity to clarify that order before the medication use process continues. Poor Prescription writing is commonly cited as a cause for medication errors. Prescriber should ensure proper use of medications by consulting with pharmacists, other physicians, or the medical literature.
- *Education and training:* Lack of knowledge among all health care practitioners is commonly associated with medication errors. Health care professionals should stay abreast of current medical literature.
- *Reporting:* Health care professionals should recognize the necessity of medication error reporting. To enable other organizations and professionals to avoid the mistakes of others, reporting must be carried out consistently and routinely.

Health System Strategies

The medication error literature emphasizes the importance of health system involvement in minimizing medication errors. It is not good enough for health systems to tell their employees to be more careful or to try to minimize errors. The medication use process involves multiple professional and nonprofessional staff that is prone to errors. Health systems must recognize that even the most highly trained and proficient practitioners will commit errors as a result of being human. In addition to individual responsibility, health systems must ensure that they provide the tools needed by all parties involved to help prevent medication errors. A medication error that reaches a patient is not the result of error committed by a single person, but a flaw in the medication use process. The following identifies some of the things health systems can do to help minimize medication errors.

- *Environmental factors:* As discussed, there are numerous work place factors that may contribute to performance lapses and medication errors. Low lighting, high levels of noise, high temperatures, and stressful work environments are examples. Health systems should ensure that their facilities do not contribute to the commission of errors.
- *Policy:* Health systems should implement policies supportive of the effort to minimize medication errors. For example, policies that support the employment of adequate personnel for staffing and supervision should be implemented. There is a direct correlation with high workloads and inadequate staffing and medication errors. Policies that demand multiple checks prior to dispensing or administering medication should also be implemented. Health systems must define medication errors and their classifications, and implement policies for monitoring and correcting such errors. Policies for medication error reporting should minimize risk to reporters of error and allow for the development of a system that supports improvement of the system rather than punishment of employees.
- *Failure mode and effect analysis:* This is a system of identifying potential errors and adverse outcomes before they occur. It has been adapted from the aerospace industry and can be applied to the medication use process. With the use of failure mode and effect analysis, health systems should be able to design and implement medication use processes that have a significantly lower incidence of medication error.
- *Drug and patient information:* Lack of information has been frequently cited as a cause of medication errors, particularly prescribing errors. Health systems should ensure that all health care providers have ready access to necessary patient specific information and general drug information. Health systems may implement technology that allows viewing of a patient chart over a computer terminal or provides electronic medical references. Health systems may establish a drug information center where pharmacists are readily available to answer drug therapy questions. Considerable success has also been found in reducing medication errors when a knowledgeable pharmacist participates on medical rounds.
- *Training:* It is important for health care professionals to stay up to date regarding drug therapy. Health systems should contribute to this effort by supporting educational programs for their employees.

- *Technology:* The health care industry seems to be behind other industries in the area of informatics. To significantly improve quality of care and minimize medication errors, health systems need to make a substantial investment in information technology. Health care practitioners need to have ready access to medical and drug information, patient data, and an automated medication order system. The lack of drug and patient information, as described, has been associated with a large number of prescribing errors. Implementation of automated medication orders, also known as physician order entry, would save time for pharmacists and physicians. Furthermore, physician order entry has been shown to significantly reduce the number of serious medication errors. Other types of technology that may minimize errors include automated dispensing equipment and software that screens for drug-drug interactions and proper dosing.
- *Reporting:* Health systems should implement nonpunitive systems for medication error reporting. Accurate error monitoring will help organizations implement successful medication use processes that minimize adverse outcomes associated with medication errors.

Precautions and Directions

Proper drug administration contributes to better patient health care by assisting the physician in treatment. Improper drug use owing to either lack of understanding or gross abuse by the patient is detrimental to both himself and society. Negligence or failure to comply with instructions obstructs and delays treatment; often the physician is unaware of these failures to follow his directions. Effective drug therapy is a result not only of the medication itself, but largely the patient's attitude toward the therapy and himself.

By explaining the medication rationale to the patient and the medicine's role in his treatment, as well as the proper method of taking the drug, the pharmacist helps to reduce greatly the number of patients who do not take their prescribed medications. Failure to comply with directions is frequently due to confusion and error; thus the patient will usually welcome information and advice about his medications.

Precautions and special directions applicable to various medications need to be relayed to the patient by the pharmacist. Instructions that might seem unnecessary to the pharmacist should not be overlooked, such as removing the wrapping on suppositories before use. The route of administration, particularly when not obvious, should be specified. A proper patient counseling can avoid / reduce certain of the medication errors.

Table 13.2 Common reasons for medication related problems in patients

Reasons
Needed drug therapy
A new medical condition
Preventive therapy needed
Return of an old medical condition
Use of wrong drug
More effective drug available
Drug not indicated for condition
Contraindication present
Dosage form inappropriate
Condition refractory to drug
Dosage is too high
Wrong dose
Frequency inappropriate
Duration inappropriate
Drug interaction
Not Receiving the drug
Forgets to take drug
Cannot afford the drug
Side effects
Prefers not to take drug
Administration error
Unnecessary drug therapy
No medical indication
Non drug therapy more appropriate
Duplicative therapy
Treating avoidable adverse reactions
Substance abuse
Dosage is too low
Wrong dose
Frequency inappropriate
Duration inappropriate
Incorrect storage
Incorrect administration
Drug interaction

Table 13.2 *Contd...*

Adverse reaction
Allergic reaction
Unsafe drug for patient
Incorrect administration
Drug Interaction
Dose increased or decreased too fast
Drug causes decrease in second drug
Drug causes increase in second drug
Effect of two drugs are canceled
Drug-food interaction
Drug interference with laboratory test

Conclusion

Medication errors are a serious problem in the health care system. Recognition of the problem is one of the important first steps in developing strategies to minimize their occurrence. Pharmacists have the responsibility of ensuring the safe and effective use of medications by minimizing the medication errors. They must take the lead role in the medication use process. Pharmacists can provide tremendous benefit to patients through reduction of medication errors. Pharmacists need to contribute in improving patient care by actively participating and pursuing improvements in the medication use process.

Study Outline

The term medication misadventure includes iatrogenic hazard/incident, all adverse drug reactions and medication errors.

Medication errors in prescribing, dispensing, administering and monitoring are responsible for significant number of drug related deaths. Hence it is the responsibility of all health care professionals and health systems to contribute to minimize the medication errors.

Medication error is defined as any preventable event that may cause or lead to inappropriate medication use or patient harm while the medication is in the control of the health care professional, patient or consumer.

ASHP defines 11 categories of medication errors based on type of error which can begin during prescribing, during administration or during patient compliance.

The factors responsible for medication errors can be categorized into

- performance lapses
- lack of knowledge
- lack or failure of safety systems

Institutions must develop systems for collecting reports to medication errors and see that better systems are implemented to prevent medication errors.

To minimize medication errors individual practitioners can implement the following strategies

- patient communication
- intra professional communication
- education and training
- reporting

Health Institutions can adopt the following strategies to minimize medication errors:

- Improve environmental factors that help to minimize medication errors
- Implement policies supportive to minimize medication errors
- Failure mode and effect analysis
- Drug and patient information
- Training to employees / health care professionals
- Adopt technology which can help prevent errors
- To develop reporting systems that are non punitive

CHAPTER 14

Adverse Drug Reactions and Management

Objectives

After reading this chapter the student should be able to:

- Define and classify adverse drug reactions
- Understand various mechanisms of adverse drug reactions
- Evaluate an adverse drug reaction and understand its management
- Initiate a adverse drug reaction reporting program and implement the program
- Define the term pharmacovigilance and understand its importance.

14.1 Introduction

The consequences of adverse drug reactions, including increased patient morbidity and mortality, have been well documented. Patients experiencing adverse drug reactions also suffer economic consequences resulting from hospital admissions, increased hospital stay, and treatment of complications. Adverse drug reactions (ADRs) contribute to over all health care costs by increasing morbidity and even mortality in severe cases. Huge amounts are being spent annually on ADR screening and treatment functions. Medicinal substances are used for their ability to affect biological processes in the body. There is always a risk associated with the use of medicines such as unwanted or unintended effects. The physician assesses the risk-benefit ratio before prescribing a medicine or drug to a patient.

Adverse reactions may limit the therapeutic potential of a drug. A better understanding of a drug's relative benefit-to-risk balance allows the clinician to make better therapeutic decisions. Not all ADRs are known at the time of marketing; therefore, there is a continual need for drug surveillance.

Definitions

There is no single definition of an ADR that has been accepted, which may be due partly to the diverse interests of manufacturers, investigators and regulators.

Unintended or undesired effects are not always unfavorable, but should obviously be so to qualify as adverse drug reactions. Whether a reaction is "unexpected" depends partly on the knowledge of the attending physician. But such terms as "unexpected" or "unusual" also present difficulties because they mean different things to different individuals. Thus, "unusual" may include the ambit of a phenomenon never previously observed to a reaction that occurs in 30 to 40 per cent of the patients treated. These synonyms of "adverse" (unintended, undesired, unexpected, and unusual) are, therefore, rather vague concepts, and in the absence of clearly definable meanings, contribute relatively little.

There is a confusion regarding the terms adverse drug reactions, adverse drug events, side effects and drug allergy. The terms "drug allergy," "drug hypersensitivity," and "drug reaction" are often used interchangeably. *Drug reactions* encompass all adverse events related to drug administration, regardless of etiology. *Drug hypersensitivity* is defined as an immune-mediated response to a drug agent in a sensitized patient. *Drug allergy* is restricted specifically to a reaction mediated by IgE.

According to WHO ADR is defined as *any response to a drug which is noxious and unintended, and which occurs at doses used in man for prophylaxis, diagnosis, or treatment*. This definition of an ADR includes an exaggerated drug response, an unwanted effect on an organ system different from that being treated, an allergic or hypersensitivity reaction, an idiosyncratic reaction or a drug interaction that causes either an increase or diminished response.

A side effect and a drug allergy are both types of ADRs. A side effect is an example of a dose related, predictable reaction to a drug. A side effect of a drug is known to occur in a given percentage of the population and has been observed with regular frequency. A side effect is also expected based on the pharmacologic activity of the agent in question.

A drug allergy is an example of a non-dose related, unpredictable adverse effect to a drug. Some side effects that are not drug allergies are inappropriately classified as such. For example, nausea secondary to narcotic use is not immunologically mediated and should not be considered an allergy; however, an anaphylactic reaction to penicillin is an adverse reaction that should be categorized as a true allergic reaction.

Karch and Lasagna gave the following definitions for drug, an adverse event and a patient drug exposure as

Drug: A chemical substance or product available for an intended diagnostic, prophylactic or therapeutic response.

Adverse drug reaction: Any response to a drug which is noxious and unintended and which occurs at doses used in man for prophylaxis, diagnosis or therapy, excluding therapeutic failures.

Patient drug exposure: A single patient receiving at least one dose of a given drug.

The FDA definition of an ADR is *any adverse event associated with the use of a drug in humans, whether or not considered drug related, including the following: adverse event occurring in the course of the use of a drug product in professional practice; an adverse event occurring from drug overdose whether accidental or intentional; an adverse event occurring from drug abuse; an adverse event occurring from drug withdrawl; and any significant failure of expected pharmacologic action.*

This definition is broad and includes overdose situations as well as situations involving abuse.

Naranjo and associates gave the following definitions to assist in determining the probability of an ADR.

Definite ADR is a reaction which: (1) follows a reasonable temporal sequence from administration of the drug, or in which the drug level has been established in body fluids or tisses; (2) follows a known response pattern to the suspected drug; and (3) is confirmed by dechallenge; and (4) could not be reasonably explained by the known characteristics of the patient's clinical state.

Conditional ADR is a reaction which: (1) follows a reasonable temporal sequence from administration of the drug; (2) does not follow a known response pattern to the suspected drug; and (3) could not be reasonably explained by the known characteristics of the patient's clinical state.

Doubtful ADR is any reaction which does not meet both the above criteria

14.2 Classification

Several classifications of undesirable drug effects have been suggested. One of these classifications is explained below.

- ***Misdosage:*** This is concerned only with those deleterious reactions that are the result of erroneous administration.
    - *Deliberate Misuse:* This designation delineates all illicit uses.

- *Medication Error:* This demarcation speaks for itself, including unintentional errors.
- *Titration:* This term describes the reactions occurring while attempting to establish the proper dosage of a given medication for a particular individual, e.g., occurrence of diarrhea while treating acute gouty arthritis with colchicine.

- ***Pharmacologic:*** This terminology is intended to include objectionable reactions due to pharmacologic action.
  - *Undesired Expected Effects*-The classification here addresses itself to all true side-effects, e.g., sedative effects with the use of antihistamines.
  - *Desired Excessive Effects*-These are enhanced pharmacologic actions beyond that those are normally associated with a particular drug, e.g., the antihistamine, Benadryl, used in increased dosages for sedative effects.
  - *Undesired Unexpected Effects*-These are those effects seen only in relatively few patients, which do result from a basic pharmacologic action of the drug, e.g., atrioventricular block during administration of cardiotonic glycoside.
- ***Non-pharmacologic:*** Emphasis here is upon those undesirable reactions unrelated to a drug's pharmacologic action.
  - *Allergic*-These reactions comprise the bulk of objectionable effects in the third category. Such reactions are, for the most part, unrelated to the dosage and difficult to predict, e.g., anaphylactic reactions caused by penicillin.
  - *Idiosyncratic*-These are the dosage unrelated reactions occurring only in certain individuals. Such reactions are generally anomalous; however, in a few cases they are well understood.

Drug hypersensitivity results from interactions between a pharmacologic agent and the human immune system. These types of reactions constitute only a small subset of all adverse drug reactions. Allergic reactions to medications represent a specific class of drug hypersensitivity reactions mediated by IgE (Immunoglobulin E). Immune mediated drug reactions may be discussed generally in the Gell and Coombs classification system, a widely accepted conceptual framework for understanding complex immune reactions. However, some reactions involve additional, poorly understood mechanisms that are not easily classified.

Drug reactions can also be classified into *immunologic* and *nonimmunologic* etiologies (Table 14.1). The majority (75 to 80 percent) of adverse drug reactions are caused by predictable, nonimmunologic effects. The remaining 20 to 25 percent of adverse drug events are caused by unpredictable effects that may or may not be immune mediated. Immune-mediated reactions account for 5 to 10 percent of all drug reactions and constitute true drug hypersensitivity, with IgE-mediated drug allergies falling into this category.

Table 14.1 Immunologic and nonimmunologic drug reactions.

Type	*Example*
Type I reaction (IgE-mediated)	Anaphylaxis from β-lactam antibiotic
Type II reaction (cytotoxic)	Hemolytic anemia from penicillin
Type III reaction (immune complex)	Serum sickness from anti-thymbocyte globulin
Type IV reaction (delayed, cell-mediated)	Contact dermatitis from topical antihistamine
Specific T-cell activation	Morbilliform rash from sulfonamides
Fas/Fas ligand-induced apoptosis	Stevens-Johnson syndrome Toxic epidermal necrolysis
Other	Drug-induced, lupus-like syndrome Anticonvulsant hypersensitivity syndrome
Non-immunologic	
Predictable	
Pharmacologic side effect	Dry mouth from antihistamines
Secondary pharmacologic side effect	Thrush while taking antibiotics
Drug toxicity	Hepatotoxicity from methotrexate
Drug-drug interactions	Seizure from theophylline while taking erythromycin
Drug overdose	Seizure from excessive lidocaine (Xylocaine)
Unpredictable	
Pseudoallergic	Anaphylactoid reaction after radio contrast media
Idiosyncratic	Hemolytic anemia in a patient with G-6-PD deficiency after primaquine therapy
Intolerance	Tinnitus after a single, small dose of aspirin

G-6-PD = glucose-6-phosphate dehydrogenase

Table 14.2 Gell and Coombs Classification of Drug Hypersensitivity Reactions.

Immune reaction	*Mechanism*	*Clinical manifestations*	*Timing of reactions*
Type I (IgE-mediated)	Drug-IgE complex binding to mast cells with release of histamine, mediators	Urticaria, angioedema, bronchospasm, inflammatory pruritus, vomiting, diarrhea, anaphylaxis	Minutes to hours after drug exposure
Type II (cytotoxic)	Specific IgG or IgM antibodies directed at drug-hapten coated cells	Hemolytic anemia, neutropenia, thrombocytopenia	Variable
Type III (immune complex)	Tissue deposition of drug-antibody complexes with complement activation and inflammation	Serum sickness, fever, rash, arthralgias, lymphadenopathy, urticaria, glomerulonephritis, vasculitis	1 to 3 weeks after drug exposure
Type IV (delayed, cell-mediated)	MHC presentation of drug molecules to T cells with cytokine and inflammatory mediator release	Allergic contact dermatitis, maculopapular drug rash	2 to 7 days after cutaneous drug exposure

MHC = major histocompatibility complex

The Gell and Coombs classification system describes the predominant immune mechanisms that lead to clinical symptoms of drug hypersensitivity (Table 14.2). This classification system includes:

- Type I reactions (IgE-mediated)
- Type II reactions (cytotoxic)
- Type III reactions (immune complex) and
- Type IV reactions (delayed, cell-mediated).

However, some drug hypersensitivity reactions are difficult to classify because of the lack of evidence supporting a predominant immunologic mechanism. These include certain cutaneous drug reactions (i.e., maculopapular rashes, erythroderma, exfoliative dermatitis, and fixed drug reactions) and specific drug hypersensitivity syndromes (Table 14.3).

Unpredictable, nonimmune drug reactions can be classified as pseudoallergic, idiosyncratic or intolerance. Pseudoallergic reactions are the result of direct mast cell activation and degranulation by drugs such as opiates, vancomycin and radio contrast media. These reactions may be clinically indistinguishable from Type I hypersensitivity, but do not involve drug-specific IgE. Idiosyncratic reactions are qualitatively aberrant reactions that cannot be explained by the known pharmacologic action of the drug and occur only in a small percent of the population. A classic example of an idiosyncratic reaction is drug-induced hemolysis in persons with glucose-6-phosphate dehydrogenase (G-6-PD) deficiency. Drug intolerance is defined as a lower threshold to the normal pharmacologic action of a drug, such as tinnitus after a single average dose of aspirin.

Table 14.3 Specific Drug Hypersensitivity Syndromes Caused by Non-IgE Immune Mechanisms.

Causative drug	*Syndrome*
Hydralazine (Apresoline) Procainamide (Pronestyl)	Lupus-like syndrome
Carbamazepine (Tegretol) Phenytoin (Dilantin)	Anticonvulsant hypersensitivity syndrome
Sulfonamides Anticonvulsants	Stevens-Johnson syndrome, Toxic epidermal necrolysis

Table 14.4 Patient Risk Factors for Adverse Drug Reactions.

General drug reactions (nonimmune)	**Hypersensitivity drug reactions (immune)**
Female gender	Female gender
Serious illness	Adult
Renal insufficiency	HIV infection
Liver disease	Concomitant viral infection
Polypharmacy	Previous hypersensitivity to chemically-related drug
HIV infection	
Herpes infection	Asthma
Alcoholism	Use of beta blockers
Systemic lupus erythematosus	Specific genetic polymorphisms
	Systemic lupus erythematosus

Another way of classifying Adverse Drug Reaction can be based on the "Severity of the Reaction" developed by Lasagna and Karch into the following categories.

- *Minor* : No antidote, therapy or prolongation of hospitalization required
- *Moderate*: Requires a change in drug therapy, specific treatment or an increase in hospitalization by at least one day.
- *Severe*: Potentially life-threatening causing permanent damage or requiring intensive medical care.
- *Lethal*: Directly or indirectly contributes to the death of the patient.

ADRs can also be classified as definite, probable, possible, conditional, or doubtful. This classification is based on the following criteria. First, is there a reasonable temporal relationship between the administration of the drug and the suspected ADR? Second, did the patient improve when the drug was withdrawn? This criterion is known as *dechallenge*. Third, did the suspected ADR recur when the drug was restarted? This is known as *rechallenge*. Finally, are there common clinical conditions that might explain the patient's symptoms? It is frequently difficult to rechallenge a patient just to document an ADR. This is especially true if the ADR is particularly severe; therefore, the evaluation of a possible ADR is often made by the other three criteria. As a result, many ADRs are reported as probable or possible. Table 14.5 presents the classification of ADRs based on fulfillment of criteria.

Table 14.5 Classification of ADRs Based on Fulfillment of Criteria.

	Type			
Documentation	**Definite**	**Probable**	**Possible**	**Conditional**
Temporal relationship	X	X	X	X
Known response	X	X	X	
Not explained clinically	X	X		X
Dechallenge	X	X		
Rechallenge	X			

14.3 Epidemiology

Adverse drug reactions caused by immune and nonimmune mechanisms are a major cause of morbidity and mortality worldwide. They are the most common iatrogenic illness, complicating 5 to 15 percent of therapeutic drug courses. 3 to 6 percent of all hospital admissions are because of adverse drug reactions, and 6 to 15 percent of hospitalized patients experience a serious adverse drug reaction. Epidemiologic data support the existence of specific factors that increase the risk of general adverse drug reactions, such as female gender, or infection with human immunodeficiency virus (HIV), or herpes (Table 14.4). Factors associated with an increased risk for hypersensitivity drug reactions include asthma, systemic lupus erythematosus, or use of beta blockers (Table 14.4). Although atopic patients do not have a higher rate of sensitization to drugs, they are at increased risk for serious allergic reactions.

The most important drug-related risk factors for drug hypersensitivity concern the chemical properties and molecular weight of the drug. Larger drugs with greater structural complexity (e.g., nonhuman proteins) are more likely to be immunogenic. Heterologous antisera, streptokinase, and insulin are examples of complex antigens capable of eliciting hypersensitivity reactions. Most drugs have a smaller molecular weight (less than 1,000 Daltons), but may still become immunogenic by coupling with carrier proteins, such as albumin, to form simple chemical-carrier complexes (hapten).

Another factor affecting the frequency of hypersensitivity drug reactions is the route of drug administration; topical, intramuscular, and intravenous administrations are more likely to cause hypersensitivity reactions. These effects are caused by the efficiency of antigen presentation in the skin, the adjuvant effects of repository drug preparations, and the high concentrations of circulating drug antigen rapidly achieved with intravenous therapy. Oral medications are less likely to result in drug hypersensitivity.

Identifiable risk factors for drug hypersensitivity reactions include age, female gender, concurrent illnesses, and previous hypersensitivity to related drugs.

14.4 Mechanism of Adverse Drug Reactions

Karch and Lasagna described various mechanisms for adverse drug reactions. These mechanisms are related to the pharmacologic or pharmacodynamic aspects of drugs and can be used to classify the type of reaction that occurs.

- *Idiosyncrasy*: an uncharacteristic response of a patient to a drug, usually not occurring on administration.
- *Hypersensitivity*: a reaction, not explained by the pharmacologic effects of the drug, caused by altered reactivity of the patient and generally considered to be an allergic manifestation.
- *Intolerance*: a characteristic pharmacologic effect of a drug produced by an unusually small dose, so that the usual dose tends to induce a massive over action.
- *Drug interaction*: an unusual pharmacologic response that could not be explained by the action of a single drug, but was caused by two or more drugs.
- *Pharmacologic*: a known, inherent pharmacologic effect of a drug, directly related to dose.

14.5 Variables Affecting ADR Incidence and Severity

Certain variables predispose individuals to developing ADRs. These variables can be patient or drug focused. Patient variables like age, underlying disease, and genetic factors and drug variables like route of administration, product formulation, and duration of therapy can predispose individuals to develop ADRs.

Patient Variables:

- *Elderly* : As the hepatic and renal functions decline with age, the elderly are subject to changes in metabolism that affect the clearance of drugs and active metabolites.

- *Neonates* : Neonates experience ADRs due to several reasons, which include the following :
    - placental transfer of drugs, which results in exposure in utero
    - a lack of information on drug use in neonates
    - altered drug disposition, metabolism and excretion profiles
- *Patients with Immunodeficiency virus disease (HIV)*

  The incidence of ADRs in patients infected with HIV appears to be higher than the incidence occurring in the general population. Severe immunosuppression, development of drug specific antibodies, and impaired capacity to clear drugs and unchanged metabolites results in an increased sensitivity to drug toxicity.
- *Genetics*: The rates of metabolism and elimination of various substances may be influenced by genetic factors (e.g., G-6-PD deficiency, acetylator status and drug induced SLE).

Drug Variables:

- *Route of Administration*: Intravenous administration may be associated with side effects local to the site of injection, such as phlebitis and extravasation, as well as with systemic adverse effects secondary to rapid increase in drug blood levels and accelerated clinical response. Oral administration will have milder adverse events.
- *Product formulation*: Product formulations that alter the extent and the rate of absorption may also affect the incidence of ADRs. For example, sustained release products may avoid the potential for adverse effects due to excessive peaks and inadequate troughs associated with immediate release products.
- *Duration of therapy*: The duration of therapy can also cause ADRs. For example, in patients greater than 60 years of age, an increase in duration of therapy with nonsteroidal anti-inflammatory drugs (NSAIDs) is associated with an increased risk of upper gastrointestinal toxicity.

14.6 Clinical Manifestations

True hypersensitivity adverse drug reactions are great imitators of disease and may present with involvement of any organ system, including systemic reactions such as anaphylaxis (Table 14.2). Drug reactions commonly manifest with dermatologic symptoms caused by the metabolic and immunologic activity of the skin. The most common dermatologic manifestation of drug reaction is morbilliform rashes. Typically, an erythematous, maculopapular rash appears within one to three weeks after drug exposure, originates on the trunk, and eventually spreads to the limbs. Urticaria is typically a manifestation of a truly allergic Type I reaction, but it may appear with Type III or pseudoallergic reactions as well. Severe nonallergic, hypersensitivity cutaneous reactions (i.e., erythema multiforme, Stevens-Johnson syndrome, and toxic epidermal necrolysis) represent bullous skin diseases that require prompt recognition because of their association with significant morbidity and mortality. Eczematous rashes are most commonly associated with topical medications and usually represent contact dermatitis, which is classified as Type IV reaction to a drug exposure.

14.7 Clinical Evaluation

Drug hypersensitivity reactions not only should be included in the differential diagnosis for patients who have the typical allergic symptoms of anaphylaxis, urticaria, and asthma, but also for those with serum sickness-like symptoms, skin rash, fever, pulmonary infiltrates with eosinophilia, hepatitis, acute interstitial nephritis, and lupus-like syndromes. A diagnosis of drug hypersensitivity depends on identifying symptoms and physical findings that are compatible with an immune drug reaction.

The initial history should include a recording of all prescription and nonprescription drugs taken within the last month, including dates of administration and dosage. The temporal relationship between drug intake and the onset of clinical symptom is critical. Unless the patient has been previously sensitized to a drug, the interval between initiation of therapy and the onset of reaction is rarely less than one week or more than one month. Patients should be asked about previous drug exposures and reactions.

The physical examination may provide further information to support drug hypersensitivity. A prudent initial step is an evaluation for signs and symptoms of an immediate generalized reaction, because this is the most severe life-threatening form of an adverse drug reaction. Warning signs of impending cardiovascular collapse include urticaria, laryngeal or upper airway edema, wheezing, and hypotension. Signs suggestive of serious adverse drug reactions include the presence of fever, mucous membrane lesions, lymphadenopathy, joint tenderness and swelling, or an abnormal pulmonary examination. A detailed skin examination is essential, because the skin is the organ most frequently and prominently affected by adverse drug reactions. Distinguishing between the various types of skin lesions is important, because this may provide substantial clues to the possible immune-mediated mechanism of drug reaction (Table 14.6).

Table 14.6 Cutaneous Symptoms of Drug Hypersensitivity Reactions.

Type of skin lesion	Associated immune-mediated mechanism of the drug reaction
Exanthematous or morbilliform eruption originating on trunk	Classic "drug rash"; most common
Urticaria	IgE antibody-mediated or direct mast cell stimulation
Purpura	Vasculitis or drug-induced thrombocytopenia
Maculopapular lesions with distribution on the fingers, toes, or soles	Serum sickness
Blistering lesions with mucous membrane involvement	Stevens-Johnson syndrome or toxic epidermal necrolysis
Eczematous rash in sun-exposed areas	Photo allergic reaction
Solitary circumscribed erythematous raised lesion	Fixed drug eruption
Papulovesicular, scaly lesion	Contact dermatitis

14.8 Laboratory Evaluation

The goal of diagnostic testing is to evaluate biochemical or immunologic markers that confirm activation of a particular immunopathologic pathway to explain the suspected adverse drug effect. Laboratory evaluation is guided by the suspected pathologic mechanism (Table 14.7).

Table 14.7 Diagnostic Testing and Therapy for Drug Hypersensitivity.

Immune reaction	Laboratory tests	Therapeutic considerations
Type I(IgE-mediated)	Skin testing RAST Serum tryptase	Discontinue drug. Consider epinephrine, antihistamines, systemic corticosteroids, bronchodilators. Inpatient monitoring, if severe
Type II (cytotoxic)	Direct or indirect Coombs' test	Discontinue drug. Consider systemic corticosteroids. Transfusion in severe cases
Type III (immune complex)	ESR C-reactive protein Immune complexes Complement studies Antinuclear antibody, antihistone antibody Tissue biopsy for immunofluorescence studies	Discontinue drug. Consider NSAIDs, antihistamines, or systemic corticosteroids; or plasmapheresis if severe.
Type IV (delayed, cell-mediated)	Patch testing Lymphocyte proliferation assay	Discontinue drug. Consider topical corticosteroids, antihistamines, or systemic corticosteroids if severe.

RAST = radioallergosorbent test; ESR = erythrocyte sedimentation rate; NSAIDs = Nonsteroidal anti-inflammatory drugs.

Confirmation of suspected Type I hypersensitivity reactions require the detection of antigen-specific IgE. Skin testing is a useful diagnostic procedure in these patients. Skin testing protocols are standardized for penicillin, and are well described for local anesthetics and muscle relaxant agents. It also may be informative when testing high-molecular-weight protein substances such as insulin, vaccines, streptokinase, polyclonal or monoclonal antibodies, and latex. Positive skin testing to such reagents confirms the presence of antigen-specific IgE and is supportive of the diagnosis of a Type I hypersensitivity reaction in the appropriate clinical setting. Negative skin testing is helpful only in penicillin skin testing because the test specificity has been adequately established. With other drug agents, a negative skin test does not effectively rule out the presence of specific IgE. In vitro testing for IgE is available for a limited number of drugs in the form of radioallergosorbent tests that are historically less sensitive than skin testing for determining specific IgE levels. In addition, the immunogenic determinants of many drugs are undefined, which makes the predictive value of in vitro tests poor.

Laboratory tests measuring mast cell activation may be helpful if obtained within four hours of onset of the suspected allergic reaction. While serum histamine levels peak five minutes after anaphylaxis and return to baseline within 30 minutes, serum tryptase levels peak one hour after anaphylaxis and remain elevated for two to four hours after the event. Histamine, tryptase, and beta-tryptase levels have proved useful in confirming acute IgE-mediated reactions, but negative results do not rule out acute allergic reactions. Type II cytotoxic reactions to a drug result in hemolytic anemia, thrombocytopenia, or neutropenia evident with a complete blood count. Hemolytic anemia may be confirmed with a positive direct and/or indirect Coombs' test, reflecting the presence of complement and/or drug-hapten on the red cell membrane.

In Type III immune complex reactions to a drug, elevation of nonspecific inflammatory markers such as erythrocyte sedimentation rate and C-reactive protein may occur. If available, more specific laboratory testing for complement levels (CH50, C3, C4) or circulating immune complexes can be conducted. Positive tests help confirm the clinical diagnosis; negative tests do not exclude the diagnosis of immune complex disease. Systemic vasculitides induced by medication may be detected by autoantibody tests such as antinuclear antibody or anti-histone antibody.

Type IV immune reactions usually present as allergic contact dermatitis caused by topical medications. In such instances, patch testing for specific drug agents, as outlined in Table 14.7, is an appropriate diagnostic step. Features of erythema, induration, and a pruritic vesiculopapular rash developing 48 hours after patch application support the diagnosis of a Type IV immune reaction.

14.9 Diagnosis

The diagnosis of drug hypersensitivity is usually based on clinical judgment, because definitive, confirmatory drug-specific testing is often difficult. Table 14.8 outlines the general criteria for the diagnosis of drug hypersensitivity reactions.

Table 14.8 General criteria for the diagnosis of drug hypersensitivity reactions.

The patient's symptomatology is consistent with an immunologic drug reaction.
The patient was administered a drug known to cause such symptoms.
The temporal sequence of drug administration and appearance of symptoms is consistent with a drug reaction.
Other causes of the symptomatology are effectively excluded.
Laboratory data are supportive of an immunologic mechanism to explain the drug reaction (not present or available in all cases).

Once the diagnosis has been established, appropriate documentation should be included in the medical record specifying the causative drug and the nature of the adverse effect. Immune-mediated drug hypersensitivity reactions typically pose a predictable, more serious health risk with re-exposure to a drug. Nonimmune drug reactions tend to be less severe and less reproducible. The continued use of an offending drug may be appropriate if the risk of not treating the underlying disease is greater than the risk of continuing the drug, and if no suitable alternative exists. In these cases, it is essential that the patient be closely monitored by an experienced physician. When discontinuing a drug, the patient should be provided with a list of substitute medications for future use.

14.10 Therapy and Management

The most important and effective therapeutic measure in managing drug hypersensitivity reactions is the discontinuation of the offending medication, if possible. Alternative medications with unrelated chemical structures should be substituted when available. The clinical consequences of medication cessation or substitution should be closely monitored. In the majority of patients, symptoms will resolve within two weeks if the diagnosis of drug hypersensitivity is correct.

Additional therapy for drug hypersensitivity reactions is largely supportive and symptomatic (Table 14.7). Systemic corticosteroids may speed recovery in severe cases of drug hypersensitivity. Topical corticosteroids and oral antihistamines may improve dermatologic symptoms. The severe drug reactions of Stevens-Johnson syndrome and toxic epidermal necrolysis require additional intensive therapy.

Evaluation and Management of Drug Reaction

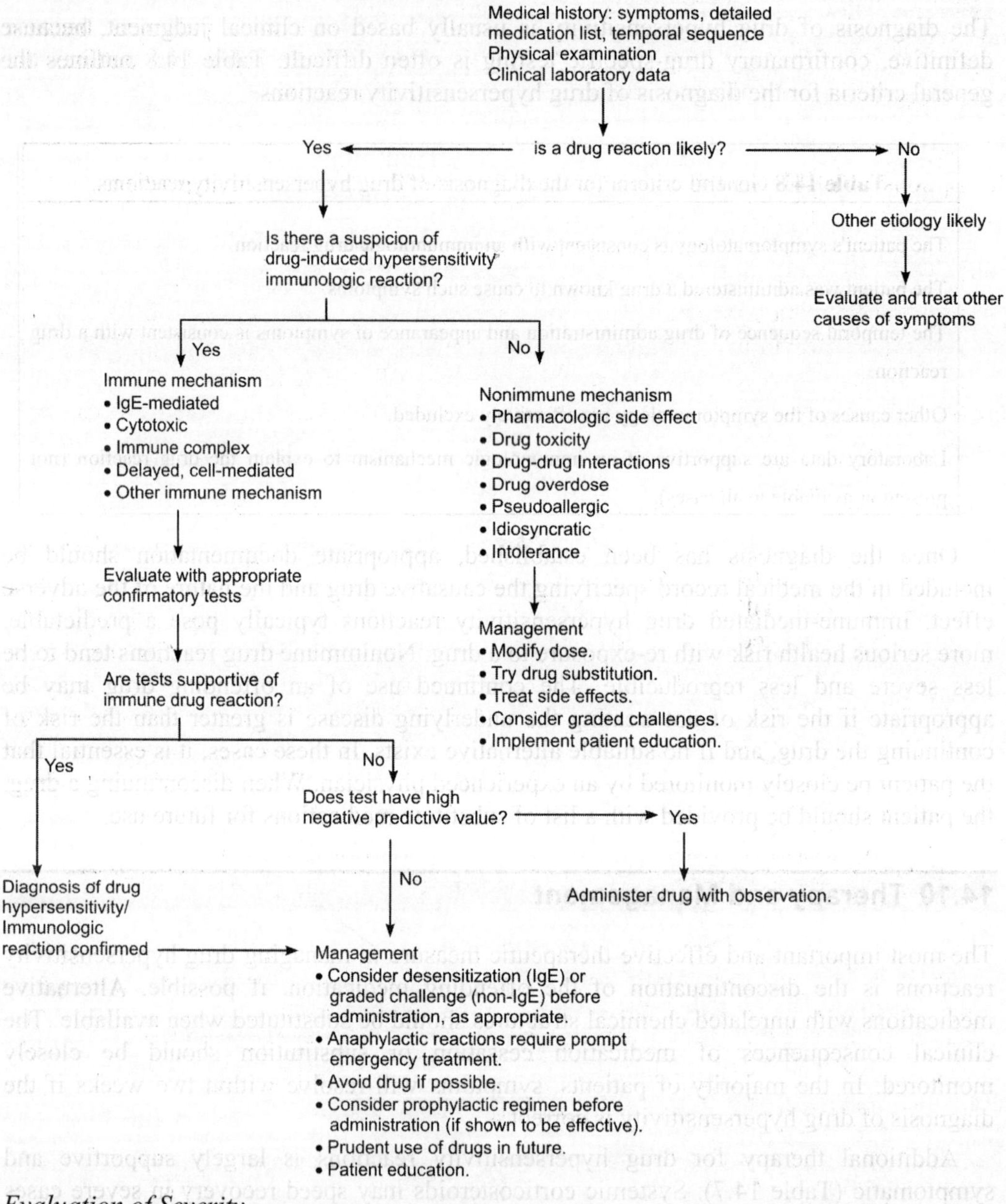

Evaluation of Severity

The management of an ADR requires an evaluation of the severity and the benefit-to-risk ratio. ADRs range from mild and tolerable to life-threatening and intolerable. The pharmacist must evaluate the patient to determine whether the reaction is mild, moderate, severe, or life-threatening. The same reaction in different patients may have a different severity. For example, an anticholinergic response resulting in dry mouth may be mild and well-tolerated in a young patient, but may lead to ill-fitting dentures and mouth irritation in an older patient. Consequently, this reaction would be severe and intolerable to the older patient.

Options for Management

The options available in the management of an ADR depend on the severity of the reaction. Obviously, the drug must be discontinued if the ADR is life-threatening; however, for less severe ADRs, discontinuation of the drug is not always necessary or desirable. Many ADRs can be managed by a dosage adjustment to achieve the appropriate therapeutic range rather than by discontinuing the drug. This is especially true for ADRs resulting from a failure to adjust the dose based on renal failure. If the therapeutic benefit exceeds the consequences of the ADR, the drug should be continued unless a less toxic, but equally efficacious, drug is available. Frequently, the ADR can be managed simply or the ADR may not severely impair the patient. Sometimes an ADR is treated with another drug. This process should be discouraged if a less toxic agent is available; however, in some cases another medication may be preferable to discontinuing the original medication. The development of an ADR, therefore, does not automatically dictate discontinuation of the drug. All of these options must be assessed and decisions made on an individual basis. The interrelation of steps in the identification and management of suspected adverse drug reactions is illustrated in Figure 14.1.

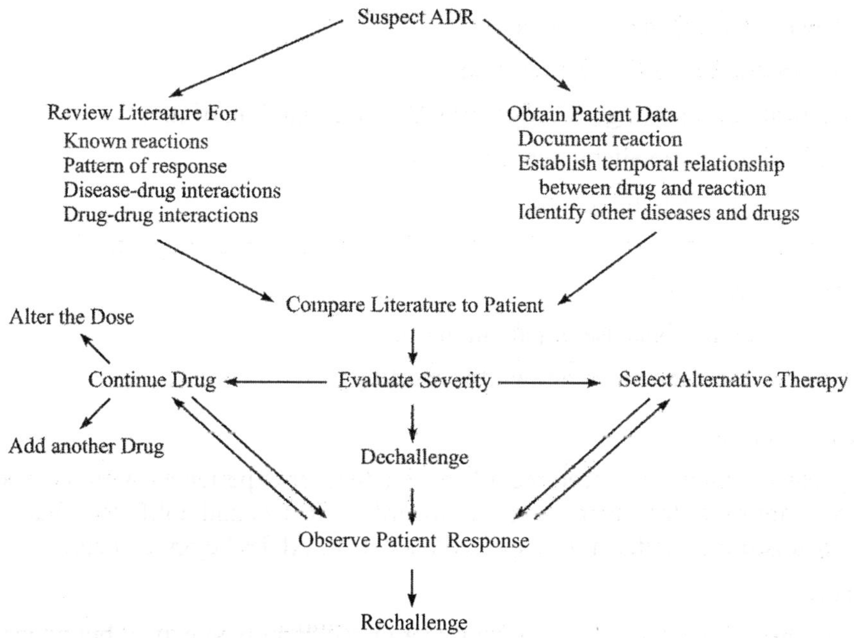

Fig. 14.1 Identification and management of adverse drug reactions.

14.11 Reporting

After the ADR has been well documented, it should be reported to those who have a special interest in ADRs. They may include the DCGI (Drug Controller General of India), CDSCO (Central Drugs Standard Control Organization), the individual pharmaceutical manufacturer, publishers of pharmaceutical or medical literature, and the medical staff and administration of the individual hospital.

Central Drugs Standard Control Organization (CDSCO)

The CDSCO program has primary interest in unexpected, significant adverse reactions to drugs and in increased frequencies of serious, known reactions. The CDSCO has less interest in common ADRs such as dehydration secondary to diuretics. The CDSCO program monitors ADRs that may be probable or possible as individual reports and combines many individual reports to establish trends or to identify rare ADRs.

Lack of ADR reporting by physicians is due to the following reasons:

- Failure to detect the reaction due to a low level of suspicion.
- Fear of potential legal implications.
- Lack of training about drug therapy.
- Uncertainty about whether the drug causes the action.
- Lack of clear responsibility for reporting.
- Paper work and time involved.
- No financial incentive for reporting.
- Unaware of reporting procedure or little understanding of it.
- Lack of readily available reporting forms.
- Desire to publish the report.
- Fear that a useful drug will be removed from the market or given a bad name.
- Complacency and lethargy.
- Guilty feelings because of patient harm.
- Opinion that reaction is not worth reporting.

Drug Manufacturer

The drug manufacturer must keep records of practitioner experiences with its products. It is the responsibility of the manufacturer to record ADR data and notify the pharmacy and medical professions by letter if unsuspected clusters of ADRs begin to occur.

Publication

For adverse drug reactions that are carefully validated in a given patient but which are not defined in the literature, publication is the best approach to raising the index of suspicion among practitioners. Once an ADR is clearly documented in the literature, other practitioners are more likely to observe it in their patients. Reporting increases the level of suspicion.

Internal reporting

Some ADRs are so predictable that the main use of the reports of their occurrence is internal. These are ADRs that could be prevented with careful monitoring techniques. Their detection may indicate the need for inservice presentations, newsletters, or increased pharmacist involvement in drug therapy monitoring.

In all ADR reporting, patient confidentiality must be maintained. If the prescribing physician does not fill out the report, the individual who does so should notify the physician that a report is being made. Copies of the final evaluation should be sent to any person notifying the ADR pharmacist of a potential reaction.

Spontaneous reporting

There is a need for continuous post-marketing drug surveillance after a drug is released for use in the general population. Intensive post marketing surveillance programs are useful in surveying drug use. While they provide numerator and denominator data so that an incidence can be postulated, they are expensive, do not reflect drug use in all patient types, and may not detect rare, delayed, or unusual ADRs. There remains the need for the individual practitioner to review drug use for the detection, assessment, and reporting of ADRs. Individual spontaneous reporting frequently alerts all practitioners to clinically important but unreported ADRs. The spontaneous report may lead to more detailed study to define the incidence, mechanism, and significance of a given ADR.

Voluntary reporting

The voluntary reporting system utilizes forms that are available on the nursing unit or are available upon request from the pharmacy. These may be the forms supplied by the CDSCO or those designed by a particular hospital. Individual practitioners must suspect an ADR, request the form, fill it out, and send it to the pharmacy. While this method does result in some reports, it is a low-yield program. It requires that the individual physician must suspect an ADR and be motivated to report the reaction. Some physicians may not want to spend the time necessary to complete these forms but may use an alert system in which the practitioner notifies the pharmacy that an ADR has occurred and the pharmacist goes to the patient unit and completes the necessary forms. Another way of increasing utilization of the voluntary reporting system by physicians is to solicit oral requests for completion of the forms. The drug information center may be utilized to promote and receive ADR evaluation requests.

Nurses are also valuable resources in detecting ADRs. They see patients under a variety of conditions and may be the first and only individuals to suspect an ADR. They may initiate the alert system either in writing or verbally. If individual pharmacists serve as liaisons with individual nursing units, the relationship can be utilized to explain the ADR program and to solicit evaluations of suspected ADRs.

14.12 Initiation of an ADR Program

An ADR program is a good way to begin clinical services. The program can start with advertising the voluntary reporting system and progress to prospective monitoring and prevention. After deciding to participate in an ADR program, a protocol should be developed which can be presented to the proper hospital committees. The pharmacy and therapeutics committee is an appropriate place to start.

Pharmacy and Therapeutics Committee

The program description presented to the pharmacy and therapeutics committee should be tailored to each institution but should contain certain basic components. These include:

- A standard protocol on ADR reporting
- A brief description of the significance and incidence of ADRs
- A description of the current program and how well this program is functioning
- A description of the proposed changes in the system
- How and by whom the new program will be implemented
- The personnel, time, and costs of the system
- How ADRs will be detected
- To whom the ADRs will be reported and
- How the program will upgrade patient care in that hospital.

The proposal should be positive, emphasizing the importance of detecting ADRs so that current and future patient care may be improved.

The initial step would be to encourage the voluntary reporting of ADRs. The pharmacist should ensure that appropriate forms are available at all nursing units and follow up with a memorandum or presentation to all professional staff (e.g., physicians, nurses, pharmacists, etc.) on the importance of reporting ADRs, together with an explanation as to how the reporting forms should be used. Anyone suspecting an adverse drug reaction should notify the ADR pharmacist and request a complete review of the patient's drug therapy plan with concomitant ADR reporting.

It may be necessary to raise the level of awareness to the importance of ADRs and to the reporting mechanism. This can be done through articles in the department of pharmacy newsletters, memoranda, and presentations. It may also be necessary to repeat periodically the awareness program as initial enthusiasm wanes or new staff begins practice in the institution.

In addition, the ADR pharmacist could arrange with the medical records department to hold all patient records indicating iatrogenic disease or ADR.

A particular diagnosis that might be drug-induced, e.g., hyperkalemia, could be monitored. The results from these detection systems should be reported back to the pharmacy and therapeutics committee and publicized in the pharmacy department's newsletters. Particularly interesting or significant ADRs should be described in newsletters or in conferences. Trends in ADRs would indicate an area for an educational program.

Audit Committee

The ADR pharmacist might also want to coordinate activities with the audit committee. This would allow individual agents to be studied intensively for short periods of time.

With the data generated by the detection system, the activities of the ADR pharmacist could be expanded to include ADR prevention. There may be several approaches to ADR prevention. If pharmacists are not available to review every patient and every drug, it may be desirable to monitor drugs with narrow therapeutic ranges. For example, all patients receiving aminoglycoside antibiotics could be monitored. The laboratory would alert the ADR pharmacist to any high drug serum levels that could potentially represent an ADR. An alternative to single drug monitoring is to monitor all of the patients on a single team or admitted by a single physician. The pharmacist could identify a physician who is favorably predisposed to pharmacy input and initiate ADR surveillance and monitoring of that physician's patients. The move to prevention rather than just detection will be a greater benefit to patient care. If an ADR program is to be successful, the ADR pharmacist must be dedicated to making it work. It will require that the pharmacist follow up on reports of suspected ADRs and provide feedback to the reporter. All of this may require that the pharmacist devote time to the ADR program that is outside of normal working hours.

If successful, an ADR program can be of considerable benefit to patient care. It can be professionally rewarding and can lead to greater involvement of the pharmacist in patient care. Figure 14.3 illustrates the interrelationships of activities involved in the initiation of an ADR program.

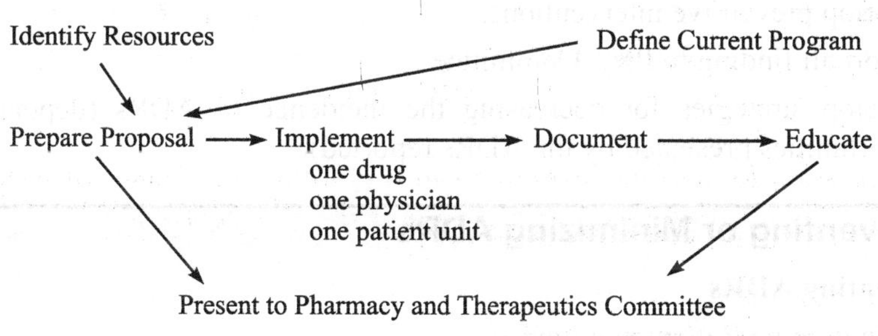

Fig. 14.3 Initiation of an ADR Program.

14.13 Implementing a Program

Prior to implementing an ADR program, the health care facility must educate its staff on the importance and significance of the program. The pharmacy department is in an excellent position to provide this education because of its involvement in the pharmacy & therapeutics committee (P&T Committee), pharmacokinetic dosing, drug utilization evaluation (DUE), and drug distribution. The pharmacy department can be an excellent resource for developing an ADR program, as well as providing data about ADRs to the P&T Committee.

Guidelines for starting a program include the following.

- Develop definition and classifications for ADRs that work for the institution.
- Assign responsibility for the ADR program within the pharmacy and throughout other key departments. A multidisciplinary approach is an essential factor.
- Develop a program with approval from the pharmacy department, medical staff, nursing department, as well as other appropriate areas within the facility. Co-operation is essential in initiation of a successful program.
- Promote awareness of the program.
- Promote the awareness of ADRs and the importance of reporting such events.
- Develop policies and procedures for handling ADRs being sent to the CDSCO. Indicate who is responsible for sending them.
- Establish mechanisms for screening ADRs. These mechanisms should include retrospective reviews, concurrent monitoring, as well as prospective planning for high-risk groups.
- Develop forms for data collection and reporting or other mechanisms for reporting.
- Establish procedures for evaluating ADRs.
- Routinely review ADRs for trends.
- Monitor ADRs continuously and concurrently.
- Develop preventive interventions.
- Report all finding to P&T Committee.
- Develop strategies for decreasing the incidence of ADRs (depending on the opportunities presented by the ADRs reported).

14.14 Preventing or Minimizing ADRs

(i) Preventing ADRs

Anticipation by Patient monitoring

It is preferable to prevent or minimize the consequences of an adverse drug reaction. This can be done by assessing the patient and anticipating the possible

ADRs that may occur in that patient. For example, certain drugs cause hemolytic anemia in patients with glucose-6-phosphate dehydrogenase (G-6-PD) deficiency. Patients at high risk for this condition could be screened for G-6-PD activity prior to administering a potentially offending agent.

Anticipation of dosage reduction

Dosage reduction prior to initiating therapy should be anticipated for certain patients. For example, patients with impaired renal function, whether due to disease or to advanced age, should receive a reduced dose of any drugs excreted unchanged in the urine.

Monitoring of serum levels

Many ADRs are associated with high drug serum levels. Examples of these drugs are theophylline, anticonvulsants, antiarrhythmics, aspirin, and aminoglycosides. Appropriate monitoring of serum levels, using basic pharmacokinetic principles, will prevent many ADRs which result from levels outside the therapeutic range.

Monitoring of pharmacologic activity

The ADRs associated with many drugs are an extension of their pharmacologic properties. For example, diuretics are given to promote salt and water loss but may cause electrolyte depletion and dehydration. Warfarin is given as an anticoagulant but may cause bleeding. Prevention of such toxic effects involves setting therapeutic endpoints and selecting appropriate monitoring techniques and frequency to ensure that the endpoint is not exceeded.

The key to the prevention and minimization of common or predictable ADRs is anticipation. As described below, many ADRs can be prevented if the individual patient is evaluated prior to the initiation of therapy for the potential of developing an ADR during therapy. Based on patient-specific information and a thorough knowledge of drug, appropriate endpoints and monitoring techniques can be selected before the patient actually receives the drug. For this reason, many ADRs can be prevented or detected and quickly corrected.

(ii) Minimizing non-preventable ADRs

Adverse drug reactions that are idiosyncratic or hypersensitive reactions are not as preventable; however, anticipation can minimize the consequences of these types of reactions. A thorough knowledge of the drug and an observation of the patient can help minimize ADRs. If reported idiosyncratic reactions occur or unusual patient symptoms are correlated with drug administration, the dose of the drug may be reduced or discontinued before the complications are severe. The reaction may be minimized also by anticipating a response and providing more frequent monitoring of the patient. If particularly severe reactions are anticipated, the consequences could be minimized by having antidotes or agents to reverse the effects on hand prior to the initiation of therapy. For example, if it is decided that a patient with a life-threatening infection such as meningitis should be treated with penicillin, although the patient has a history of penicillin allergy, diphenhydramine, epinephrine, and corticosteroids should be available. Then, if the patient is carefully monitored, the allergic reaction if it occurs may be quickly recognized, treated, and minimized.

14.15 Legal Aspects of ADR Detection

Reactions to drugs may be the basis for law suits, and every ADR program must consider this potential problem. The careful recording of adverse drug reactions and the attendant rectification of prescribing problems may be used to document quality control efforts. In addition, if the ADR program includes prevention as well as detection, it can further exemplify quality of care.

14.16 Benefits of a Surveillance Program

An adverse drug reaction surveillance program benefits current and future patients individually, it affords educational benefits to the institution, improves prescribing practice, and facilitates for overall improved patient care.

- *Benefits to Current Patients:* A successful ADR program can benefit an individual patient by preventing or minimizing the consequences of ADRs. Diagnosis may be made faster and the duration of hospitalization shortened.
- *Benefits to Future Patients:* Future patients benefit from an ADR program through improved understanding about the benefits and limitations of drug therapy. Better therapeutic decisions can be made for future patients based on knowledge and experience gained through the treatment of current patients.
- *Improved Prescribing:* Individual practitioners raise their level of suspicion about drug-induced disease through ADR programs. Individual and institutional prescribing problems can be identified and resolved. The ability to make therapeutic decisions will be measurably enhanced.
- *Educational Benefit:* The ADR program offers an educational experience for the entire hospital. It offers the opportunity for interdisciplinary cooperation and recognition of abilities.

- *Pharmacist Involvement in Patient Care:* Individual pharmacists may become more involved in direct patient care as a result of participating in an ADR program. Chart review allows the pharmacist to become familiar with laboratory tests, medical terminology, and medical jargon. Prospective monitoring offers the ADR pharmacist the opportunity to have input in patient care.

14.17 Computer Applications in ADR Monitoring

Computers have been routinely used in the epidemiological evaluation of ADRs. Programs for determining numerator and denominator data are in wide use. More recently, however, computer programs have been developed to aid in the monitoring and prevention of ADRs. Patient profiles can be entered into a computer which may be programmed to search for recognized drug-drug, drug-disease, drug-nutrient, or drug-laboratory interactions. The pharmacist is alerted if all baseline patient data needed to dose a drug properly has been obtained. Computer programs have also been developed to match patient history of ADRs and allergic reactions to prescribing. Thus, the same or similar medications can be avoided. Since a growing number of hospitals are using computers to store and process patient data, the pharmacist will find the computer increasingly helpful in patient monitoring. The computer can quickly review data and alert pharmacists to irregularities in prescribing or patient responses; however, clinical judgment will still be necessary to resolve the irregularities on an individual patient basis.

Table 14.9 Methods of detecting adverse drug reactions.

1.	Patient Chart Check-Off	An adverse drug reaction notification slip is completed by the physician when he completes the patient chart.
2.	Chart Scanning	Discharge summary sheets are scanned to obtain information relating to an adverse drug effect.
3.	Voluntary Physician Reporting	The physician completes an adverse reaction form after noting a reaction.
4.	Review of Physician Orders	Drug orders are monitored by a pharmacist.
5.	Adverse Reaction Rounds	Pharmacy students and practitioners participate in ward survey patients receiving drugs.
6.	Form Notification System	The Physician who observes a reaction completes a form that alerts the adverse reaction team to follow through on reporting.

Table 14.10 Some important Adverse Drug Reactions.

Sl.No	Class of Drugs	Adverse Drug Reactions or Effects
A	DRUGS ACTING ON CENTRAL NERVOUS SYSTEM	
1	**Narcotic Analgesics**	
(i)	Morphine	Dysphoria, constipation, dryness of mouth, mental clouding, headache and fatigue, intolerance, respiratory depression
(ii)	Pethidine and Methadone	Sweating, euphoria, dizziness, dry mouth, weakness and palpitation, anaphylactic shock leading to circulatory collapse and bronchospasm, coma or tremors
2	**Hypnotic Sedatives**	
(i)	Barbiturates	Headache, nausea, vomiting, allergic skin, lesion like urticaria, slurred speech, ataxia, impaired reflexes, anxiety, restlessness, tremors, abdominal cramps, CNS depression, particularly respiratory and circulatory collapse, rapid pulse
3	**Antipyretic Analgesics**	
(i)	Salicylates	Skin rashes, urticaria, angioneurotics edema, GI problems such as dyspepsia, nausea, vomiting and sometimes GI bleeding, reduction in plasma prothrombin level and interference with prostaglandin synthesis
(ii)	Paracetamol	Skin reactions, anemia, haemolysis, liver damage due to large doses
4	**Non-steroidal Anti-inflammatory Drugs (NSAIDs)**	
(i)	Phenylbutazone	Peptic ulcer, hemolytic reactions such as anemia, agranulocytosis, edema, displacement of anticoagulants due to high protein binding, leukemia
(ii)	Other NSAIDs like Indomethacin, Ibuprofen, Naproxen, Piroxicam, etc.,	Headache, mental confusion, blurring of vision, depression, peptic ulcer, liver damage, renal damage
5	**Anti-convulsants or Anti-epileptics**	
(i)	Hydantoins, Succinimides and Oxazolidine diones	Urticaria, skin rashes, drowsiness, fatigue, blurring of vision, GI irritation, megaloblastic and aplastic anemia, hypertrophy of gums
6	**Tranquilizers**	
(i)	Phenothiazines	Skin eruption, photosensitivity, ANS effects like tachycardia, blurred vision, CNS effects like drowsiness, tremors, muscular rigidity, agranulocytosis in 0.5% patients, obstructive jaundice, long term use may lead to irregularities in menstrual cycle, impotence and weight gain

Table 14.10 *Contd....*

7	**Anti- depressant drugs**	
(i)	Tricyclic compounds like Imipramine, Amitriptyline, MAO inhibitors like Phenelzine, Iproniazide	Dryness of mouth, tachycardia, impotence, delayed ejaculation, tremors, ataxia, disturbed sleep, orthostatic, hypotension, hyperpyrexia, convulsions
8	**Antihistaminic Drugs**	
(i)	Diphenhydramine HCl, Cetrizine, etc.,	Drowsiness and sedation, hypotension, dry mouth, blurred vision, delirium, nausea and vomiting, toxicity gives rise to respiratory collapse and coma
B	**DRUGS ACTING ON AUTONOMIC NERVOUS SYSTEM**	
1	**Adrenergic Drugs**	
(i)	Epinephrine, Isoproterenol, Amphetamine, Ephedrine, Nor-Adrenaline, etc.,	Palpitaion, tachycardia, arrhythmia, headache and flushing, tremors, psychosis, insomnia, anginal pain-especially in asthmatic patients, GI upset and confusion
2	**Adrenergic Blockers**	
(i)	α-Adrenergic Blockers, Tolazoline, Phentolamine, etc.,	Cardiac and GI stimulation, tachycardia, arrhythmias and anginal pain, sensation of cold, hypotension, high doses cause myocardial infarction
(ii)	Beta adrenergic blockers, Propranolol, Nadolol, Atenolol	Hypotension, bradycardia, constipation, nausea, vomiting, bronchospasm
3	**Other Cardiovascular Drugs**	
(i)	Centrally acting Hydralazine, Clonidine, Guanethidine, et.,	Drowsiness, vertigo, dry mouth, palpitation, tachycardia, dizziness, flushing, anorexia, postural hypotension, mental depression, reduction in renal blood flow, GI bleeding
(ii)	Calcium Channel Blockers like Verapamil, Nifedipine, Diltiazem	Headache, fatigue, orthostatic hypotension, forgetfulness, mental depression, parkinsonism, altered liver functions, leg cramps, skin rashes
(iii)	Vasodilators like Organic Nitrates, Isosorbide	Giddiness, weakness, postural hypotension, heart block
(iv)	Anti-inflammatory Drugs, Quinidine	Vertigo, ringing in ears, skin rash, conduction blocks, bradycardia, light headedness
4	**Cholinergic drugs**	
(i)	Carbachol, Pilocarpine, Eserine, Malathion, Parathion	GI irritation, flushing, bronchospasm, heavy chest, abdominal, cramps, myasthenia gravis, epigastric distress, skeletal muscle paralysis
5	**Cholinergic Blockers**	
(i)	Atropine, Scopalamine, Semi-synthetic atropine analogs	Dry mouth, constipation, dermatitis, postural hypotension, urinary retention, impotence, euphoria, neuromuscular blockade, psychosis, restlessness

Table 14.10 *Contd....*

C	**Diuretics**	
(i)	Acetazolamide, Furesemide, Ethacrynic acid	Hypokalemia, hypochloremic alkalosis, weakness, fatigue, cramps, vertigo, orthostatic hypotension, deafness, metabolic acidosis, skin rash
D	**Local Anesthetics**	
(i)	Procaine etc,	Dermatitis, fall in blood pressure, hypoxia, medullary depression, anorexia, hallucinations, sexual dysfunction, arrhythmia, myocardial infarction
E	**Anticoagulant Drugs**	
(i)	Warfarin etc.,	Haemorrhage, bleeding of gums, haematuria, renal damage, agranulocytosis, edema, fever, diarrhea
F	**Hypoglycemic Agents**	
(i)	Tolbutamide, Glipizide, Glibenaclamide, Phenformin	Skin rash, bone marrow depression, goitrogenic reactions, anorexia, bitter taste, cholestatic jaundice
G	**Chemotherapeutic Agents**	
(1)	**Antibiotics**	
(i)	Penicillins, Ampicillin, Cloxacillin, etc.,	Anaphylactic shock causing cardiovascular collapse, bronchospasm or edema of larynx, platelet aggregation
(ii)	Aminoglocoside Antibiotics like Streptomycin, Gentamycin	Ototoxicity, neuromuscular blockage, nephorotoxicity, optic neuritis, albuminuria, dizziness
(iii)	Tetracyclines	Erythemia, GI irritation, liver dysfunction, formation of chelates with calcium and have adverse effect on bones and teeth, local thrombosis, renal damage
(iv)	Cephalosporins, Cephalexin, Cephalothin	Serum sickness, anaphylactic reactions, dose related nephrotoxicity
(v)	Sulphonamides, Sulphadiazine, Sulphasalazine	Hemolytic anemia, aplastic anemia, fever, serum sickness, crystaluria, arthritis, peripheral neuritis, hepatitis, skin and mucus lesions and hypothyroidism
H	**Antileprotic Drugs**	
(i)	Dapsone, Clofazimine	Haemolysis, methaemoglobin, anorexia, nausea, vomiting, dermatitis, jaundice, insomnia, red and black pigmentation
I	**Antitubercular Drugs**	
(i)	Isoniazid, Ethambutol, Rifampicin, Pyrazinamide	Convulsions, optic neuritis, jaundice, loss of self control, hepatitis, dermatitis, joint pain, dry mouth, urinary retention, anorexia, nausea
J	**Antimalarial Drugs**	
(i)	Chloroquine, Primaquine, Quinine	GI upset, pruritis, ringing in the ear, visual disturbances, ventricular tachycardia, cramps, epigastric distress
K	**Anti-amoebic and Antihelminthetics**	
(i)	Emetine, Metronidazole, Di-iodohydroxyquin, Iodochlorohydroxyquine, Diloxanide furoate	Myocardial effects, metallic taste, flushing, pruritis, urticaria, glossitis, stomatitis, dizziness, vertigo, muscle weakness, chills, fever, diarrhea, itching, abdominal pain, myelitis like illness, anal irritation

Conclusion

The choice of a drug for the patient is a calculated risk, since no drug is without adverse effects. In the professional judgment of the health team, however, a particular drug may be the drug of choice. In such situations, careful monitoring of the patient may allow alterations in therapy or modification of the dose before serious adverse effects occur. In these instances, the variables and intricacies will challenge the pharmacist to the full extent of his professional competence and expertise.

The detection of an adverse drug reaction requires a lot of experience, alertness and knowledge on part of every member of a health care team. The pharmacist, however, should always be alert for the contingency of these perplexities. Moreover, he can also fulfill a valuable administrative role in coordinating adverse drug reaction data collection, reporting, and storage.

Study Outline

Adverse Drug reactions contribute to overall health care costs by increasing morbidity and even mortality in severe cases. ADR is defined as one which is noxious, unintended, and occurs at dosages normally used in man for prophylaxis, diagnosis and therapy of disease or for modification of physiological function.

ADR may include any of the following:

- an exaggerated drug response
- an unwanted effect on an organ system different from that being treated
- an allergic or hypersensitivity reaction
- an idiosyncratic reaction
- a drug interaction that causes either an increase or decrease in response

Classification

Misdosage - here ADRs result due to erroneous administration

Pharmacologic – ADRs are objectionable reactions due to drugs pharmacologic action

Non Pharmacologic – Allergic, idiosyncratic

Another classification is based on severity of reaction

- Minor
- Moderate
- Severe
- Lethal

Epidemiology – 5 to 6 % of all hospitals admissions are because of ADRs

Certain factors like HIV infection, asthma, use of Beta blockers etc., are associated with increased risk for ADR.

Mechanism of Adverse Drug Reactions:

- Idiosyncrasy
- Hypersensitivity
- Intolerance
- Drug interaction
- Pharmacologic

Variables affecting ADR incidence and severity

Patient variables – age, immune status, genetics

Drug variables – route of administration, formulation, duration of therapy

Clinical manifestations

Dermatologic symptoms – rashes, urticaria to severe erythema multiforme and toxic epidermal necrolysis, eczematous rashes, contact dermatitis to systemic reactions such as anaphylaxis.

Clinical Evaluation

- History
- Physical examination
- Laboratory evaluation
- Diagnosis

Therapy and Management

- discontinuation of offending medication
- alternative medications with unrelated chemical structures
- additional therapy for reactions, systemic corticosteroids

Adverse Drug Reaction Form

ADR Submission # _____ MEDICATION(S):_____
ADMIT DATE: __-__-__ DOSAGE/ROUTE/FREQUENCY: _____

Probability from Naranjo Scale (see below):
☐ ≥ 9 (definite) ☐ 5-8 (probable) ☐ 1-4 (possible) ☐ 0 (doubtful)

Severity: ☐ 1 (minor temporary) ☐ 3 (major temporary) ☐ 5 (potential continuing)
☐ 0 (no disability) ☐ 2 (minor permanent) ☐ 4 (major permanent) ☐ 6 (death)

Was the ADR preventable? ☐ Yes ☐ No

Outcome? (Briefly describe management of patient/drug therapy change. Seventy-five space limit.)

_____

FDA reportable? ☐ Yes ☐ No (If reported, do not send this form.)

Reporter's name: _____ Preceptor's name:_____ date:__-__-__

NARANJO ADVERSE DRUG REACTION PROBABILITY SCALE

Purpose of the Naranjo scale: To provide a systematic method for assessing the probability of an adverse drug reaction in a clinical setting

Read each question to determine the correct response, check the box, and place the number corresponding to that response in the appropriate box in the score column. Total the numbers in the score column to determine the probability that a particular medication was responsible for the reported adverse event.

NARANJO SCALE				
Question	**Yes**	**No**	**NA**	**Score**
• Are there previous *conclusive* reports?	+1☐	0☐	0☐	
• Did the adverse event appear after the suspected drug was administered?	+2☐	-1☐	0☐	
• Did the adverse event improve when drug was discontinued or *specific* antagonist was administered?	+1☐	0☐	0☐	
• Reaction was more severe with increased dose or less severe with decreased dose?	+1☐	0☐	0☐	
• Did the reaction appear when the drug was readministered?	+2☐	-1☐	0☐	
• Are there other nondrug causes for the adverse event?	-1☐	+2☐	0☐	
• Did the reaction appear when a placebo was given?	-1☐	+1☐	0☐	
• Was a toxic serum concentration noted?	+1☐	0☐	0☐	
• Does patient have a history of similar reaction with drug or drug class?	+1☐	0☐	0☐	
• Adverse event confirmed by any objective evidence?	+1☐	0☐	0☐	
			Total Score	

Adapted from Naranjo CA, Busto U, Sellers EM et al. A method for estimating the probability of adverse drug reactions. *Clin Pharmacol Ther.* 1981; 30:239-45.

Major determinants of causality:
- Timing of event
- Other causes for the reaction
- Dechallenge information
- Previous experience with the drug or similar drug
- Objective evidence (e.g. serum concentration)
- Rechallenge information

Problems with causality assessment:
- Confounding factors
- Inter-reviewer variability

SUSPECTED ADVERSE DRUG REACTION REPORTING FORM

CDSCO

Central Drugs Standard Control Organization

Directorate General of Health Services,
Ministry of Health & Family Welfare, Government of India,
Nirman Bhawan, New Delhi - 110011
www.cdsco.nic.in

For VOLUNTARY reporting of Adverse Drug Reactions by health care professionals

Report #

To be filled in by Pharmacovigilance centres receiving the form.

A. Patient information

1. Patient identifier initials ________ In confidence

2. Age at time of event: ________ or Date of Birth:

3. Sex: ☐ M ☐ F

4. Weight_____ Kgs

B. Suspected Adverse Reaction

5. Date of reaction started (dd/mm/yy):

6. Date of recovery (dd/mm/yy):

7. Describe reaction or problem

12. Relevant tests/ laboratory data, including dates

13. Other relevant history, including pre-existing medical conditions (e.g., allergies, race, pregnancy, smoking alcohol use, hepatic/ renal dysfunction, etc.)

14. Seriousness of the reaction

☐ Death (dd/mm/yy)__________
☐ Life threatening
☐ Hospitalization-initial or prolonged
☐ Disability
☐ Congenital anomaly
☐ Required intervention to prevent permanent impairment/ damage
☐ Other (specify)__________

15. Outcomes

☐ Fatal
☐ Continuing
☐ Recovering
☐ Recovered
☐ Unknown
☐ Other (specify)__________

C. Suspected medication(s)

Sl. No.	8. Name (brand and / or generic name)	Manufacturer (if known)	Batch No. / Lot No. (if known)	Exp. Date (if known)	Dose used	Route used	Frequency	Therapy dates (if unknown, give duration) Date started	Date stopped	Reason for Use or prescribed for
i										
ii										
iii										
iv										

Sl. No. As per C	9. Reaction abated after drug stopped or dose reduced Yes	No	Unknown	NA	Reduced dose	10. Reaction reappeared after reintroduction Yes	No	Unknown	NA	If reintroduced, dose
i										
ii										
iii										
iv										

11. Concomitant medical products and therapy dates including self medication and herbal remedies (exclude those used to treat reaction)

D. Reporter (see confidentiality section in first page)

16. Name and Professional Address: __________

Pin code: __________ E-mail: __________

Cell No. / Tel. No. with STD Code: __________

Speciality: __________ Signature: __________

17. Occupation

18. Date of this report (dd/mm/yy)

ADVICE ABOUT REPORTING

- **Report adverse experiences with medications**

- **Report serious adverse reactions. A reaction is serious when the patient outcome is:**
  - death
  - life-threatening (real risk of dying)
  - hospitalization (initial or prolonged)
  - disability (significant, persistent or permanent)
  - congenital anomaly
  - required intervention to prevent permanent impairment or damage

- **Report even if:**
  - You're not certain the product caused adverse reaction
  - You don't have all the details although point nos. 1, 5, 7, 8, 11, 15, 16 & 18 (see reverse) are essentially required.

- **Who can report:**
  - Any health care professional (Doctors including Dentists, Nurses and Pharmacists).

- **Where to report:**
  - After completing, please return this form to the same Pharmacovigilance centre from where you received.
  - A list of countrywide Pharmacovigilance Centres is available at: www.cdsco.nic.in

- **What happens to the submitted information:**
  - Information provided in this form is handled in strict confidence. Peripheral Pharmacovigilance Centres will forward this form to the Regional Pharmacovigilance Centres, where the causality analysis is carried out and the information is forwarded to the Zonal Pharmacovigilance Centres. Finally the data is statistically analysed and forwarded to the Global Pharmacovigilance Database managed by WHO Uppsala Monitoring Center in Sweden.
  - Data is periodically reviewed by the National Pharmacovigilance Advisory Committee constituted by the Ministry of Health and Family Welfare. The Committee is entrusted with responsibility to review the data and suggest any interventions that may be required.

Suspected Adverse Drug Reaction Reporting Form

For VOLUNTARY reporting
of suspected adverse drug reactions by
health care professionals

CDSCO

Central Drugs Standard Control Organization

Directorate General of Health Services,
Ministry of Health & Family Welfare, Government of India.
Nirman Bhawan, New Delhi-110011
www.cdsco.nic.in

ATTENTION
HEALTH CARE PROFESSIONALS

Your 5 Minutes Can Help Us Ensure Safer Medications

Please return this form to:

Confidentiality: The patient's identity is held in strict confidence and protected to the fullest extent. Programme staff is not expected to and will not disclose the reporter's identity in response to a request from the public. Submission of a report does not constitute an admission that medical personnel or manufacturer or the product caused or contributed to the reaction.

Chapter 15

Total Parenteral Nutrition

Objectives

After reading this chapter, the student should be able to:

- Define and understand the term Total Parenteral Nutrition
- Discuss the various indications for a Total Parenteral Nutrition
- Understand the various constituents involved in Total Parenteral Nutrition, prepare a TPN and know the storage conditions
- Explain the various complications associated with Total Parenteral Nutrition usage
- Know the role of Pharmacist in Total Parenteral Nutrition Program

15.1 Introduction

With the advent of total parenteral nutrition, interest in and knowledge of the nutritional status and nutritional therapy of patients has increased immensely. It has been shown that malnutrition is a contributing factor in depressed immunocompetence, decreased response to chemotherapy, poor wound healing, increased duration of hospitalization, and increased morbidity and mortality. Clearly, malnutrition in hospitals is a major disease entity which requires prompt recognition and appropriate therapy. Much of the malnutrition seen in the hospitalized patient is iatrogenic in nature. Several cases were presented to illustrate the potential morbidity from hospital acquired malnutrition. In addition to the support necessary to prevent hospital acquired malnutrition, many disease states require nutritional support as adjunct therapy for a successful recovery. The literature supports the use of nutritional support in patients with severe burns, cancer, Crohn's disease, other gastrointestinal disorders, liver failure, acute and chronic renal failure, respiratory failure, short-bowel syndrome, extensive abdominal surgery, and trauma.

It is a known fact that there is a strong relationship between malnutrition and morbidity (and mortality). Experience in nutrition support pharmacy practice reveals that malnutrition is prevalent in most hospitals, and that it is not only a problem in surgical wards but also in medical wards where severity is directly proportional to length of hospitalization. The best route for providing nutrients is the gastrointestinal tract. However, in cases where the use of this route is precluded, parenteral nutrition should be employed. Parenteral nutrition is the provision of required nutrients by intravenous routes. It is commonly referred to as total parenteral nutrition (TPN) or hyper alimentation. TPN should be considered when oral or enteral feeding is impossible, or when gastrointestinal absorption and other functional activities are impaired. The TPN regimen is designed to provide, in addition to fluid (water), six essential groups of nutrients, which are necessary for tissue synthesis and energy balance. These are carbohydrates, essential fatty acids, nitrogen, vitamins, electrolytes and trace elements.

The two primary goals of nutritional intervention are: I) to meet the energy demands of the individual patient so that no energy deficit exists, and 2) to provide amino acids in sufficient amounts to support optimal rates of protein synthesis. Carbohydrates and fats are the nutritional substrates currently used to provide sufficient energy, while amino acids and protein isolates are used to provide adequate protein. Nutritional intervention can be provided by the intravenous or enteral route. Generally, if a patient has an intact gastrointestinal tract, oral alimentation or tube feeding is the preferred route. Enteral methods of nutrition are nasogastric, nasoenteric, gastrostomy and jejunostomy feeding. If the gastrointestinal tract cannot be used, the nutritional substrates will be provided by the intravenous route. Methods of parenteral nutrition delivery include central and peripheral vein administration. Techniques for the preparation and administration of nutritional substrates involve very complex processes. Since these techniques require a high degree of sophistication, patient morbidity and mortality can be increased if the strict protocols required for safe administration are not adhered to. As the trend today is to individualize nutritional regimens, taking into account the patient's primary disease state, secondary complications, drug therapy, and nutritional status, this process is even more complex. Patients receiving nutritional support by intravenous and enteral methods must be monitored on a daily basis for the mechanical, septic, and metabolic complications that may occur. Once these complications are recognized, corrective measures must be taken to alleviate these problems. As patient monitoring becomes more sophisticated and clinical experience improves, many of these complications can be anticipated, and therefore, prevented.

15.2 History

The most significant advance in nutrition has been the demonstration of the feasibility of providing complete nutrition solely by the intravenous route. This would not have been possible were it not for the description of the circulatory system by William Harvey in 1616. Harvey's concept of blood circulating through the body and transporting nutrients to the cells and carrying waste products away paved the way for the classical experiment in 1665 in which Escholtz administered intravenous infusion to animals. During this period the administration of medication by intravenous injection in three patients was reported. By 1831, Thomas Latta had successfully infused a large volume of salt solution into a human for the purpose of rehydration. Two very important discoveries took place before the use of parenteral nutrition became well established. First, there was Joseph Lister and Louis Pasteur's theory of microbial infection and second in 1966 Dudrick demonstrated that beagle puppies receiving only intravenous nutrients grew and developed normally for periods of several months. Similar results were observed in patients using hyperosmolar solution containing protein hydrolysate, glucose, electrolytes, minerals and vitamins through an indwelling catheter placed in the superior Vena Cava. Infusion into such vessel brings about quick dilution of the hyperosmolar solution due to the rapid blood flow while aseptic preparation of the infusate and the use of an intravenous line filter help prevent microbial contamination.

By the late 1960s, Rhoads and Dudrick had documented continued growth and improvement in nutritional markers in humans with the use of central intravenous nutrition. As the use of intravenous nutrition became more wide spread, reports of complications increased. During the next 15-20 years, clinical experience and research resulted in the development of standard protocols which promoted better patient care and a decline in complications associated with parenteral nutrition (PN) therapy. The scope of the practice or specialized nutrition support may utilize specially formulated parenteral or enteral nutrients to maintain or restore optimal nutrition status depending on the level of nutritional intervention required based on a patient's nutrition assessment. The pharmacist's role in providing nutrition support has been recently defined. A clear understanding of the principles of patient selection, initial therapy design and outcome monitoring is essential to provide safe and effective care to those who require nutrition support.

Successful techniques for providing intravenous nutrition support were introduced for clinical use in humans during the early 1960s. Dilute nutrient solutions containing glucose with or without hydrolyzed protein were infused peripherally along with intravenous fat emulsion to provide adequate calories. However, fat emulsions were withdrawn from commercial availability in the United States in 1965 following several reports of serious adverse effects associated with infusions of the cottonseed oil products. Without lipid emulsions, larger volumes of nutrient solutions were required to provide the patient's energy requirements. Patients receiving intravenous nutrition solution volumes of up to 5 L/d were often given concomitant diuretic therapy to manage fluid status. Metabolic complications associated with fluid overload and electrolyte imbalances stimulated the investigation of central venous access. These larger vessels permitted infusion of more concentrated formulas which decreased the fluid volume required and avoided the phlebitis that commonly occurred when hypertonic infusions were given peripherally.

15.3 Indications for Total Parenteral Nutrition

Total parenteral nutrition is potentially life saving, experience has shown that very severe metabolic, mechanical, and infectious complications can occur during its use. Therefore, patient selection for total parenteral nutrition must be done with care. Although desirable, the immediate results of TPN, such as improving patient's response to therapy of specific diseases, prolonging patient survival, and decreasing complications, should not be the main criteria for patient selection. Patients should be selected for TPN, based primarily on the need for maintenance and/ or repletion of their nutritional status in the face of injury, disease and or inability to consume adequate nutrients by other routes (TPN should be used only when oral or enteral support is impossible). It is definitely indicated in the absence or failure of the GIT. Thus indications for TPN include the following:

- Inability to absorb nutrients via the gastrointestinal tract because of one or more of the following:
  - Massive small bowel resection
  - Intractable vomiting when adequate external intake is not expected for 5-7 days.
  - Severe diarrhea not expected to resolve in 5-7 days.
  - Inflammatory bowel disease (Crohn's disease, ulcerative colitis)

    Parenteral Nutrition may benefit patients with acute exacerbations of ulcerative colitis when surgery is being considered and when preservation of lean body mass and functional capacity with enteral nutrition is impossible.
  - Bowel obstruction.
- Cancer – antineoplastic therapy, radiation therapy, bone marrow transplantation.
  - Enteral tube feeding and parenteral nutrition support may benefit some severely malnourished cancer patients or those in whom gastrointestinal or other toxicities are anticipated to preclude adequate oral nutritional intake for more than 1 week. Patients who are candidates for nutrition intervention

under these circumstances should receive nutrition support, if possible in conjunction with the initiation of oncologic therapy.

- Specialized nutrition support is not routinely indicated for well-nourished or malnourished patients undergoing surgery, chemotherapy or radiation therapy

- Moderate to serve pancreatitis when adequate enteral intake is not expected for 5-7 days.

  Parenteral Nutrition should be used when enteral feeding exacerbates abdominal pain, ascites or fistula output in patients with pancreatitis and limited oral intake.
- Severe malnutrition with a temporary (5-7 days) nonfunctional gastrointestinal tract.
- Critical care situations

  Moderate to severe catabolism with or without malnutrition when the gastrointestinal tract is nonfunctional for 5-7 days (e.g., major surgery, trauma, sepsis).
- Organ failures – liver, renal, respiratory

  Moderate to severe catabolism with or without malnutrition when enteral feeding is contraindicated
- Preoperative malnutrition when the gastrointestinal tract is not functional and surgery is not expected for at least 7 days.
- Hyper emesis gravidarum
- Eating disorders - Parenteral Nutrition should be considered for patients with anorexia nervosa who require compulsory feeding but who cannot tolerate enteral support for physical or emotional reasons.

15.4 Constituents of Total Parenteral Nutrition Solution

TPN solutions are composed of a variety of constituents such as carbohydrate (e.g., dextrose), protein (e.g., crystalline amino acids), fat, electrolytes, trace elements, vitamins and water. Other additives that are sometimes added to TPN solutions are insulin, heparin, and albumin.

Water: Water functions as solvent for biological systems. Water is distributed in the intracellular space and extracellular space. Water is essential to the body. For a patient on TPN the intake of water is from the TPN mixture and from tissue metabolism plus the oxidation of food substrates in the body.

Carbohydrates: This is the main source of energy provided during TPN. The monohydrate form of glucose is the primary source of carbohydrates used in TPN. Each gram of dextrose used in TPN, provides 3.4 kcal of energy. Other carbohydrate source such as ethanol, fructose, galactose and sorbitol should not be used as energy sources in TPN. Dextrose is commercially available as 5%, 10%, 20%, 50% and 70% w/v solution in water. The amount of glucose provided in TPN is limited by the weight of the patient, glucose tolerance, and the route of administration and the required osmolality of the solution.

Fat: This is the primary source of essential fatty acid (linoleic acid) in TPN. Linoleic acid is useful as precursors of prostaglandin and in the synthesis of other fatty acids which are essential for cell membrane integrity. Fat is obtained from lipid emulsions which are available as 10% and 20% w/v solutions. Fat supplies 9 kcal/g. However, intravenous lipid emulsions supply 1.1 kcal/ml and 2 kcal/ml from 10% and 20% lipid emulsions respectively.

Protein: Protein is provided by crystalline amino acids (CAA). They are used to prevent nitrogen loss or in the treatment of negative nitrogen balance. Although crystalline amino acids have a calorific value of 4 kcal/gm, they are not counted towards the supply of energy to the patient as carbohydrates and fat are used for this purpose. The principal use of CAA is protein synthesis. 1 gm of nitrogen is produced by 6.25 gm of protein (amino acids). There are many commercial preparations of amino acids, most of which are regarded as standard solutions.

Electrolytes: These include sodium (Na), potassium (K), calcium (Ca), magnesium (Mg), chloride (Cl), phosphate and acetate. Ca, Mg and phosphorous are sometimes referred to as minerals. Electrolytes form an essential part of TPN regimens. They are used to maintain normal body metabolism.

Trace elements: These are zinc (Zn), copper (Cu), chromium (Cr), manganese (Mn), molybdenum (Mo), selenium (Se), Iodine (I), iron (Fe).

Vitamins: Water and lipid soluble vitamins are required for the metabolism of carbohydrate, protein, and fat. Fat soluble vitamins include vitamins A, D, E and K. The water soluble vitamins are vitamins B_1, B2, B_6, B_{12}, and C. Also included in this group are pantothenic acid, niacin, and biotin.

15.5 Calculating the Parenteral Nutrition Regimen

Although computer software for calculating volumes of base solutions for Parenteral Nutrition regimens is now widely available, the steps for manual calculations are briefly reviewed. There are several guidelines or clinical rules of thumb that may help the pharmacist calculate a Parenteral Nutrition regimen after a patient's nutritional requirements have been decided. For example, patients receiving only Parenteral Nutrition therapy will likely need larger volumes of fluid to provide maintenance requirements and replace extra renal losses. However, patients requiring other intravenous drug therapy will likely receive adequate fluids through the use of a standard intravenous maintenance solution such as 0.45% w/v NaCl in 5% w/v dextrose and piggy-backed medications. Depending on individual institutional practices, maximally concentrating the Parenteral Nutrition solution and utilizing an inexpensive maintenance fluid to manage hydration may provide a cost-effective regimen that requires fewer adjustments. Another guideline that may be helpful in designing a parenteral nutrition regimen where the CAA/dextrose base is infused separately from the IVFE (Intravenous fat emulsion) is to allow a volume of approximately 50-100 mL/L of base solution for electrolytes and other additives. Given this guideline, two clinically useful and highly concentrated base solutions are (final concentration) 7% w/v CAA / 15% w/v dextrose, which can be prepared from 10% CAA and 70% dextrose stock solutions, or 8% w/v CAA / 25% w/v dextrose compounded from 15% CAA and 70% dextrose stock solutions. Parenteral nutritional regimens for patients who require very small amounts of additives such as those with renal failure, may be further concentrated.

15.6 Ordering the Parenteral Nutrition Regimen

Ordering Parenteral Nutrition solutions may be accomplished by several methods that are generally institution specific. Some institutions may require the entire formula to be written in individual components and additives. More commonly, institutions have simplified the ordering process by implementing order forms designed specifically for parenteral nutrition. These standardized order forms promote education of practitioners by providing brief guidelines for initiating parenteral nutrition and foster cost-efficient, compounding, and administration. Standardized order forms may also include options for ordering certain related procedures, laboratory tests, protocols for patient management or consultation with other medical services related to the patient's nutrition support. Standardized forms and protocols should be reviewed and updated periodically to reflect changes in the practices and patient population of an institution and also advances in technology that may effect provision of nutrition support.

15.7 Compounding, Storage and Infection Control

Several considerations are necessary when preparing and storing parenteral nutrition solutions. In general, the type of solution being prepared will dictate methods of compounding, storage, and infusion. Currently, the two major types of parenteral nutrition solutions most commonly used are the traditional CAA/dextrose combination with or without IVFE piggybacked into the parenteral nutrition line, and TNAs (total nutrient admixture). Use of TNA solutions offers several potential advantages including reduced inventory (infusion pumps, tubing, and other related supplies), decreased time for compounding and administration, potential decrease in manipulations of the infusion line, which should correspond with a decreased risk of catheter contamination, and case of delivery and storage for patients receiving home parenteral nutrition. Potential disadvantages are associated with infectious, stability, and compatibility concerns. For example, stability of TNA solutions may be less predictable compared to CAA/dextrose solutions. In addition, the opaque solution that results after the addition of IVFE makes detection of particulate matter difficult, and TNAs solutions cannot be filtered with a bacterial retentive 0.22 μm filter. Methods for compounding parenteral nutrition solutions vary based on an institution's size, patient population, and medical practices. Some institutions prepare Total parenteral nutrition base solutions by transferring CAA stock solutions to partially filled bags of concentrated dextrose stock solutions. Other institutions may use commercially prepared CAA/dextrose products that are separated in a single bag and then mixed prior to use. Recent advances in compounding technology have facilitated use of automated compounders in the hospital setting. Automated compounders are computer based systems that perform the calculations necessary to determine volumes of nutrient stock solutions for preparation of parenteral nutrition solutions. In addition, most automated compounder systems include software that directly communicates the determined calculations to a transfer pump device. The pump delivers appropriate volumes of stock solutions to an empty intravenous bag by converting volume to weight based on the specific gravity of the stock solution. Advantages associated with automated compounders include reduction in personnel time and compounding materials and improved accuracy of compounding. Disadvantages include the potential for equipment failure and power cuts.

Assurance of solution sterility during compounding, storage, and administration is very important in reducing the risk of infection and related complications in patients receiving parenteral nutrition. Several studies of microbial growth in CAA/dextrose Parenteral Nutrition solutions have demonstrated that these solutions are poor media for bacterial growth. The acidic pH and hyper tonicity of CAA/dextrose solutions hinder bacterial growth. However, fungi such as *Candida albicans* may continue to proliferate in CAA/dextrose solutions for 7-10 days. Refrigeration at 4°C suppresses growth of both bacteria and *C. Albicans* and should be the routine storage temperature. The National Coordinating Committee on Large Volume Parenterals (NCCLVP) recommends immediate refrigeration of admixed solutions that are not administered within 1 hour after admixing. If refrigerated, admixed solutions should be used within 24 hours of compounding. The addition of albumin to parenteral nutrition solutions also increases the potential for fungal and bacterial growth. Intravenous lipid emulsions support growth of gram-positive and gram-negative bacteria as well as fungi. Visual changes may or may not occur even with high degrees of microbial contamination. Currently the centers for Disease control and Prevention recommends a maximum hang time of 12 hours for IVFE after 12 hours. In general, TNA solutions appear to support growth of bacteria less than IVFE but more than CAA/dextrose solutions. However, investigations of TNA used in a clinical setting have demonstrated safe administration over 24 hours without greater risk of contamination than is reported with CAA/dextrose solutions.

Use of aseptic technique during compounding and administration is prerequisite to ensure that the patient receives an uncontaminated Parenteral Nutrition solution. Solutions should be prepared in the aseptic environment provided by a properly maintained laminar flow hood. The hood should be situated such that the contaminant potential of normal work traffic and air currents is minimized. Personnel must be adequately trained and must practice strict aseptic technique. Supervision by a pharmacist experienced in compounding intravenous solutions and knowledgeable about stability, compatibility, and storage of Parenteral Nutrition solutions is also necessary. Quality assurance procedures should be developed to maintain safe and accurate admixture preparation. The potential risk of sepsis associated with parenteral nutrition solution contamination can be greatly decreased when pharmacy based admixture programs follow specific guidelines developed for compounding of parenteral nutrition solutions.

15.8 Stability and Compatibility

Because of their complex compositions, parenteral nutrition solutions are prone to problems with stability and compatibility. Comprehensive sources of current information about compatibilities and stability of parenteral nutrition solutions is *Trissel's handbook on injectable drugs*, which is published every 2 years with supplements during alternating years, and the *Guide to parenteral admixtures*, which is updated quarterly. In many cases, the exact answer to a compatibility question may not be readily available and a review of the primary literature may be necessary. When information is not available, clinical judgment and experience must be used carefully to resolve the situation.

CAA/dextrose solutions are generally stable for 1-2 months if refrigerated at 4°C and protected from light. Many studies have investigated stability of solutions containing various amounts of CAA, dextrose, and IVFE. Several factors affect stability of TNA solutions including pH, electrolyte charges, temperature, and time after compounding. Because of differences in pH among various CAA products and differences in phospholipid content among IVFE products, specific manufacturers should be consulted for compatibility and stability information prior to routine mixing of components. In general, electrolytes (except phosphate) and trace elements should be added to the dextrose solution, phosphate should be added to the CAA solution, and finally, the amino acid solution should be added to the IVFE prior to or simultaneously with dextrose solution. While TNA solutions should be infused within 24-48 hours after compounding, investigations of certain TNA solutions have reported acceptable stability for 10-28 days when refrigerated at 4-5°C.

The precipitation of calcium and phosphorus is a common interaction that is potentially life threatening. Factors that enhance the risk of precipitate formation include high concentrations of calcium and phosphorus salts, use of the chloride salt of calcium, decreased amino acid concentrations, and increased solution temperature, increased solution pH, use of improper sequence when mixing calcium and phosphorus salts and the presence of other additives including IVFE. Electrolyte stability in TNA solutions is of greater concern because of poor visualization of a precipitate when it occurs. Alternative methods of delivering electrolytes or other medications should be pursued in clinical situations where compatibility information involving a TNA solution is lacking. Although some published compatibility data suggest otherwise, the addition of sodium bicarbonate to parenteral nutrition solutions is not recommended. Addition of bicarbonate to acidic parenteral nutrition solutions may result in the formation of carbon dioxide gas and insoluble calcium and magnesium carbonates. Use of a bicarbonate precursor salt such as acetate is usually preferred.

Vitamins may be adversely affected by changes in solution pH, presence of other additives, storage time, solution temperature, and exposure to light. Variable but significant losses of vitamin A have been reported secondary to adsorption to intravenous administration tubing and polyvinyl chloride intravenous bags. Thiamine may be subject to degradation in solutions containing bisulfite. Because of variable stabilities of individual vitamins, intravenous vitamin solutions should be added to the parenteral nutrition solution as near to the time of administration as is clinically feasible and should not be in the parenteral nutrition solution longer than 24 hours.

Many patients receiving parenteral nutrition at home or in a hospital also receive other intravenous medications. The compatibility of parenteral nutrition and other intravenous solutions is an important concern in delivering safe and effective drug and nutritional therapy. Intravenous medications are most often infused as a separate admixture piggybacked in the parenteral nutrition line. However, some medications may be added directly to the parenteral nutrition solution and administered at the same rate as the parenteral nutrition infusion. Because of the potential for ineffective drug therapy or other complications associated with physiochemical incompatibility and stability of the parenteral nutrition solution, specific criteria should be considered before one adds a medication directly to the parenteral nutrition solution. The dosage regimen should be stable for each 24-hour period and should have pharmacokinetic properties appropriate for continuous infusion. There should be documented chemical and physical compatibility of the medication with parenteral nutrition mixture components and other medications that may be concomitantly piggybacked into the parenteral nutrition line. Finally, the parenteral nutrition regimen should be infused continuously over 24 hours. Advantages of using parenteral nutrition admixtures as drug vehicles include consolidation of dosage units, improved pharmacotherapy for certain drugs, conservation of fluid in volume restricted patients, fewer venous catheter violations and decreased compounding and administration time. However, a major disadvantage to use of parenteral nutrition solutions as drug delivery vehicles is the lack of compatibility and stability data in the parenteral nutrition solutions, which are commonly used in clinical practice. Medications frequently added to parenteral nutrition solutions include albumin, aminophylline, regular insulin, and H_2 receptor antagonists such as cimetidine, ranitidine, and famotidine.

15.9 Administration

Vascular Access during TPN - Some form of access route is required for the provision of total parenteral nutrition. The peripheral or central veins are usually employed for this purpose.

Peripheral access - Peripheral veins are used for this purpose. Blood flow is low in these small veins, thus the infusion of hypertonic TPN solutions through them can result in pain, thrombophlebetis, and hemolysis. As a result, severe restrictions are often placed on the osmolality of TPN solutions to be infused. There is also the need for frequent change of the infusion site especially for patients on long term nutrition support therapy.

Central access - This route is reserved especially for patients whose metabolic requirements are high. With this technique hyperosmolar TPN solutions do not present a problem, as these large veins have a high blood flow resulting in the solution being diluted about 1000 times. Although there are many central access routes cited in the literature, the most common method is the cannulation of the superior vena cava via the subclavian vein. Percutaneous puncture of the subclavian vein by the infraclavicular route is the procedure of choice for TPN.

The parenteral nutrition solution is infused through special tubing for intravenous administration that connects the parenteral nutrition bag or bottle with the intravenous catheter. PN solutions should be administered with an infusion pump to ensure consistent and controlled delivery of the solution. The intravenous administration line may include an in-line filter at a point prior to connection to the catheter. A 0.22 µm filter is recommended for use with CAA/dextrose solutions to remove particulate matter, air, and any microorganism that may be present in the solution from prior manipulations of the admixture or the administration line. Because the average size of IVFE particles is approximately 0.5 µm IVFE administered separately from the CAA/dextrose solution must be piggybacked into the parenteral nutrition line at a site beyond the in-line filter. Routine use of in-line filters (>0.22 µm) with TNA solutions is controversial. However, the Food and Drug Administration recommends use of a 1.2 µm filter which may be effective in preventing catheter occlusion due to precipitates or lipid aggregates. This filter size is also reported to remove *C.albicans*. Others support use of a 5 µm filter to minimize occlusion alarms from infusion pumps while maintaining filtration of particles capable of obstructing pulmonary capillaries.

Continuous Versus Intermittent Infusions

Parenteral nutrition solutions may be infused continuously or intermittently. The concentration of dextrose in the formula and the patient's history of glucose tolerance will dictate the infusion rate at which the parenteral nutrition solution should be initiated. Protocols for initiating parenteral nutrition differ widely among institutions. Many institutions begin infusions slowly and gradually increase the rate over 24-48 hours to the desired rate. The rate is also lowered in a stepwise fashion when parenteral nutrition therapy ends. This protocol is used to prevent development of hyperglycemia, respectively.

Cyclic parenteral nutrition is the infusion of parenteral nutrition over a period of time less than 24 hours, usually for 12-18 hours each day. Cyclic parenteral nutrition is useful in hospitalized patients with limited venous access where administration of multiple other medications requires interruption of the parenteral nutrition infusion. Cyclic parenteral nutrition may also prevent or treat hepatotoxicities associated with continuous parenteral nutrition therapy. In addition, cyclic parenteral nutrition allows patients receiving parenteral nutrition at home the ability to resume a relatively normal lifestyle. Recommendations for administration of cyclic parenteral nutrition are similar to those for continuous parenteral nutrition. Various protocols have been reported that suggest incremental increases to the maximum infusion rate for a desired period of time followed by a gradual taper to discontinue the solution. However, metabolically stable patients receiving lipid based parenteral nutrition regimens are likely candidates for abrupt initiation and discontinuation of the cyclic parenteral nutrition regimen. Cyclic parenteral nutrition may not be well tolerated by patients with severe glucose intolerance of diabetes, or by those patients with unstable fluid balance.

15.10 Monitoring

Thorough and consistent monitoring of patients receiving parenteral nutrition is necessary to ensure that the desired nutritional outcomes are achieved and to prevent the occurrence of adverse effects or complications associated with parenteral nutrition therapy. Routine evaluation should include the assessment of the patient's clinical condition with a focus on nutritional and metabolic effects of the parenteral nutrition regimen. Serial documentation of a patient's response to a particular regimen is a helpful guide for determining appropriate adjustments in fluid, electrolyte, and nutrient therapies.

A variety of biochemical and clinical measurements are necessary for effective monitoring of patients receiving parenteral nutrition. Important clinical laboratory measurements include serum concentrations of electrolytes, hematologic indices, and biochemical markers for renal function, liver function, and nutrition status. Other important clinical measurements include vital signs, weight, total fluid intake and losses, and nutritional intakes. The frequency of clinical laboratory measurements is usually dependent on the stability of a patient's clinical condition.

The intensive monitoring required for patients receiving nutritional support has opened the doorway for an interdisciplinary approach to this effort. The busy physician will often not have the time to collect and assess all the necessary data for effective monitoring of patients receiving aggressive nutritional support. Monitoring parameters for patients receiving nutritional support are listed below.

- Temperature
- Weight
- intake/output
- Urine checks
- Sodium
- Potassium
- Phosphorus
- Magnesium

- Calcium
- Glucose
- BUN/Cr
- Trace elements
- Serum proteins
- Total lymphocyte count
- Liver function tests
- Prothrombin time
- Nitrogen balance
- Subjective data

Collecting and/or interpreting the monitoring data are another important activity in which the clinical pharmacist may become involved. The pharmacist who is well trained in the use of fluids and electrolytes can significantly contribute to the nutritional support of the hospitalized patient. Patient monitoring is done for several reasons in the practice of nutritional support: problem detection, (such as electrolyte abnormalities and fluid overload), problem prevention, and documentation of the effectiveness or failure of a nutritional support regimen.

- *Temperature*

  Since infectious complications are common with central intravenous lines, daily temperature evaluation is mandatory for the central TPN patient. Centers with considerable TPN experience will draw blood cultures when a patient spikes a temperature of 101°F (38.3°C) or greater. If other potential sources of infection prove negative (e.g., urine and sputum cultures), the central catheter may have to be removed and the patient treated for sepsis. Daily temperature evaluation will be performed to monitor for insensible water loss in both parenteral and enteral nutrition patients. This is especially important for a patient who is unconscious or who has depressed mental status and cannot express thirst. Patients will lose approximately 600 to 900 ml of water per day when afebrile, but this loss can be increased to 2000 ml per day with continuous high fever. Recognition of this increased need for free water and the appropriate supplementation can prevent the patient from becoming dry and having a decreased urine output.

- *Weight*

  Monitoring weight gain can be an effective way to document whether or not a patient is receiving adequate nutritional support. Consider these items when monitoring this parameter: 1) the extremely malnourished patient may lose a little weight shortly after aggressive nutritional support is begun; 2) the patient's extracellular fluid compartment is usually expanded, and the intracellular fluid compartment is contracted with prolonged starvation; 3) once nutritional support is begun, the body will lose water from the extracellular fluid compartment faster than the gain of water by intracellular compartment resulting in a slight weight loss; 4) after the first few days of therapy, a gain of approximately 0.3 to 0.5 kilograms per day can represent an increase in lean body mass, whereas any gain over this amount probably represents an increase in fluid; therefore, monitoring fluid balance can often explain abrupt changes in weight.

- *Intake and Output*

  Monitoring fluid balance is extremely important for the critically ill patient who cannot express thirst or regulate oral intake. The patient receiving nutritional support should be monitored daily to ensure that prescribed intake is actually being delivered to the patient. The intake should be separated into TPN, enteral tube intake, oral intake, and intravenous fluid intake. In this way the actual number of calories and the amount of protein taken in can be determined. Output should be monitored also, including urine, stool, nasogastric suction fluid, and any type of drain (gastrostomy, chest tube, and fistula). Stool output during enteral nutritional support is an important indicator of gastrointestinal intolerance. Excessive losses of gastrointestinal fluids through drains may cause large losses of various electrolytes and acid-base disorders. These losses must be replaced in the nutrient solutions or standard intravenous solutions. Urine electrolytes are often useful in determining approximate losses by this route and help explain abnormal serum values. Increased free water can be delivered to the patient by increasing the intravenous solution rate, bolusing water down a nasogastric or nasoenteric tube, increasing oral fluid intake, or by diluting the tube feedings with water and increasing the rate. Fluid restriction with TPN can be achieved by using more concentrated solutions of dextrose, crystalline amino acids, and fat emulsions. Enterally, fluid restriction may be attained by using a more concentrated product, such as one which delivers 2 kcal/ml instead of the conventional 1 kcal/ml. The stable patient who is able to drink oral fluids and remain in a good state of hydration may not have to be monitored as strictly as the critically ill patient.

- *Urine checks for sugar/acetone*

  This is a mandatory monitoring parameter for the patient who is started on central TPN. The most feared complication of central TPN is hyperglycemic, hyperosmolar, non-ketotic dehydration (HHND). As with an uncontrolled diabetic HHND results from the osmotic diuresis which occurs with uncontrolled hyperglycemia as glucose is excreted renally. Close monitoring of the urine sugar and a sliding scale with regular insulin will usually prevent this serious complication. Urine glucose spillage should be corrected before the rate of the TPN solution is advanced. Subcutaneous or intramuscular injections of regular insulin are effective in controlling glycosuria, as is the addition of regular insulin to the TPN solution itself. Once the patient has reached maximum rate and is not spilling glucose into the urine, the urine checks may be decreased to every eight hours. A patient on TPN who has been very stable and then begins spilling glucose in the urine may be showing early signs of stress (probably sepsis). This glucose intolerance will often occur before clinical signs of sepsis are manifest (i.e., fever, hypotension, and tachycardia).

- *Laboratory Monitoring*

The clinical condition of the patient will dictate which laboratory parameters need to be checked, and with what frequency. The critically ill patient receiving aggressive nutritional support (central TPN, tube feeding) will require frequent lab checks because of the multitude of potential complications that can occur.

- *Sodium:* The usual sodium requirement is 50 to 200 mEq per day. For the patient with adequate sodium balance, the sodium requirement equals the sodium loss. This means that the patient with excessive losses from nasogastric suction or gastrointestinal drains will have increased sodium requirements. The patient with total body sodium and water overload (as with congestive heart failure, ascites, renal failure) should be sodium restricted unless he has orthostatic hypotension or has severe hyponatremia, where seizures are a potential complication. Hyponatremia is almost always dilutional, and fluid restriction will usually correct the abnormality; treatment with exogenous sodium will not be required in this case. Hypernatremia is rare and usually reflects a state of free water loss in excess of sodium loss (dehydration). Administration of free water or intravenous dextrose in water will usually correct this problem. Sodium should be measured daily for the first few days of nutritional support and then one to two times weekly.

- *Potassium:* The usual potassium requirement is 60 to 150 mEq per day; however, a patient with acute renal failure may not require any potassium when initially given nutritional support. Hypercatabolic patients may require greater than 150 mEq per day. Aggressive nutritional support will cause the potassium ions to be driven intracellularly, which lowers the serum level during the first few days of therapy. If hypokalemia occurs secondary to refeeding, supplemental potassium should be administered to the patient. Patients receiving TPN can be treated with additional potassium added to the parenteral solution, and those receiving tube feeding can be treated by adding potassium to the enteral product.

- *Phosphorus:* The usual requirement for phosphorus is 30 to 45 mMol per day; however, requirements may vary widely depending on the disease state. Phosphate is one of the major intracellular anions, and like potassium, will be driven intracellularly with vigorous nutritional support as glycogen stores are repleted. This will lower the serum phosphorus level in the first few days of feeding. Because death from severe hypophosphatemia secondary to refeeding has been reported, it is advisable to monitor the serum phosphorus daily for the first three to four days of nutritional support. Follow-up serum phosphorus should be measured one to two times per week thereafter. Concomitant antacid therapy will bind ingested phosphorus and secreted phosphorus in the gut, which may contribute to the hypophosphatemia of refeeding. If vigorous antacid therapy must be continued, phosphorus will probably have to be supplemented by the intravenous route. The TPN patient's phosphate can be supplemented by adding potassium or sodium phosphate to the parenteral solution.

- *Magnesium:* The usual intake of magnesium is 8 to 20 mEq per day. Like potassium, magnesium is an intracellular cation. Serum magnesium may be lowered with refeeding, but the decrease is not as profound as in the case of phosphorus and potassium. Hypomagnesaemia is common in nutritionally supported patients, but prolonged poor intake with vomiting may be a more important etiology than refeeding. Vigorous diuretic therapy and large losses of gastrointestinal fluids can also cause a magnesium deficiency. Baseline and twice weekly serum magnesium levels are necessary for initial monitoring. When the patient is stable, once weekly monitoring of magnesium is satisfactory.
- *Calcium:* The usual intake of calcium is 5 to 20 mEq per day; however, specific requirements during nutritional support are not known at the present time. Many institutions do not add calcium to peripheral TPN solutions, but most add *5* to 10 mEq to each liter of central TPN. Hypocalcaemia is a very common finding in the hospitalized patient. Most institutions measure both ionized and protein-bound calcium when a blood sample is drawn. These hospitalized patients often have a depressed serum albumin level which would decrease the albumin-bound calcium even though ionized calcium would be normal. Hypomagnesaemia may cause hypocalcaemia because the parathyroid hormone response is dependent on the magnesium ion; therefore, bone resorption may be impaired, and serum calcium levels in the blood will remain depressed. Correction of the magnesium deficiency corrects the serum calcium. Hypercalcemia is also a common finding in hospitalized patients with bone metastases. When serum calcium is abnormally high, it should be withheld from the TPN solution. Calcium should be monitored one to two times weekly during nutritional support.
- *Glucose:* Serum glucose should be monitored at least daily on all central TPN patients during the first few days of nutritional support. Diabetic and stressed (burns, trauma, sepsis) patients will often require that regular insulin be added to the TPN solution when this method of nutritional support is required. Enterally fed patients who are stressed or diabetic and have significant hyperglycemia will have to be treated with intravenous, intramuscular, or subcutaneous insulin. Once a patient begins to recover from stress, the insulin requirements will often markedly decrease and the dose will have to be reduced to prevent hypoglycemia. Once a patient is stable, urine glucose checks will suffice and serum glucose can be checked once or twice a week.

- *Blood Urea Nitrogen (BUN) and Creatinine (Cr):* Blood urea nitrogen and serum creatinine are parameters commonly used to assess renal function. Parenteral or enteral nutritional support should not significantly change BUN or Cr in a patient with adequate renal function. Blood urea nitrogen, like serum sodium, can be used as a parameter for fluid status. Dehydrated patients will have an increased BUN with a stable creatinine. Free water liberalization will usually correct this disorder. Over hydrated patients will have a decreased BUN, often mandating fluid restriction.
- *Trace Elements:* Monitoring a patient's trace element status is a fairly new concept. Zinc is required for wound healing, immunocompetence, taste acuity, and many enzymatic functions of the body. It is also known that zinc requirements are supranormal in a malnourished patient who is being aggressively fed parenterally or enterally. Patients who have large nasogastric suction losses, gastrointestinal fistula losses, and significant diarrhea lose large amounts of zinc. Many hospitals are now able to run assays for serum zinc. These serum levels are not often a reflection of total body stores, making it difficult to assess the need for supplementation. Clinical judgment may be preferred in determining the need for zinc supplementation. Since zinc is available as a single entity intravenous product, supplemental zinc can be added to TPN solutions.
- *Serum Proteins:* Serum albumin has been one of the hallmarks in assessing nutritional status. Being one of the proteins synthesized in the liver, it is assumed that adequate circulating albumin is a reflection of adequate substrate for protein synthesis. Since the half-life of albumin is twenty days, immediate increases are not seen, even with aggressive nutritional support; therefore, serum albumin is a very poor parameter to use as a guide for optimal nutritional repletion. Some patients who are in positive nitrogen balance will actually show a decrease in serum albumin secondary to an increased extracellular fluid compartment.
- *Total Lymphocyte Count and Cell-Mediated Immunity:* These parameters measure lymphocyte number and function. It should be pointed out that many disease states (cancer, sarcoidosis, Cushing's) and drugs (steroids, azathioprine) will either decrease total lymphocytes or impair cell-mediated immunity or both. In these types of patients, skin testing will not be an accurate assessment of nutritional status and energy may not convert even with adequate nutritional support.
- *Liver Function Tests.* A frequent complication of TPN is liver dysfunction secondary to hepatic steatosis and, occasionally, cholestasis. Whether this abnormality is caused by essential fatty acid deficiency, over-feeding with dextrose, or amino acid deficiencies is not clear at the present time. Once to twice weekly monitoring of alkaline phosphatase, serum glutamic oxaloacetic

transaminase, serum glutamic pyruvic transaminase, and total bilirubin is recommended for patients receiving central TPN. Preventive therapy includes two to three administrations of intravenous fat emulsions per week to avert essential fatty acid deficiency. Patients who develop this disorder may also be treated by lowering the dextrose concentration of the TPN or cycling the nutritional regimen.

- *Prothrombin Time:* Most standard TPN regimens do not contain vitamin K because it is not included in the available parenteral vitamin products. Many nutritional support teams administer vitamin K prophylactically on a weekly basis (5 to 10 mg IM or SC) while others will monitor the prothrombin time (PT) and administer vitamin K only when the PT is greater than three seconds. Patients receiving broad-spectrum antibiotics concurrently with TPN usually require vitamin K sooner than patients receiving TPN without antibiotics. Gut flora are reduced when antibiotics are administered, impairing *in vivo* synthesis of vitamin K.
- *Nitrogen Balance:* Nitrogen balance is a commonly used parameter to assess nutritional adequacy. It requires a 24-hour urine collection for urea nitrogen to calculate the grams of nitrogen lost renally. A concurrent collection for urine creatinine is also done to ensure that the collection is accurate. Two of the commonly used formulas are shown below.
    - Nitrogen Balance Nitrogen in - (UUN + 4)
    - Nitrogen Balance Nitrogen in - (UUN + 20% UUN ± 2)

$$\text{Nitrogen in} = \frac{\text{Grams of Protein}}{6.25}$$

UUN = Grams of urea nitrogen excreted in a 24-hour urine collection

A nitrogen balance of 0 to + 1 is adequate for maintaining nutritional status. For successful repletion of severely malnourished patients, a nitrogen balance of + 4 to + 6 has been suggested. A calculated negative nitrogen balance suggests failure to meet the patient's energy (carbohydrate and fat) or protein requirements or both. Obviously, the stressed patient (sepsis, trauma, burns) will require more calories and protein compared to the unstressed patient.

- *Bedside monitoring*

The patient receiving nutritional support should be seen by the nutritional support service each day. This can be the person doing the monitoring or the entire nutritional support team during rounds. Enteral tube patency and proper pump operation can be verified at this time. Subjective complaints by the patient can also be obtained and communicated to either the attending physician or the physician on the nutritional support team.

All of the above may be performed by a pharmacist as a clinical pharmacy activity. As expertise in monitoring is gained, interpretation of the data and appropriate interventions by recommendation will follow. The pharmacist who serves on the nutritional support service can be a vital link between the physician writing the nutritional support orders and the personnel preparing these formulas in the pharmacy and dietary departments. Being present on rounds or monitoring patients will reveal to the pharmacist the primary disease state, secondary complications, chronic diseases, drug therapy, and nutritional status of each one. These must all be considered when making recommendations for a nutritional regimen. The pharmacist involved with the nutritional care of complex patients will recognize the special nutritional and electrolyte requirements in this population and be able to communicate this information to the personnel preparing the TPN solutions or tube feedings. This may save a telephone call to the physician by the pharmacy for an explanation of the unfamiliar orders.

Table 15.1 Routine monitoring data for parenteral nutrition.

Every Day	2-3 Times/Wk.	Every Week.
Weight	Complete blood count	Nitrogen balance
Vital signs (temperature	Clotting studies (PT/PTT, platelets)	Total protein
Pulse, respirations)		
	Creatinine	Albumin
Fluid	Calcium	Transferin or prealbumin
Nutritional intake	Phosphorus	Liver biochemical tests
Kcal, protein, fat	Magnesium	Alkaline
Phosphatase		
Electrolytes, vitamins		AST
Trace elements		ALT
Serum electrolytes		LDH
Sodium		Bilirubin
Potassium		Other tests as warranted
Chloride		
Bicarbonate		
Glucose		
BUN		
Urine glucose, acetone (every 6h)		
Output		
Urine		
Gastrointestinal		
Other losses		

Key: PT, prothrombin time, PTT, partial thromboplastin time, AST, aspirate aminotransferase (SGOT); ALT, alanine aminotransferase (SGPT); LDH, lactate dehydrogenase; BUN, blood urea nitrogen.

15.11 Complications of Parenteral Nutrition

Parenteral nutrition can be a safe effective therapy when appropriate patients have been selected and the course of therapy is correctly monitored and adjusted as a patient's metabolic condition dictates. However, parenteral nutrition support is a complex therapy that is associated with numerous complications. These complications may be divided into four categories:

- mechanical or technical,
- infectious,
- metabolic, and
- Nutritional.

Mechanical/Technical

Mechanical or technical complications include malfunctions in the system used for intravenous delivery of the solution. Examples of such malfunctions include infusion, pump failure, problems with administration sets or tubing, and problems with the catheter. Catheter related complications are often of concern because they are potentially life-threatening. Pneumothorax, catheter misdirection into the wrong vein or ill-positioned within the cardiac chambers, arterial puncture, bleeding, and hematoma formation may occur during surgical placement of the catheter. Many of these complications in addition to venous thrombosis and air embolism may occur after insertion as well. Catheters occasionally occlude or break during use. If these problems cannot be easily rectified, the catheter may need to be surgically replaced.

Table 15.2 Complications of Central venous catheters

Complication	Description
Arterial injury	Puncture of subclavian or carotid artery during catheter insertion
Pneumothorax	Perforation of the pleura or lung during insertion, which results in air collection in the pleural space.
Air embolism	Introduction of air into the catheter, which subsequently enters thc vcnous circulation.
Catheter embolism	A portion of the catheter fragments and enters the venous circulation.
Venous thrombosis	Formation of thrombosis inside the lumen of the catheter and/or inside the vessel around the catheter or vessel occlusion.
Chylothorax	Injury to the thoracic duct during catheter insertion.
Brachial plexus injury	Injury to the nerve during catheter insertion, or injury secondary to catheter malposition or extravasation of a hypertonic solution.

Infections

Infectious complications can be a major hazard in patients receiving central parenteral nutrition. Often these patients are predisposed to infection as a result of compromised immunity and/or concomitant infection already present in the urinary tract, wounds, or lungs. Frequent use of broad-spectrum antibiotic therapy and malnutrition are also predisposing factors for development of infection. Bacterial translocation across the wall of the GI tract has also been implicated as a source of sepsis in patients receiving Parenteral Nutrition for prolonged periods without enteral feeding. Infection may develop secondary to solution contamination. However, strict adherence to specific protocols for preparation of parenteral nutrition solutions has minimized this occurrence. A more common source of infection is catheter related infections. Catheter related sepsis is defined as the presence of bacterial or fungal growth from the catheter tip and peripheral blood cultures. Catheter infection is defined as microbial growth from the catheter tip or from a blood culture drawn from the catheter with no growth of the same organism in the peripheral blood culture. Patients with catheter related infections may exhibit signs of sepsis-syndrome such as fever, chills, mental status, changes, hypotension, or glucose intolerance. These infections occur when the catheter becomes colonized by direct microbial invasion of the skin at the insertion site or at the infusion site of the catheter. For example, colonization may occur after multiple manipulations of the line used for parenteral nutrition administration, which can occur when the parenteral nutrition line is used to administer other medications. Other examples include failure of in-line bacterial filters, poor technique used in placement of the catheter, and poor care of the insertion site.

When no other source of infection is apparent in symptomatic patients, the catheter should be evaluated as the potential source. Blood cultures are drawn from a peripheral site and from the central catheter. In many institutions the suspected catheter is removed, the tip is quantitatively cultured, and a new central catheter is inserted. If bacterial or fungal growth of the same organism occurs from the catheter tip and the peripheral blood culture, the exchanged catheter is removed and another is placed in a different anatomic site. If bacterial or fungal growth occurs from the catheter tip or from a blood culture drawn from the catheter with no growth of the same organism in the peripheral culture, the catheter may be removed and replaced with another in the same anatomic location. However, because the clinical value of frequent central catheter replacement in patients with sepsis secondary to catheter elated infection is controversial, other treatment protocols have been suggested.

Metabolic/Nutritional

Metabolic complications associated with parenteral nutrition therapy are numerous and if left untreated, may be potentially fatal. Common metabolic abnormalities are related to substrate intolerance and fluid, electrolyte, and acid-base disorders. Predisposing factors and general strategies for intervention are also included. The etiology, mechanisms, and implications of individual metabolic abnormalities are multifactorial and have been summarized.

Hepatic dysfunction, as evidenced by elevation in serum liver function measurements such as total bilirubin, AST, ALT and alkaline phosphatase, is well documented in the literature. The most commonly reported abnormalities are fatty liver, cholelithiasis, and cholestasis. In most patients, these complications are reversible by manipulations of substrate intake. Progressive liver injury in patients who have received long term parenteral nutrition has been reported in a small number of patients. However, the relationship between the long-term parenteral nutrition and development of chronic liver disease is not clear.

Nutritional complications of parenteral nutrition therapy generally develop over a prolonged course of therapy (weeks to months) as a result of inappropriate intake of a particular nutrient. Certain conditions such as metabolic stress in a previously malnourished patient, may elicit symptoms of deficiency much earlier if a nutrient is not appropriately provided. For this reason, at least maintenance doses of vitamins, trace elements, and essential fatty acids should be provided to all patients receiving Parenteral Nutrition.

Clinical symptoms of trace element deficiencies, although rare, have been reported in patients receiving parenteral nutrition. More commonly, decreased serum trace element concentrations have been reported in a variety of patient populations. However, the clinical significance of decreased concentrations of many trace elements is not known because serum concentrations often do not correlate with total body stores. Zinc deficiency has been observed in both children and adults who have received shorter courses of parenteral nutrition and long term parenteral nutrition. Patients with large ostomy losses or severe chronic diarrhea are at highest risk for development of zinc deficiency. Clinical signs of zinc deficiency include hair loss, periorbital seborrheic dermatitis, dysgeusia, and sometimes ileus. Chromium deficiency presents as a diabetes like syndrome, while copper deficiency may appear as hypochromic, normocytic anemia with neutropenia. Selenium deficiency may develop during the course of parenteral nutrition therapy as cardiomyopathy and muscle pain.

15.12 Role of Pharmacist

A pharmacist is usually included on most organized nutritional support teams. The role of the pharmacist in home TPN programs and as a potential leader of the nutritional support team is well documented. The responsibilities of the pharmacist in the delivery of nutritional support can be divided into two categories: absolute and potential. Although all pharmacist responsibilities could be considered clinical pharmacy activities, those listed under potential responsibilities meet the strict criteria of clinical services.

- *Absolute Responsibilities.* The pharmacist's role in nutritional support initially began with the preparation, storage, and delivery of the parenteral nutrition products. Since most hospitals stock parenteral solutions in the pharmacy, the pharmacist was the logical person to assume responsibility for the meticulous steps involved in preparation of the TPN solutions. Because of the high potential for infection associated with TPN delivery, it is essential that these solutions remain sterile. The quality control needed to ensure sterility is provided by the pharmacist. Many hospital pharmacies are responsible for priming the tubing before the TPN solution is administered, adding the inline filter to the TPN infusion system, and maintaining the infusion pumps in acceptable working order.

  The pharmacist is also responsible for maintaining an adequate inventory of the products needed for successful delivery of nutritional support. As more commercial manufacturers enter into the lucrative nutritional products market, the pharmacist must become very familiar with the available products and be prepared to make decisions on inventory to be stocked in the pharmacy. Although differences among these amino acid solutions do exist, clinical superiority of any one over the others has not been demonstrated to date.

  It is also important for the pharmacist to know which drugs can be administered in the TPN solutions, since this may be the only venous access patients have available. Many antibiotics, cimetidine, trace minerals, and other drugs may be administered safely and efficaciously via the TPN solution. Other drugs, such as insulin, bind to the intravenous tubing, bag, or bottle, which may dramatically affect the patient's clinical response to the drug's administration.

- *Potential Responsibilities.* As the need for specially trained health care personnel has increased, the pharmacist's role has expanded into patient management. This increase in responsibility in the area of nutritional support is evidenced by the recent evolvement of specialty residencies and fellowships.

  Pharmacist involvement with nutritional support is one of the areas in which the efforts of clinical pharmacists have been well accepted by other professionals. The nutritional support team pharmacist should serve as liaison between the physician ordering the nutritional support solutions and the pharmacy department. Many nutritional support teams are responsible for the daily management of nutritional support patients, and the pharmacist may be present when the orders are written. This allows the pharmacist to be involved in the decision making process and alerts the pharmacy department when orders that differ markedly from the "standard" TPN solution are written. If the nutritional support service serves in a consulting role, the nutrition pharmacist is the one to notify the physician about orders that need clarification. The pharmacist should also make the pharmacy department aware of patients receiving nutritional support whose clinical status is fluctuating, as this may warrant the use of special solutions. The nutritional support pharmacist is the logical person to provide in service instruction to the pharmacy staff on fluid and electrolyte therapy and parenteral and enteral nutritional support. The nutritional support pharmacist may also instruct nurses about different nutritional products and their proper administration.

The identification of significant drug-nutrient interactions is a clinical pharmacy activity and provides a unique contribution to the nutritional care of the patient. Many drugs have significant effects on the fluid and electrolyte status of patients and must be monitored during nutritional repletion. Several antibiotics are prepared as the sodium salt, and this intake must be considered when assessing a patient's electrolyte status. Diuretics and non-reabsorbable anions may have profound effects on serum potassium, and antacids will often decrease serum phosphate during a period of supranormal requirements. Several drugs have been reported to stimulate or suppress appetite, induce taste dysfunction, and cause gastrointestinal abnormalities which may interfere with normal intake of nutritional substrates. Drug induced vitamin deficiencies may occur quite often in the malnourished patient. It is also known that nutritional therapy may have some effect on drug therapy. Food can interfere with the absorption of many drugs. Other concerns to the nutrition pharmacist are: altered drug therapy secondary to nutritional status (e.g., theophylline clearance), drug failure secondary to nutrients (e.g., warfarin and enteral products containing large amounts of vitamin K), and adverse drug reactions caused by nutrients (e.g., MAO inhibitors and tyramine-containing foods). Considering the growing body of knowledge about potential drug-nutrition interactions, drug therapy given concurrently with nutritional support should be monitored closely by the pharmacist.

The pharmacy's involvement with the preparation, storage, and delivery of enteral tube feeding products is a rather controversial area of nutritional support. Many dietary departments consider this their responsibility; yet others have relinquished this responsibility to the pharmacy. There is no reason why a progressive dietary department could not undertake this responsibility and achieve the same results. Whether or not the pharmacy is involved with the preparation of enteral tube feedings will be institution dependent. Obviously, the most important factor is that the patient receives the correct product in a safe and efficacious manner. Pharmacy involvement with enteral products at any level requires the nutritional support pharmacist to become very familiar with the available products and the situations in which to administer them appropriately.

Table 15.3 Scope of practice for nutrition support pharmacists

Activities		Description
Assessment of the patient's nutrition care needs	*	Determine nutrient requirements based on patient's data. Prevent and /or identify nutrient-nutrient, drug – nutrient, drug-drug and drug-disease/condition interactions. Assess suitability for specialized nutrition support.
Development of a nutrition care plan	*	Define goals and objectives of specialized nutrition support therapy Select the preferred route for administration of nutrition support therapy. Design patient specific feeding formulations.
Implementation of the nutrition care plan	*	Obtain or write prescriptions for feeding formulations Be proficient with techniques of compounding feeding formulations. Perform or supervise the compounding and dispensing of parenteral feeding formulations.
Monitoring the patient's response to the nutrition therapy	*	Evaluate laboratory data to determine the parent's clinical, nutritional, and metabolic responses to specialized nutrition support. Prevent and or identify nutrient –nutrient, drug-nutrient, drug-drug and drug-disease/condition interactions Evaluate continued need for specialized nutrition support.
Administrative management	*	Participate in development of policy and procedures for patient care and operational aspects of specialized nutrition support.
Quality care	*	Develop and implement quality improvement activities directed at the process of nutritional and metabolic care.
Advancement of nutrition support pharmacy practice	*	Contribute to the professional development of Pharmacists and other health care professionals and to the education of patients through presentations, publications, and research.

15.13 Team Approach

Providers of TPN services should have a basic understanding of nutrition, biochemistry, anatomy, pathology, physiology, bacteriology, epidemiology, pharmaceutical technology and pharmacology. Although it is a well known fact that TPN can be lifesaving, careless use, due to inadequate knowledge can result in very severe complications. Therefore, it is now becoming apparent that a multi disciplinary approach involving well trained and highly skilled medical personnel incorporated into a consultative "nutrition support team" is vital to the safety and therapeutic effectiveness of TPN. A TPN team should include physicians, clinical pharmacists, nurses, and dietitians. Other specialists who may be considered periodically are the infectious disease consultants and physiotherapists.

Shortly after total parenteral nutritional (TPN) became popular, the team approach, with members from several disciplines (physician, pharmacist, nurse, dietitian), was recognized to serve the patient best and ensure proper and safe delivery of these nutritional substrates. Mechanical, septic, and metabolic complications were markedly reduced in the team-managed patients. Team approach, using a protocol with rigid guidelines for the administration of TPN, diminishes the risk and rate of complications. It would seem reasonable to assume that these complication rates would also decrease in patients receiving properly monitored and managed enteral nutritional support.

- Physicians

  The physician is usually the head of the team. He assumes the responsibility for the implementation of policy and procedures for the delivery of nutritional support at that institution, and serving as "back-up" if not involved with the patient's management on a daily basis. Their immediate role is to evaluate potential candidates for nutrition support. They also place a central line if so indicated and, with the assistance of the clinical pharmacists, review metabolic data and place orders for TPN. Physicians also make daily rounds on patients on TPN and should be available on a 24 hour basis for evaluation and management of any complication.

- Clinical Pharmacists

  Clinical pharmacists should be knowledgeable regarding interpretation of laboratory data, and the formulation, compounding, delivery and monitoring of TPN solutions since they are expected to carry out these functions. They are responsible for obtaining laboratory data and reviewing each patient's clinical outcome, after which they should write the TPN order for the next 24 hours. The pharmacist is responsible for the storage, preparation, and delivery of the parenteral nutrition solutions. The pharmacist may also help monitor the patients and serve as the liaison between the nutritional support team and the pharmacy department.

- Nurses

  The nutrition nurse may perform all dressing changes needed for patients on central TPN, assists in the placement of central TPN lines, maintains permanent records, and serves as the liaison between the nutritional support service and the nursing department. The nutrition support nurses see all patients referred to the TPN team and review care plans. They interpret team objectives and help determine the appropriateness of TPN. Ward nurses are not part of the TPN team. However, they are the vital link between the TPN team and the patient. They perform primary patient care through monitoring of vital signs, ensuring constant infusion of the TPN solutions. Ward nurses should be knowledgeable regarding the early signs and symptoms of possible complications.

- Dietitians

  Dietitians are essential to the TPN team. However, they should be knowledgeable in special oral and dietary formulas. Patients referred to the team are first evaluated by the dietitians, who perform an initial nutritional assessment in order to define nutritional status of the patient, determine the degree of stress, estimate nutritional needs and recommend supplemental nutritional support if needed. The dietitian also maintains the records of calorie counts, and makes recommendations for tube feedings and oral diets. These professionals share the information from their individual area of specialty that contributes to the overall quality of patient care.

  The responsibilities of the different members of the nutritional support service may vary somewhat among different institutions, depending on which disciplines are represented, the number of patients seen by the service, and whether or not the members serve on a part-time or full-time basis. Representation from all four disciplines would appear to be politically wise to avoid conflicts between the different departments and the nutritional support service.

15.14 Developing and Involving in Nutritional Support Team

Functioning Nutrition Support team

If a nutritional support team already exists in the institution, the goals of the team and the services it offers will be fairly well established. In order for a pharmacist or any other practitioner to be accepted on the team, it will have to be shown that he has some special knowledge or talent which will assist the team in achieving its purposes.

The Pharmacist may have to take the initiative in explaining the value of having a pharmacist on the team. Several qualifications unique to pharmacists have been mentioned earlier in this unit, including knowledge about parenteral nutrition products, incompatibilities of intravenous products, drug-nutritional substance interactions, and costs of parenteral nutrition products and drugs. Another important reason for having a pharmacist on the nutritional support team is to provide a communication link between the team and the pharmacy department. This is an important consideration in coordinating the preparation of TPN solutions with administration times and with changes in orders. Considerable waste is avoided by having good coordination between the team and the pharmacy department. A number of articles in the literature demonstrate the importance and cost-effectiveness of pharmacist involvement in the delivery of nutritional support.

Developing a nutritional Support Team

The establishment of a nutritional support service may be initiated by an interested physician or, as is often the case, by other hospital personnel interested in clinical nutrition as a specialty (pharmacists, dietitians). A stepwise plan for establishing a nutritional support team has been described.

- *Assessing the Level of Practice in the Institution:* The initial step in developing a nutritional support team should be to assess the level of nutritional support practice in the institution / hospital and to identify individuals or departments interested in developing a formal nutritional support service. The number of patients receiving aggressive nutritional support and the number of patients receiving suboptimal nutrition for prolonged periods of time should be noted, and an evaluation of the nutritional care of critically ill patients should be undertaken. The results of such an assessment will speak to the need for a nutritional support team in your institution.

  Obviously, an interested and qualified physician is vital for the success of the team, and it may be that such an individual would have to be recruited to head up the team. The physician team leader will be responsible for communications needed between the nutritional support team and the rest of the medical staff, and between the team and the hospital administration.

- *Building a Foundation of Support:* Success in establishing a nutritional support team will depend on a foundation of support from the medical staff, hospital administration, and other key individuals in the institution. There must be acceptance of the fact that a team is needed as well as agreement on what specific nutritional support services the team should provide. It may be necessary to invite experts in nutritional support to conduct educational programs for the medical staff, nurses, dietitians, and others. Visits to other institutions with established nutritional support teams and attendance at national conferences will also be helpful.

- *Developing a Proposal:* A proposal for a nutritional support team might consist of the following four parts: a) statement of need, b) delineation of functions to be performed by the team, c) analysis of available resources, and d) a description of the benefits to be derived.

  - *Need:* The statement of need should be based on the results of an assessment of the level of nutritional support currently provided by the institution. Specific deficiencies or weaknesses in patient care should be pointed out.

- *Functions:* Most would agree that the major goal of a nutritional support service is to provide optimal nutrition to all patients at all times, and to provide this support safely and effectively. A proposal to establish a nutritional support team should address the envisioned functions of the team in terms of such a statement of purpose.

  The specific objectives for a nutritional support team might be divided into two groups: immediate and long-range objectives. Immediate objectives might include decreasing the incidence of malnutrition in the hospital through appropriate intervention, in service education on nutritional support delivery techniques, and establishment of a quality control program for the preparation of TPN solutions. Long range objectives might include expanding enteral nutrition to modular feeding programs, developing home feeding programs with TPN and enteral nutrition, conducting clinical evaluations, and participating in nutritional support research protocols.

- *Available resources:* The written proposal should include a description of the resources needed to implement a nutritional support program (personnel, space, equipment, and supplies), with an indication of which resources already exist within the institution. It is quite possible that all the professional talent required to start a team is already available. Many of the physical requirements (office space, intravenous infusion pumps, enteral infusion pumps, laminar flow hoods, special preparation area for enteral nutrition products) may likewise be available. It will be important to remember, in preparing a proposal, that most nutritional support services are financially self-sufficient, so that start-up costs can be recovered once revenue begins to be generated.

- *Benefits.* The written proposal should include a summary of the benefits to be gained by the addition of a nutritional support service. Patient care, from a nutritional standpoint, should be improved through the safe, rational, and effective use of nutritional products. Further, the energy and protein needs of the total patient population are more apt to be met, regardless of the patient's disease state or metabolic problems.

• *Delivering Services:* The next step in establishing a nutritional support service is to decide how to identify patients who may be candidates for nutritional support. Mass screening of the entire patient population in the hospital would likely be an inefficient use of time. Many institutions rely on a consultation request from primary physicians, but this method may prove to be inadequate, especially when the team is just being set up. Screening patients known to have nutritional problems is a good way to get started. Likely candidates are patients with cancer, sepsis, trauma, or burns. Routine patient nutritional assessments or metabolic profiles will be very helpful in identifying candidates. Evaluating stress state (fever, sepsis, long-bone fractures, etc.) will help to identify patients who have special energy and protein requirements. Special monitoring forms will be needed for these purposes. It would be wise to obtain several forms from other institutions to help you in developing those which best suit the needs of your institution.

- *Establishing the Roles of Team Members:* The final step in establishing a nutritional support service is to define the roles of the different members of the team. It should be emphasized again that these roles may somewhat overlap, so working together is very important. The pharmacist's roles may include monitoring patients, writing formal consultations, and making appropriate recommendations concerning the care of the patient. In some institutions the pharmacist is allowed to write the nutritional support and laboratory orders for the patients followed by the service. These should be signed by the physician on the service as soon as possible. Obviously, this responsibility should be approved by the medical staff.

Conclusion

Parenteral nutrition is not a benign therapy. Appropriate patient selection, assessment, and monitoring are key to successful nutritional therapy, helping in prevention of unnecessary complications or harm to the patient. Standardized order forms and monitoring protocols are useful tools to ensure appropriate administration and monitoring of parenteral nutrition therapy. Pharmacists have been involved in the provision of parenteral nutrition at many levels including direct patient care, education, and research. The field of pharmacy nutrition support has grown into a well-defined area of pharmacy practice with formally defined standards of practice. The use of parenteral nutrition therapy and the role of the nutrition support pharmacist will be affected primarily by new insights from clinical research and economic challenges in the health care environment.

Study Outline

Malnutrition in hospitals is a major disease entity which requires prompt recognition and appropriate therapy. TPN is the provision of required nutrients by i.v route, designed to provide in addition to water, six essential groups of nutrients necessary for tissue synthesis and energy balance,

Indications for TPN

- inability to absorb nutrients via GIT
- cancer
- moderate to severe pancreatitis
- severe malnutrition with temporary non functional GIT

- critical care needing situations like major surgery, sepsis
- preoperative malnutrition
- organ failures hyper emesis gravidarum
- eating disorders

Constituents of TPN

- water – as solvent for biological systems
- carbohydrates – main source of energy
- fat – primary source of essential fatty acids (linoleic acid)
- protein – to treat negative nitrogen balance
- electrolytes – Na, K, Ca, Mg, Cl, Phosphate, Acetate
- Trace elements – Zn, Cu, Cr, Mn, Mo, Se, I , Fe
- Vitamins - Fat soluble vitamins like A,D, E and K
  - Water soluble like B complex and C

Calculations

The TPN requirements depend upon individual institutional practices.

Ordering, compounding, storing, stability, compatibility and other aspects of TPN to be monitored.

CHAPTER 16

Drugs in Pregnancy and Lactation

Objectives

After reading this chapter, the student should be able to:

- Understand the effect of drugs on fetus in pregnancy and the risks involved in using drugs during pregnancy
- Explain the role of various social and illicit drugs in pregnancy
- Discuss the effect of drugs on fetus during lactation
- Know which drugs that can be used safely during lactation, drugs that can be used under medical supervision and drugs that are contraindicated during lactation.

16.1 Drugs in Pregnancy

More than 90% of pregnant women take prescription or non-prescription (over-the-counter) drugs or use social drugs (such as tobacco and alcohol) or illicit drugs at some time during pregnancy. In general, drugs, unless absolutely necessary, should not be used during pregnancy because many can harm the fetus. About 2 to 3% of all birth defects result from the use of drugs other than alcohol.

Sometimes drugs are essential for the health of the pregnant woman and the fetus. In such cases, a woman should talk to the doctor or other health care practitioner about the risks and benefits of taking drugs. Before taking any drug (including over-the-counter drugs) or dietary supplement (including medicinal herbs), a pregnant woman should consult her health care provider. A health care provider may recommend that a woman take certain vitamins and minerals during pregnancy.

Drugs taken by a pregnant woman reach the fetus primarily by crossing the placenta, the same route taken by oxygen and nutrients, which are needed for the fetus's growth and development.

Drugs that a pregnant woman takes during pregnancy can affect the fetus in several ways:

- They can act directly on the fetus, causing damage, abnormal development (leading to birth defects), or death.
- They can alter the function of the placenta, usually by causing blood vessels to narrow (constrict) and thus reducing the supply of oxygen and nutrients to the fetus from the mother. Sometimes the result is a baby that is underweight and underdeveloped.
- They can cause the muscles of the uterus to contract forcefully, indirectly injuring the fetus by reducing its blood supply or triggering preterm labor and delivery.

How a drug affects a fetus depends on the fetus stage of development and the strength and dose of the drug. Certain drugs taken early in pregnancy (within 20 days after fertilization) may act in an all-or-nothing fashion, killing the fetus or not affecting it at all. During this early stage, the fetus is highly resistant to birth defects. However, the fetus is particularly vulnerable to birth defects between the 3rd and the 8th week after fertilization, when its organs are developing. Drugs reaching the fetus during this stage may have no effect, or they may cause a miscarriage, an obvious birth defect, or a permanent but subtle defect that is noticed later in life. Drugs taken after completion of organ development are unlikely to cause birth defects, but they may alter the growth and function of organs and tissues.

The Food and Drug Administration (FDA) classifies drugs according to the degree of risk they pose the fetus if they are used during pregnancy. Some drugs are highly toxic and should never be used by pregnant women because they cause severe birth defects. A classic example is thalidomide. Several decades ago, this drug caused phocomelia, which is as extreme underdevelopment of arms and legs and defects of the intestine, heart, and blood vessels in the babies of women who took the drug during pregnancy. Some drugs cause birth defects in animals, but the same effects have not been seen in people. One example is meclizine, frequently taken for motion sickness, nausea, and vomiting.

Table 16.1 Categories of Risk for Drugs during Pregnancy

Category	Description
A	These drugs are the safest, well-designed studies in people show no risks to the fetus.
B	Studies in animals show no risk to the fetus, and no well-designed studies in people have been done. OR Studies in animals show a risk to the fetus, but well-designed studies in people do not.
C	No adequate studies in animals or people have been done. OR In animal studies, use of the drug resulted in harm to the fetus, but no information about how the drug affects the human fetus is available.
D	Evidence shows a risk to the human fetus, but benefits of the drug may outweigh risks in certain situations. For example, the mother may have a life-threatening disorder or a serious disorder that cannot be treated with safer drugs.
X	Risk to the fetus has been proved to outweigh any possible benefit.

Often, a safer drug can be substituted for one that is likely to cause harm during pregnancy. For an overactive thyroid gland, propylthiouracil is usually preferred. For prevention of blood clots, the anticoagulant heparin is preferred. Several safe antibiotics, such as penicillin, are available.

Some drugs can have effects after they are stopped. For example, isotretinoin, a drug used to treat skin disorders, is stored in fat beneath the skin and is released slowly. Isotretinoin can cause birth defects if women become pregnant within 2 weeks after the drug is stopped. Therefore, women are advised to wait at least 3 to 4 weeks after the drug is stopped before they become pregnant.

Vaccines made with a live virus (such as the rubella and varicella vaccines) are not given to women who are or might be pregnant. Other vaccines (such as those for cholera, hepatitis A and B, plague, rabies, tetanus, diphtheria, and typhoid) are given to pregnant women only if they are at substantial risk of developing that particular infection. However, all pregnant women who are in the 2nd or 3rd trimester during the influenza (flu) season should be vaccinated against the influenza virus.

Drugs to lower high blood pressure (antihypertensives) may be needed by pregnant women who have had high blood pressure before pregnancy or who develop it during pregnancy. Either type of high blood pressure increases the risk of problems for the woman and the fetus. However, antihypertensives can markedly reduce blood flow to the placenta if they lower blood pressure too rapidly in pregnant women. So pregnant women who have to take these drugs are closely monitored. Two types of antihypertensives—angiotensin-converting enzyme (ACE) inhibitors and thiazide diuretics—are usually not given to pregnant women because these drugs can cause serious problems in the fetus.

Digoxin, used to treat heart failure and some abnormal heart rhythms, readily crosses the placenta. But it typically has little effect on the baby before or after birth.

Most antidepressants appear to be relatively safe when used during pregnancy.

Table 16.2 Some Drugs That Can Cause Problems during Pregnancy*

Type	Examples	Problem
Antianxiety drug	Diazepam	When the drug is taken late in pregnancy, depression, irritability, shaking, and exaggerated reflexes in the newborn
Antibiotics	Chloramphenicol	Gray baby syndrome, In women or fetuses with glucose-6-phosphate dehydrogenase (G6PD) deficiency, the breakdown of red blood cells
	Fluoroquinolones (such as ciprofloxacin, ofloxacin, levofloxacin, and norfloxacin)	Possibility of joint abnormalities (seen only in animals)
	Kanamycin	Damage to the fetus's ear, resulting in deafness
		In women or fetuses with G-6-PD deficiency, the breakdown of red blood cells
	Streptomycin	Damage to the fetus's ear, resulting in deafness
	Sulfonamides (such as sulfasalazine and trimethoprim – sulfamethoxazole)	When the drugs are given late in pregnancy, jaundice and possibly brain damage in the newborn (much less likely with sulfasalazine), In women or fetuses with G-6-PD deficiency, the breakdown of red blood cells
	Tetracycline	Slowed bone growth, permanent yellowing of the teeth, and increased susceptibility to cavities in the baby Occasionally, liver failure in the pregnant woman

Table 16.2 *Contd..*

Type	Examples	Problem
Anticoagulants	Heparin	When the drug is taken for long time, osteoporosis and a decrease in the number of platelets (which help blood clot) in the pregnant woman
	Warfarin	Birth defects, Bleeding problems in the fetus and the pregnant woman
Anticonvulsants	Carbamazepine	Some risk of birth defects, Bleeding problems in the newborn, which can be prevented if pregnant women take vitamin K orally every day for a month before delivery or if the newborn is given an injection of vitamin K soon after birth
	Phenobarbital	Same as those for carbamazepine
	Phenytoin	Same as those for carbamazepine
	Trimethadione	Increased risk of miscarriage in the woman, High (70%) risk of birth defects, including a cleft palate and defects of the heart, face, skull, hands, or abdominal organs
	Valproate	Some (1%) risk of birth defects, including a cleft palate and defects of the heart, face, skull, spine, or limbs
Antihypertensives	Angiotensin-converting enzyme (ACE) inhibitors	When the drugs are taken late in pregnancy, kidney damage in the fetus, a reduction in the amount of fluid around the developing fetus (amniotic fluid), and defects of the face, limbs, and lungs
	Beta-blockers	When some beta-blockers are taken during pregnancy, a slowed heart rate and low blood sugar level in the fetus and possibly slowed growth
	Thiazide diuretics	A decrease in the levels of oxygen, sodium, and potassium and in the number of platelets in the fetus's blood, Slowed growth

Table 16.2 *Contd...*

Type	Examples	Problem
Chemotherapy drugs	Actinomycin	Possibility of birth defects (seen only in animals)
	Busulfan	Birth defects such as underdevelopment of the lower jaw, cleft palate, abnormal development of the skull bones, spinal defects, ear defects, and clubfoot, Slowed growth
	Chlorambucil	Same as those for busulfan
	Cyclophosphamide	Same as those for busulfan
	Mercaptopurine	Same as those for busulfan
	Methotrexate	Same as those for busulfun
	Vinblastine	Possibility of birth defects (seen only in animals)
	Vincristine	Possibility of birth defects (seen only in animals)
Mood-stabilizing drug	Lithium	Birth defects (mainly of the heart), lethargy, reduced muscle tone, poor feeding, underactivity of the thyroid gland, and nephrogenic diabetes insipidus in the newborn
Nonsteroidal anti-inflammatory drugs (NSAIDs)	Aspirin and other salicylates Ibuprofen Naproxen	When the drugs are taken in large doses, a delay in the start of labor, premature closing of the connection between the aorta and artery to the lungs (ductus arteriosus), jaundice, and (occasionally) brain damage in the fetus and bleeding problems in the woman during and after delivery and in the newborn, When the drugs are taken late in pregnancy, a reduction in the amount of fluid around the developing fetus
Oral antihyperglycemic drugs	Chlorpropamide	A very low level of sugar in the blood of the newborn, Inadequate control of diabetes in the pregnant woman, When the drug is taken early in pregnancy by a woman with type 2 diabetes, possibility of increased risk of birth defects
	Tolbutamide	Same as those for chlorpropamide

Table 16.2 *Contd...*

Type	Examples	Problem
Sex hormones	Danazol	When this drug is taken very early in pregnancy, masculinization of a female fetus's genitals, sometimes requiring surgery to correct
	Diethylstilbestrol	Abnormalities of the uterus, menstrual problems, and an increased risk of vaginal cancer and complications during pregnancy in daughters, Abnormalities of the penis in sons
	Synthetic progestins (but not the low doses used in oral contraceptives)	Same as those for danazol
Skin treatments	Etretinate	Birth defects, such as heart defects, small ears, and hydrocephalus (sometimes called water on the brain)
	Isotretinoin	Same as those for etretinate Mental retardation Risk of miscarriage
Thyroid drugs	Methimazole	An enlarged or underactive thyroid gland in the fetus Scalp defects in the newborn
	Propylthiouracil	An enlarged or underactive thyroid gland in the fetus
	Radioactive iodine	Destruction of the thyroid gland in the fetus, When the drug is given near the end of the 1st trimester, very overactive and enlarged thyroid gland in the fetus
	Triiodothyronine	An overactive and enlarged thyroid gland in the fetus
Vaccines (live virus)	Vaccine for German measles (rubella) and chickenpox (varicella)	Potential infection of the placenta and developing fetus
	Vaccines for measles, mumps, polio, or yellow fever	Potential but unknown risks

* Unless absolutely necessary, drugs should not be used during pregnancy. However, drugs are sometimes essential for the health of the pregnant woman and the fetus. In such cases, a woman should consult her health care practitioner about the risks and benefits of taking the drugs.

Social Drugs

Cigarette (Tobacco) Smoking: The most consistent effect of smoking on the fetus during pregnancy is a reduction in birth weight. The more a woman smokes during pregnancy, the less the baby is likely to weigh. The average birth weight of babies born to women who smoke during pregnancy is 6 ounces less than that of babies born to women who do not smoke. The reduction in birth weight seems to be greater among the babies of older smokers.

Birth defects of the heart, brain, and face are more common among babies of smokers than among those of nonsmokers. Also, the risk of sudden infant death syndrome (SIDS) may be increased. A mislocated placenta (placenta previa), premature detachment of the placenta (abruptio placentae), premature rupture of the membranes (containing the fetus), preterm labor, uterine infections, miscarriages, stillbirths, and premature births are also more likely. In addition, children of women who smoke have slight but measurable deficiencies in physical growth and in intellectual and behavioral development. These effects are thought to be caused by carbon monoxide and nicotine. Carbon monoxide may reduce the oxygen supply to the body's tissues. Nicotine stimulates the release of hormones that constrict the vessels supplying blood to the uterus and placenta, so that less oxygen and fewer nutrients reach the fetus.

Pregnant women should avoid exposure to second hand smoke because it may similarly harm the fetus.

Alcohol: Drinking alcohol during pregnancy is the leading known cause of birth defects. Because the amount of alcohol required to cause fetal alcohol syndrome is unknown, pregnant women are advised to abstain from drinking alcohol regularly or on binges; avoiding alcohol altogether may be even safer. The range of effects of drinking during pregnancy is great.

The risk of miscarriage almost doubles for women who drink alcohol in any form during pregnancy, especially if they drink heavily. Often, the birth weight of babies born to women who drink regularly during pregnancy is substantially below normal. The average birth weight is about 4 pounds for babies exposed to large amounts of alcohol, compared with 7 pounds for all babies. Newborns of women who drank during pregnancy may not thrive and are more likely to die soon after birth.

Fetal alcohol syndrome is one of the most serious consequences of drinking during pregnancy. It occurs in about 2 of 1,000 live births. This syndrome includes inadequate growth before or after birth, facial defects, a small head (probably caused by inadequate growth of the brain), mental retardation, and abnormal behavioral development. Less commonly, the position and function of the joints are abnormal and heart defects are present.

Babies or growing children of women who consumed alcohol during pregnancy may have severe behavioral problems, such as antisocial behavior and attention deficit disorder. These problems can occur even when the baby has no obvious physical birth defects.

Caffeine: Whether consuming caffeine during pregnancy harms the fetus is unclear. Evidence seems to suggest that consuming caffeine in small amounts (for example, one cup of coffee a day) during pregnancy poses little or no risk to the fetus. Caffeine, which is contained in coffee, tea, some sodas, chocolate, and some drugs, is a stimulant that readily crosses the placenta to the fetus. Thus, it may stimulate the fetus, increasing the heart rate. Caffeine may also decrease blood flow across the placenta and decreases the absorption of iron, possibly increasing the risk of anemia. Some evidence suggests that drinking more than seven cups of coffee a day may increase the risk of having a stillbirth, premature birth, low-birth-weight baby, or miscarriage. Some experts recommend limiting coffee consumption and drinking decaffeinated beverages when possible.

Aspartame: Aspartame, an artificial sweetener, appears to be safe during pregnancy when it is consumed in small amounts, such as in amounts used in normal portions of artificially sweetened foods and beverages. Pregnant women with phenylketonuria, an unusual disorder, should not consume any aspartame.

Illicit Drugs

Use of illicit drugs (particularly opioids) during pregnancy can cause complications during pregnancy and serious problems in the developing fetus and the newborn. For pregnant women, injecting illicit drugs increases the risk of infections that can affect or be transmitted to the fetus. These infections include hepatitis and sexually transmitted diseases (including AIDS). Also, when pregnant women take illicit drugs, growth of the fetus is more likely to be inadequate, and premature births are more common.

Babies born to mothers who use cocaine often have problems, but whether cocaine is the cause of those problems is unclear. For example, the cause may be cigarette smoking, use of other illicit drugs, deficient prenatal care, or poverty.

Hallucinogens, such as methylenedioxymethamphetamine (MDMA, or Ecstasy), rohypnol, ketamine, methamphetamine, and LSD (lysergic acid diethylamide) may, depending on the drug, lead to an increased incidence of spontaneous miscarriage, premature delivery, or fetal/neonatal withdrawal syndrome.

Opioids: Opioids such as heroin, methadone and morphine, readily cross the placenta. Consequently, the fetus may become addicted to them and may have withdrawal symptoms 6 hours to 8 days after birth. However, use of opioids rarely results in birth defects. Use of opioids during pregnancy increases the risk of complications during pregnancy, such as miscarriage, abnormal presentation of the baby, and preterm delivery. Babies of heroin users are more likely to be small.

Amphetamines: Use of amphetamines during pregnancy may result in birth defects, especially of the heart.

Marijuana: Whether use of marijuana during pregnancy can harm the fetus is unclear. The main component of marijuana, tetrahydrocannabinol, can cross the placenta and thus may affect the fetus. However, marijuana does not appear to increase the risk of birth defects or to slow the growth of the fetus. Marijuana does not cause behavioral problems in the newborn unless it is used heavily during pregnancy.

16.2 Drugs in Lactation

Assessing the safety of breast feeding during maternal drug therapy is an individualised risk: benefit analysis. An infant's exposure depends on drug transfer into milk, daily milk intake and the bioavailability of the drug in the infant. Exposure and the potential for adverse effects are greatest in premature neonates and decreases over the first few months of life as the infant's clearance mechanisms mature. Risk should be assessed in the light of the inherent toxicity of the drug and any published data on milk transfer and infant exposure. When maternal drug therapy is necessary, the breast-fed infant should be regularly assessed for adverse effects such as sedation, failure to thrive and achievement of developmental milestones. Laboratory measurement of drug transfer into the milk and the infant's blood should be used, where possible, to confirm suspected adverse effects.

When mothers who are breastfeeding have to take a drug, they should be cautious about the following issues:

- How much of the drug passes into the milk
- Whether the drug is absorbed by the baby
- How the drug affects the baby
- How much milk the baby consumes, which depends on the baby's age and the amount of other foods and liquids in the baby's diet.

Depending on the above issues the usage of drugs in lactation can be continued or discontinued.

- ***Drug transfer into milk:*** When a breast-feeding woman takes a drug, the concentration of the drug in her plasma (Cmaternal) is determined by the dose regimen and her drug clearance.

  C maternal = dose rate / clearance

  The concentration in the milk is related to the maternal plasma concentration, reflected in the often-quoted milk to plasma concentration (M/P) ratio. This ratio is most reliable when it comes from studies where area under the concentration-time profiles has been measured over a whole dose interval. M/P data based on single time point concentration measurements in the two phases can be misleading because the time course of concentrations in milk and plasma may not parallel each other.

As almost all drugs pass into milk from maternal plasma by passive diffusion, the M/P ratio is affected by the composition of the milk (aqueous, lipid, protein and pH) and the physicochemical characteristics of the drug (protein binding, lipophilicity and pKa). Milk contains substantially more lipid and less protein than plasma, and is slightly more acidic. Therefore, drugs which tend to concentrate in milk are weak bases, with low plasma protein binding and high lipid solubility.

The composition of milk is by no means constant, with marked inter- and intra-individual variation in the characteristics and content of the lipid and protein phases. However, these fluctuations are usually not of great clinical importance.

- ***Infant dose and plasma concentration:*** It is important to remember that nearly all drugs cross into milk to some extent. The risk to the infant during breast feeding depends on the amount of drug ingested by the infant, the final concentration achieved in the suckling infant and the pharmacodynamic effects of that concentration.

The dose of drug ingested by the infant (D infant) can be calculated from the likely maternal plasma concentration (C maternal), the M/P ratio, and the volume of milk ingested (V; approximately 0.15 L/kg/day). The infant dose is usually standardised by expressing it as a percentage of the maternal dose in mg/kg.

D infant = C maternal x M/P x V
(note that the drug concentration in milk = C maternal x M/P)

The steady-state infant plasma concentration (C infant) is determined by this dose along with the oral availability (F) and clearance (Cl infant) in the infant.

C infant = F x D infant / Cl infant

It is important to remember that clearance may be substantially impaired in the neonate, especially the premature neonate. For example, Cl infant may be about 10% of Cl maternal in pre-term infants, 33% at birth, and 100% at approximately 6 months of age. However, information about specific drugs is often lacking and estimations based on first principles must be made.

- ***Assessment of risk to the suckling infant:*** The breast-fed infant usually receives no benefit from a drug taken by the mother and is largely an innocent bystander. Therefore, arbitrary decisions have to be made as to what constitutes a `safe' dose (or concentration) in the infant. A dose (concentration) of <10% of that received by the mother (on an mg/kg basis) has been suggested as a starting point for argument. A lower value should be used for drugs with greater inherent toxicity or where doses are uncontrolled (e.g.social drugs). For drugs which are particularly toxic, or have the potential for severe adverse effects, even in very small concentrations, breast feeding should be avoided unless evidence enables a positive conclusion about safety.

It has been suggested that feeding towards the end of a maternal dose interval may reduce infant exposure. The practicality of this strategy is questionable and it should be considered only when there is milk concentration data available for the whole dose interval. Milk produced earlier in the interval should be expressed.

- ***Drugs that can be safely used in Lactation:*** The term `safe' should be taken to mean that published data suggest that adverse effects are unlikely to occur in the infant because of low concentrations in the infant and because inherent toxicity is low. However, each case must be considered on its own merits as factors such as maternal dose and infant vary widely.

  Some drugs, such as epinephrine, heparin, and insulin, do not pass into breast milk and are thus safe to take. Some drugs pass into breast milk, but the baby usually absorbs so little of them that they do not affect the baby. Examples are the antibiotics gentamicin, kanamycin, streptomycin, and tetracycline.

  Drugs that are considered safe include most nonprescription (over-the-counter) drugs. Exceptions are antihistamines (commonly contained in cough and cold remedies, allergy drugs, motion sickness drugs, and sleep aids) and, if taken in large amounts for a long time, aspirin and other salicylates. Acetaminophen and ibuprofen, taken in usual doses, appear to be safe.

  Drugs that are applied to the skin, eyes, or nose or that are inhaled are usually safe. Most antihypertensive drugs do not cause significant problems in breastfed babies. Women may take beta-blockers during breastfeeding, but the baby should be checked regularly for possible side effects, such as a slow heart rate and low blood pressure. Warfarin can be taken if the baby is full-term and healthy, but its use should be monitored. Caffeine and theophylline do not harm breastfed babies but may make them irritable. The baby's heart and breathing rates may increase. Even though some drugs are reportedly safe for breastfed babies, women who are breastfeeding should consult a health care practitioner before taking any drug, even an over-the-counter drug, or a medicinal herb. All drug labels should be checked to see whether they contain warnings against use during breastfeeding.

- ***Drugs that can be used in Lactation under medical supervision:*** Some drugs require a doctor's supervision during their use. Taking them safely while breastfeeding may require adjusting the dose, limiting the length of time the drug is used, or timing when the drug is taken in relation to breastfeeding. Most antianxiety drugs, antidepressants, and antipsychotic drugs require a doctor's supervision, even though they are unlikely to cause significant problems in the baby. However, these drugs stay in the body a long time. During the first few months of life, babies may have difficulty eliminating the drugs, and the drugs may affect the baby's nervous system. For example, the antianxiety drug diazepam (a benzodiazepine) causes lethargy, drowsiness, and weight loss in breastfed babies. Babies eliminate phenobarbital (an anticonvulsant and a barbiturate) slowly, so this drug may cause excessive drowsiness. Because of these effects, doctors reduce the dose of benzodiazepines and barbiturates as well as monitor their use by women who are breastfeeding.

- ***Drugs that are contra-indicated while breast feeding:*** Some drugs should not be taken by mothers who are breastfeeding. They include amphetamines, chemotherapy drugs (such as doxorubicin, and methotrexate), chloramphenicol, ergotamine, lithium, radioactive drugs for diagnostic procedures, and illicit drugs such as cocaine, heroin, and phencyclidine (PCP). Drugs that may suppress milk production should not be taken. They include bromocriptine, estrogen, oral contraceptives that contain high-dose estrogen and progestin, and levodopa.

If women who are breastfeeding must take a drug that may harm the baby, they must stop breastfeeding. They can resume breastfeeding after they stop taking the drug. While taking the drug, women can maintain their milk supply by pumping breast milk, which is then discarded.

Women who smoke should not breastfeed within two hours of smoking and should never smoke in the presence of their baby whether they are breastfeeding or not. Smoking reduces milk production and interferes with normal weight gain in the baby.

Alcohol consumed in large amounts can make the baby drowsy and cause profuse sweating. The baby's length may not increase normally, and the baby may gain excess weight.

The following groups of drugs are discussed as many questions were raised about the safety of these drugs.

Analgesics (Table 16.3)

Codeine, paracetamol, ibuprofen, indomethacin and naproxen are poorly transferred into milk, have a low risk potential and are considered safe. Aspirin is contraindicated because of the theoretical risk of Reye's syndrome. Methadone use by mothers in maintenance programs is associated with a high incidence (approximately 60%) of withdrawal symptoms in the infants following birth. This indicates that the amount in the milk may be insufficient to prevent withdrawal; supportive therapy is often required. Sumatriptan has a very short half-life and expressing milk for 8 hours can completely avoid infant exposure to this drug.

Anthelminthics

Although there are no data on the distribution of mebendazole and pyrantel pamoate into human milk, both drugs are poorly absorbed from the gastrointestinal tract and their distribution into human milk is unlikely to be significant. Praziquantel, which is well absorbed, has an M/P ratio of 0.25-0.32 and an infant dose of 0.1%. These drugs are considered safe.

Anticoagulants (16.4)

Heparin, with a high molecular weight, does not pass into human milk; warfarin has not been detected in human milk. These drugs are considered safe. The passage of low molecular weight heparin into human milk has not been reported. However, its low oral availability would be expected to minimize risk. Phenindione passes into human milk in significant quantities and, as there has been one report of haemorrhage in an exposed infant, breast feeding should be avoided.

Anticonvulsants

There are currently no human data on the distribution into human milk of the newer anticonvulsants, vigabatrin and lamotrigine. Carbamazepine, clonazepam, phenytoin and sodium valproate are considered safe in lactation if the infant is observed carefully for sedation and central nervous system depression. Phenobarbitone is best avoided.

Antidepressants (Table 16.5)

Postnatal depression affects some 10-20% of mothers and there are also a small percentage of women in the population who will require antidepressant treatment throughout their pregnancy and during lactation. The presence of active metabolites needs to be considered for several of these drugs. Although the tricyclics have the potential to cause sedation and anticholinergic effects in the nursing infant, very few problems have been encountered and breast feeding is generally considered an acceptable risk. Doxepin use is controversial and, while it is probably safe, diligent clinical observation of the infant is recommended. Moclobemide, mianserin and the selective serotonin reuptake inhibitors (SSRIs) also appear to be safe, but more studies are needed. With some tricyclics and SSRIs, long half-lives and the potential for substantial *in utero* exposure at usual therapeutic doses suggest that there may be a significant risk of a `withdrawal syndrome', particularly in the first 1-2 weeks after birth. Long-term effects in infants have only been studied for dothiepin and cognitive development measures were normal.

Antihistamines (H_1 blockers) and cold preparations (Table 16.6)

Information on the distribution of antihistamines into human milk is limited, but there is no evidence to show that breast-milk supply may be diminished as has been speculated. Short- or medium-acting antihistamines may cause irritability or sedation in infants. Nevertheless, many consider their short-term use safe, although there are few studies to support this view. Drugs such as chlorpheniramine, dexchlorpheniramine, diphenhydramine, hydroxyzine and promethazine have been in use for many years without adverse effects being reported. The newer non-sedating antihistamines, astemizole and terfenadine, are best avoided until more human data are available; loratadine is probably safe. Cough and cold preparations frequently contain an antihistamine, a decongestant and an analgesic. Pseudoephedrine has an M/P ratio of 1.97 and an infant dose of 3% and, together with phenylephrine and phenylpropanolamine, is considered safe, although the infant should be monitored for excessive irritability. The usual short-term use of these preparations also gives some degree of safety. The possible adverse effects of oral decongestants may be reduced by using nasal sprays or drops.

Anti-infectives (Table 16.7)

Most anti-infective agents carry the risks of changes in bowel flora, and allergic sensitization. Penicillins and cephalosporins are generally considered safe, although the third generation cephalosporins are more likely to alter bowel flora. The macrolides, erythromycin and roxithromycin, are also considered safe. Tetracyclines impose a theoretical risk of teeth staining and bone growth inhibition. However, this risk is small, as they are commonly used in short courses, distributed into milk in small amounts, and most form unabsorbable complexes with calcium. Doxycycline has low binding to calcium in milk and thus its absorption by the infant may be greater. Sulfonamides are safe to use in healthy, full-term infants, but should be avoided in infants with glucose-6-phosphate dehydrogenase (G-6-PD) deficiency. Although the concentrations in human milk are low, quinolones are best avoided as they are known to cause arthropathies in immature animals.

The use of metronidazole is controversial because of mutagenicity and carcinogenicity in animal studies, although this risk has not been confirmed in humans. In one trial, no adverse effects were observed in breast-fed infants whose mothers were receiving up to 400 mg 3 times daily. However, diarrhoea and secondary lactose intolerance have been reported in one case and the drug may impart an adverse taste to the milk. Nevertheless, exposure is less than 10% of the recommended daily infant dose for metronidazole (approximately 10 mg/kg) and it is considered safe for short-term therapy. Exercise caution if therapy is single high dose (expresses and discards milk for 24 hours).

Benzodiazepines

Floppy infant syndrome with symptoms of hypotonia, lethargy and reduced suckling is a possible consequence of breast feeding while using this group of drugs. For diazepam, M/P values range from 0.1-1.3 and average infant exposure is around 5% of the maternal dose. Its active metabolite desmethyldiazepam also has an M/P of 0.13 and would contribute similarly to infant exposure. Lethargy and weight loss have been reported in breast-fed infants and diazepam is therefore not recommended. Oxazepam, nitrazepam and flunitrazepam have M/P values of 0.1, 0.27 and 0.54 and infant exposure of 1%, 2.3% and 0.6% respectively. While there are no reports of toxicity with these drugs, like diazepam, they have moderate to long half-lives in adults and are probably best avoided. If a benzodiazepine hypnotic is needed during lactation, then temazepam is the drug of choice. Although its M/P is also around 0.12, its half-life is short and it is undetectable in milk at an average of 15 hours after an evening dose.

Social drugs (Table 16.8)

The major problem with these drugs is that intake is variable, so the infant dose may be unacceptably high. There are few studies of the long-term effects on infant development. With cannabis and tobacco (nicotine) exposure, the intake of lipid-soluble carcinogens from the pyrolysis process may also be a hazard to the infant. Recent studies also show that food-derived mutagens fed to rodents are excreted in the milk and absorbed by the pups.

Summary of information needed to assess infant risk

Most product information is unhelpful because, for medico legal reasons, it often advises against breast feeding. Nevertheless, a literature search may elicit published data from which an assessment of risk can be made. The primary data required for dose estimation are

- Values for maternal milk and plasma concentrations at steady-state, or values for milk concentration alone
- M/P ratio
- Infant milk intake (approximately 0.15 L/kg/day).

Measured values are preferred, but literature estimates are adequate on many occasions. Dose for infant can then be calculated and should be considered in the light of the approximate age-related Clearance infant value. Note that a high M/P value does not necessarily translate to a high infant dose. Literature reports (without milk or plasma data) of no adverse effects in breast-fed infants of mothers taking specific medications may also be helpful.

What to do when adverse effects in the infant are suspected

- First consider the age of the infant and whether the effects could be the result of *in utero* exposure to the drug (e.g. methadone, fluoxetine).
- If possible, take milk from the mother and blood samples from both the mother and infant for laboratory analysis as this can provide definitive data.
- Make an informed decision and, if appropriate, write a case report and/or complete an adverse drug reaction blue reporting card so others can benefit from your experience.

Table 16.3 Distribution of analgesics into human milk, calculated infant dose and interpretation of data.

Drug/Group[1]	M/P ratio[2]	Infant dose[3] (%)	Comments and recommendations for breast feeding
Aspirin	0.06	3.2	Possible association with Reye's syndrome. Avoid.
Codeine	ND	ND	Trace amounts in milk. Considered safe.
Ibuprofen	_	_	Non-detectable in milk. Considered safe.
Methadone	0.45	2.6	Symptoms of withdrawal occur in the first week for 60% of infants born to mothers on methadone maintenance. Considered safe.
Naproxen	ND	2.8	Low concentrations in milk. Exposure is approximately 3.6% of pediatric dose. Probably safe, but more data needed.
Paracetamol	1.0	4.2	No adverse effects. Dose in milk is about 4.5% of therapeutic pediatric dose. Considered safe.
Sumatriptan	4.1-5.7	0.3-6.7	Probably safe. Actual dose received probably diminished by low oral bioavailability of drug. Expressing milk for 8 hours will completely avoid exposure from a single 6 mg subcutaneous maternal dose.

Table 16.4 Distribution of anticonvulsants into human milk, calculated infant dose and interpretation of data.

Drug/Group[1]	M/P ratio[2]	Infant dose[3] (%)	Comments and recommendations for breast feeding
Carbamazepine	0.24-0.69	3.6-4.1	Considered safe; observe infant for undue tiredness and poor suckling.
Clonazepam	0.33	ND	Considered safe; observe infant for CNS depression and apnoea, particularly after *in utero* exposure.
Phenobarbitone	0.4-0.6	48.2-93.6	Infant exposure too high. Sedation observed in some infants. Avoid.
Phenytoin	0.18-0.54	0.5-4.8	Considered safe. One report of methaemoglobinaemia, drowsiness and poor suckling.

Table 16.4 *Contd...*

Drug/Group[1]	M/P ratio[2]	Infant dose[3] (%)	Comments and recommendations for breast feeding
Sodium valproate	0.01-0.05	1.2	No adverse effects reported in infants. Considered safe at low dose rates. Use with caution at high doses when there is a risk of hepatitis and haemorrhagic pancreatitis.
Vigabatrin	ND	ND	No human data available. Avoid.

Table 16.5 Distribution of antidepressants into human milk, calculated infant dose and interpretation of data.

Drug/Group[1]	M/P ratio[2]	Infant dose[3] (%)	Comments and recommendations for breast feeding
Tricyclics			
Amitriptyline (nortriptyline)	1.53 (0.95)	1.1 (0.8)	Non-detectable in plasma of breast-fed infants. Probably safe.
Clomipramine	ND	ND	Non-detectable or negligible concentrations in plasma of breast-fed infants. *In utero* exposure resulted in high levels at birth in one infant. No adverse effects reported. Probably safe.
Desipramine	1.2	1.0	Non-detectable in infant plasma. No adverse effects. Probably safe.
Dothiepin (nordothiepin)	0.78-1.59 (0.85-1.36)	0.58 (0.23)	Low concentrations detected in some infant plasma/urine samples. No adverse effects reported. Cognitive development measures show no effect in breast-fed infants at age 3-5 years compared with controls. Considered safe.
Selective serotonin reuptake inhibitors			
Sertraline	0.62	0.67	Non-detectable or very low concentrations in infant plasma. No adverse effects in infants. Probably safe, but more data needed.
Others			
Venlafaxine	ND	ND	Not recommended until published data available.

Table 16.6 Distribution of antihistamines into human milk, calculated infant dose and interpretation of data.

Drug/Group[1]	M/P ratio[2]	Infant dose[3] (%)	Comments and recommendations for breast feeding
Astemizole	4.4	ND	Avoid until human data available.
Promethazine	ND	ND	Passage into milk likely to occur. Probably safe. Observe infant closely for sedation or irritability.
Loratadine (Descarboethoxyloratadine)	1.2 (0.8)	0.01 (0.02)	No adverse effects reported in infants. Probably safe.
Terfenadine (carboxylic acid metabolite)	ND (0.13)	ND (0.45)	Irritability reported in infants. Avoid the drug, pending more human data.
Trimeprazine	ND	ND	Passes into human milk in small amounts. Considered safe.
Triprolidine	0.5-0.56	0.2	Considered safe.

Table 16.7 Distribution of anti-invectives into human milk, calculated infant dose and interpretation of data.

Drug/Group[1]	M/P ratio[2]	Infant dose[3] (%)	Comments and recommendations for breast feeding
Cephalosporins			
Cefaclor	ND	ND	Low concentrations in human milk. Considered safe.
Cephalexin	0.01-0.014	ND	As above.
Cefotaxime	0.16	ND	Third generation cephalosporins have more potential to affect bowel flora. Considered safe.
Ceftriaxone	0.03-0.06	3.2-5.7	As above.

Table 16.7 ***Contd...***

Drug/Group[1]	M/P ratio[2]	Infant dose[3] (%)	Comments and recommendations for breast feeding
Macrolides			
Erythromycin	0.5	0.5	May affect bowel flora. Considered safe.
Roxithromycin	0.03-0.04	ND	Small amounts in milk. May affect bowel flora. Considered safe.
Penicillins			
Amoxycillin	0.013-0.043	ND	Trace amounts in milk. No adverse effects observed but potential problem of bowel flora modification and sensitization. Considered safe. While Amoxycillin is often given together with clavulanic acid, there are currently no data on the distribution of the latter in milk.
Penicillin G	0.06-0.57	0.2	As above.
Flucloxacillin	ND	ND	Trace amounts in human milk; similar adverse effects to other Penicillins. Considered safe. Exercise caution with high-dose parenteral use.
Tetracyclines			
Doxycycline	0.32-0.36	0.8	Theoretical risk of dental staining and some growth inhibition. Avoid.
Tetracycline	0.6-1.3	0.5	As above.
Sulphonamides			
Sulphamethoxazole and trimethoprim (as cotrimoxazole)	0.1 1.26	2-2.5 3.75-5.5	Contraindicated in infants with hyperbilirubinaemia and G6PD deficiency.
Others			
Acyclovir	0.6-4.1	1.6	Significant amount in milk. No adverse effects reported in infant. Considered safe.
Ciprofloxacin	0.85-2.14	ND	Potential for arthropathy and other serious toxicity. Avoid.

Table 16.8 Distribution of `social drugs' into human milk, calculated infant dose and interpretation of data.

Drug/Group[1]	M/P ratio[2]	Infant dose[3] (%)	Comments and recommendations for breast feeding
Alcohol	0.9	3.9-19.5	Low toxicity but prudent to limit maternal intake to one standard drink daily. However, chronic intake even at low levels may affect psychomotor development. Safe but minimal intake preferred.
Caffeine	0.61	9.6-34.3	The drug has been detected in infant plasma. Half-life of caffeine is around 80-98 hours in neonates and restlessness and irritability have been documented. Safe only when intake kept low.
Nicotine (cotinine)	2.92 (0.78)	ND ND	Both nicotine and its metabolite cotinine detected in infant plasma. No adverse effects recorded. Not recommended.
Amphetamine	2.8-7.5	ND	Has been detected in urine of breast-fed infants, but no insomnia or stimulation noted. Avoid as long-term effects unknown.

[1] active metabolites in parenthesis

[2] individual value, means or range from selected studies

[3] infant doses in mg/kg as percent maternal dose in mg/kg. Data from selected studies

ND no data available

(Adapted from "Drug distribution in milk" – 1997, Vol. 20, Australian prescriber)

Conclusion

Pregnancy and lactation are the physiological conditions which are well cared for by the natural, inherent homeostatic mechanisms of the body. Most drugs taken by the mother will reach the fetus to some extent and can cause harm to the fetus. There is only a very small patient population in whom there is an absolute necessity of using drugs during these special physiological conditions. Some women will need drug therapy for chronic diseases that existed before pregnancy such as diabetes mellitus or hypertension. It is important to assess whether the risk of a congenital defect from drug exposure exceeds the risk of a defect occurring without drug exposure. It is difficult to assess the exact probability of which a drug may harm the fetus. Information available in the literature is limited, as clinical trials are not conducted in this population. Social drugs can be avoided totally, at least during pregnancy and lactation because by doing so, the health of the new born and health of the child yet to be born is being protected and is the responsibility of all mothers and mothers to be. Lactating mothers must also be assessed as to whether they need medication or not, as many drugs will distribute into milk. If drug therapy is indicated, then a drug with low milk to plasma ratio should be chosen. Short acting drugs or drugs with short half-life are preferred over long acting medications. If drug therapy is needed the mother must be well informed of the complications or risks involved so that a well informed, ethical and educated decision is made. One has to remember that nobody has a moral right to cause any harm to the health of the fetus or the child. A clinical pharmacist can go a long way in fulfilling this obligation.

Study Outline

In general, drugs unless absolutely necessary should not be used during pregnancy, because many drugs can cause harm to the fetus.

- can act directly on fetus causing damage or death
- can alter functions of placenta resulting in underdeveloped under weight baby
- Can cause muscles of uterus to contract forcefully injuring the fetus or triggering preterm labour.

FDA classifies drugs according to degree of risk they pose for fetus as A, B, C, and D and X categories. Category X drugs are highly toxic and should never be used e.g., thalidomide

Unless absolutely necessary, drugs should not be used during pregnancy.

Certain substances like tobacco, alcohol, opioids, marijuana are called as social drugs. They are more harmful during pregnancy as along with the mother they can also affect the fetus. Hence all social drugs should be avoided during pregnancy.

Drugs in lactation

Assessing safety of breast feeding during maternal drug therapy is an individualized risk: benefit analysis.

The factors to be considered are

- how much of drug passes into milk
- whether drug is absorbed by the baby
- how does the drug affect the baby
- how much milk the baby consumes

Depending on safety of drugs during lactation, drugs can be classified into 3 categories

- drugs that can be safely used during lactation, E.g., most OTC drugs, paracetamol, ibuprofen, insulin, epinephrine
- drugs that can be used during lactation under medical supervision E.g., diazepam, Phenobarbital
- drugs that are contraindicated while lactation E.g., amphetamine, chemotherapeutic agents, chloramphenicol

When adverse effects in the infant are suspected

- milk samples from mother and blood samples from infant are to be analyzed to obtain definitive data
- Considering the age of the infant (whether exposure could be in utero) make an informed decision and report the adverse effect.

CHAPTER 17

Technology and Automation

Objectives

After reading this chapter, the student should be able to:

- Understand the need for technology and automation in Clinical Pharmacy Practice
- Explain the benefits, advantages and challenges of technology and automation
- Know different types of pharmacy automation
- Discuss the computer applications in pharmacy

17.1 Introduction

Technology has penetrated health care. The computer, like no other single equipment, has changed the way overall health care is practiced. Information technology and automation have also changed the way pharmacy is practiced.

Information technology and automation improve the medication use process and can help advance pharmacy practice and pharmaceutical care. It is important that the use of technology and automation in pharmacy practice be well thought out and used correctly.

As the complexity of the clinical practice of medicine increases, so does the need for improved information processing and communication. Use of the computer for data processing and communication allows health practitioners to have a great deal of information available in an organized form. Pharmacists will find a growing need for computers as useful applications are demonstrated and as the practice of pharmacy becomes more clinically oriented.

In the traditional practice of pharmacy, storage and retrieval of information was relatively simple. Each community pharmacy maintained a file of prescriptions in sequential order or a family record of prescriptions. Business records, such as cash register receipts, numbers of prescriptions filled per day, and inventory data were also kept and maintained.

As pharmacists become more involved in the clinical aspects of medical care, their use of the computer must and will increase. The amount of drug information in existence is increasing rapidly and its utilization becomes difficult unless a tool such as the computer is available for storage and retrieval of this information. (For example, few pharmacists can recall all pertinent data on drug interactions, and published information is outdated date as soon as it is distributed).

As medical care becomes more complex, more and more information is being collected on each patient while the traditional medical record, organized in patchwork fashion and full of illegible script, becomes difficult to use. Finally, unless computers eventually assume label typing and record keeping tasks, there will not be a sufficient number of pharmacists available to provide adequate service.

Information technology refers to the storage, access and use of information stored in a database (software) that can be accessed using computers.

Pharmacy automation is an aggregate of two or more physical components and a set of procedures in the pharmacy medication process that function together.

17.2 Need for Technology

Pharmacy should use technology and automation for several reasons:

- to improve medications safety
- to improve patient care
- to improve efficiency of the medication process and
- to improve the documentation of care.

Improved safety: Information technology and automation should improve patient safety by building into the medication process a system of checks and balances that would be humanly impossible to know, remember, and to perform. Computers can track and check hundreds of procedures and let the users know when possible problems are discovered.

Improved patient care: By incorporating various standards of practice and care plans, the computer system can track all orders and check patient results and thus track actual performance versus desired performance. The computers can also provide reminders to the users of how to improve performance.

Improved efficiency: Computers can work much faster than humans. Thus, when properly set up, computer system can process orders, provide documents and information about patients, and help prepare medication for patients. Medication orders can be processed faster, and patients can receive their medication sooner.

Improved documentation of care: The use of technology and automation can provide details on what has taken place in the drug-use process – the processing, preparation, dispensing, and administration of medication. Such details and documentation cannot be provided by manual systems.

Other reasons why pharmacy should use technology and automation are :

- *To improve the timeliness, accuracy, legibility of drug-related communications and safety:*

  Computers can process and communicate information quickly and accurately. The most important reason for using computers may be their vast information-handling capabilities. Information technology and automation should improve patient safety by building into the medication process a system of checks and balances that would be humanly impossible to know.

- *To integrate the medication system with other information and control systems in the hospital; to expand control of medications and to improve patient care:*

  Any information entered into an automated information system can be shared and utilized throughout the entire system. Pharmacists should consider the usefulness of all data collected in the hospital so that, checks and balances may be integrated into the medication system. An automated laboratory reporting system should include a report of the possible interferences of drugs with laboratory tests. Computers can also be used to analyze various aspects of the medication order, such as compatibility of intravenous drugs, interaction of drugs, correct dosages, and possible allergies.

  By incorporating various standards of practice and care plans, the computer system can track all orders and check patient results and thus track actual performance versus desired performance.

- *To help ensure that the integrity and confidentiality of drug records are maintained:*

  The computer provides a new and yet uncharted dimension in information availability and can make vast quantities of previously inaccessible data available to physicians, nurses, and pharmacists. Proper safeguards can assure that information is made available only to those persons serving the best interests of the patient. Systems have been developed that include a badge reader that accepts a plastic "credit card' to allow limited access to the system. Access could be structured to provide certain information to various hospital employees, e.g., a clerk may have access, by using her 'credit card," to census information only.

- *To collect drug utilization data so that drug therapy can be effectively monitored and improve efficiency:*

  Utilization review may include retrospective reviews of drug usage as well as epidemiologic studies to facilitate adverse drug reaction research and reporting. A number of drug utilization studies published recently have utilized computers, and it is unlikely that they could have been done without a computer.

- *To strengthen the administrative skills of the hospital pharmacist:*

  Computers have been used most frequently for administrative activities. Many systems were originally developed on unit record equipment or systematized in some way and then transferred onto electronic equipment. Purchasing, inventory control, and other accounting procedures have been computerized in business and hospitals for a number of years. Beginning the use of computers in hospitals in administrative functions therefore may be the most practical, since experience gained and equipment acquired will be helpful as patient care applications of computers are developed.

- *To decrease the pharmacist's record-keeping and paper handling chores; to help ensure that the talents of the pharmacist are utilized properly:*

  Computers can be used to type labels, maintain inventory, provide drug information, keep patient profiles, prepare the formulary, and keep narcotic records. By using such systems, the pharmacist is freed to develop his skills in clinical role which is considered important.

17.3 Information Technology

Information technology stores, accesses, and uses information in a data base that can be accessed by pharmacists using computers. This technology provides information to pharmacists about drugs, drug therapy and patients. The information may be on the internet, stored in a data base at a remote location, or stored in the memory of the pharmacy computer.

Computers and databases of information have removed the need for paper work, increased access to information, speeded up information processing, are being used to increase market share, and have freed up and made tools available for pharmacists to practice pharmaceutical care.

- *Less paperwork:* Pharmacists can use computers to reduce the paper work like prescription records, manual patient profiles, controlled substance records, and insurance information. Insurance claims had to be written, copies made, and the original sent to the third-party payer. Computer storage has nearly eliminated these procedures.

- *Faster access to Information:* Pharmacies linked to internet now have information at their finger tips almost at lightening speed. Access to information about new drugs, old drugs, drug therapy, and diseases are available with only a few clicks of the computer mouse.

- *Increased speed in processing information:* A major advantage of computers is their speed. This is important in pharmacy, where there is no end to the increased number of prescriptions to dispense and insurance claims to process. The increased processing of orders helps efficiency and hopefully improves safety.
- *Increased market share:* Community pharmacies are starting to use the computer in creative ways to increase market share. The lead taken is from *telemedicine* practiced by physicians and some hospitals. Pharmacies have started *telepharmacy,* which includes dispensing of medications and the provision of pharmaceutical care to patients from a distance.
- *Tools for pharmaceutical care:* Computers and information technology can provide tools and help free up pharmacists to practice pharmaceutical care. Computers can store patient information to help pharmacists check patients and make recommendations to physicians on the appropriate use of medication. Computers can help screen patients and provide lists of patients who might benefit from the care of a pharmacist. They also can perform complex pharmacokinetic dosing calculations and check for problems in dosage, overlapping therapy and dug interactions.
- *E-prescribing:* E-prescribing is the use of an automated data entry system to generate and send a prescription to the community pharmacist, rather than writing it on a paper and giving it to the patient. Automation of the outpatient prescribing process has many potential benefits, especially increased safety.
- *Computerized Prescriber Order Entry:* Computerized prescriber order entry (CPOE) system can improve prescribing and transcribing accuracy. CPOE allows prescribers to enter their orders directly into the hospital information system, either on a terminal in the hospital, or sometimes from their handheld palm devices or office computers.

17.4 Automation

Pharmacy automation started in the late 1960s in USA, with the use of tablet counting machines – units that held medication and had a dial for setting the number to be counted. During the 1980s the first device to automate the preparation of total parenteral nutrition (TPN) solutions became available. The first automated unit-dose filling machine was available in 1990s.

Advantages of Automation

- *Improved Speed:* Microprocessors in automated equipment are able to process information at almost lightening speeds. This speed is needed in the medication process so the time from when the physician writes the medication order until the patient receives the first dose is the shortest possible

- *Improved accuracy:* Computers are flawless at computing and processing information, unless there is a human programming or intervention error. This is needed in the medication process to remove errors.
- *Improved documentation:* The major advantage of computers and automated medication devices is their ability to document what has taken place in a clear format. Who ordered the drug, who dispensed it, who checked it, who gave it, how much they gave, and when it was given is automatically recorded.
- *Improved efficiency:* Pharmacy automation can do the work of many people. Automation can save the salary costs, can free pharmacy technicians to do other important tasks, and can free pharmacists to do pharmaceutical care.

Challenges of Pharmacy Automation

- *Cost:* The major challenge to using pharmacy automation is cost. Pharmacy automation is expensive. The benefits must outweigh the costs.
- *Space:* One problem of pharmacy automation is availability of space to accommodate the equipment in the already congested pharmacy.
- *Fear of being replaced:* Pharmacy automation can reduce the manpower needs.
- *One error can become many errors:* Pharmacy automation can either decrease errors or make them worse. If an automated preparation and dispensing device is not set up correctly, the same error can be repeated many times until the error is discovered.

Types of Pharmacy Automation

There are three general types of pharmacy automation

- Tablet counters – These devices count oral solids i.e., tablets and capsules.
- Intravenous (IV) compounders – Most of the devices are for compounding TPN solutions
- Dispensing machines – Dispensing automation is the largest category of equipment. Pharmacy automation is now categorized by where it is used: in central pharmacy, in decentralized areas, or other pharmacy automation. Devices can be divided into two basic kinds : i) systems that repackage medications from bulk and ii) systems that use over packaged, manufacturer wrapped unit-of-use.

17.5 Computer Applications in Pharmacy

- ***Drug Distribution and Information***

  The Hospital Formulary: Several hospital pharmacists have used electronic data processing to prepare the hospital formulary. Revision of the formulary can be done by the computer more accurately and quickly than by conventional means.

The computer is an excellent editing device in the preparation of a formulary.

Drug Information: Computers can be used to provide drug information in a number of ways.

Drug Dispensing: Dispensing machines have been used for a number of years to control and dispense multiple dose packages of drugs in hospitals. A method exists for linking the dispensing machine to a keypunch so that a charge card is produced as the doses are dispensed.

- ***Drug Control***

Control of Restricted Drugs: Narcotics, amphetamines, barbiturates, and investigational drugs are all subject to perpetual inventory in pharmacy practice. Systems for controlling these drugs have been developed using rather simple data processing techniques.

Drug Utilization Review: The pharmacist is responsible for monitoring drug usage in the hospital. Other than control of restricted drugs and studies of antibiotic usage, it has been difficult, if not impossible, to accomplish this task on a regular basis for most drugs. The volume of data is too great and present storage methods do not facilitate retrieval of information. Monitoring is critical for studies of adverse reactions to drugs and patterns of sensitivities of organisms to certain antibiotics, as well as studies of drug costs. Computers and information technology have a great utility in all these areas.

Business and Administrative Uses: Pharmacy inventory and patient billing systems have been the primary computer application in hospital pharmacies for many years, and are still predominant.

Outpatient and Community Practice: Automation of outpatient pharmacy practice has not progressed as rapidly as that for inpatient; very little automation in community pharmacy has even been attempted. The smaller volume and less critical need have probably contributed to this situation.

Conclusion

Computers, Information technology and automation are tools that a pharmacy should use. They improve the medication dispensing process by making it safer and more efficient. By the usage of these tools the pharmacist can get enough free time to perform pharmaceutical care and in turn improve the quality of drug therapy for patients. Pharmacists must take the responsibility and see that these systems meet the needs of the pharmacy staff and other health care workers who use them. It is also the responsibility of the pharmacists to see that these systems are helpful in improving the care of patients.

Study Outline

Information technology refers to the storage, access and use of information stored in a database (software) that can be accessed using computers. *Pharmacy automation* is an aggregate of two or more physical components and a set of procedures in the pharmacy medication process that function together.

Need for technology – Pharmacy should use technology and automation for several reasons

- to improve medication safety
- to improve patient care
- to improve efficiency of the medication process and
- to improve the documentation of care

Advantages of Pharmacy automation

- improved speed
- improved accuracy
- improved documentation
- improved efficiency

Computers have several applications in pharmacy like drug distribution and information, drug control, drug utilization review, business and administrative uses, outpatient and community practice

CHAPTER 18

Pharmacoeconomics

Objectives

After reading this chapter, the student should be able to:

- Define Pharmacoeconomics and understand the principles involved
- Explain the Scope of Pharmacoeconomics and discuss the Pharmacoeconomic models for evaluation
- Discuss the relationship between Pharmacoeconomics and drug development, Pharmacoeconomics and Quality of Life
- Explain various steps involved in designing a Pharmacoeconomic evaluation
- Understand the applications of Pharmacoeconomics in drug therapy decisions

18.1 Introduction

Many changes are taking place in the health care recently. The introduction of new technologies, including many new drugs, has been among these changes. As the number of new drugs continues to increase, so does their cost. The increase in the number of new drugs combined with the increased cost of these drugs provide a great challenge for managed care organizations as they struggle to deliver quality care while minimizing costs. Today's cost-sensitive health care environment has created a competitive and challenging workplace for clinicians. Competition for diminishing resources has necessitated that the appraisal of health care goods and services extend beyond evaluations of safety and efficacy and considers the economic impact of these goods and services on the cost of health care. A challenge for health care professionals of the 2000s is to provide quality patient care with minimal resources.

Pharmacy and Therapeutics (P & T) committee is responsible for evaluating these new drugs and determining their potential value to organizations. Evaluating drugs for formulary inclusion can often be an overwhelming task. The application of pharmacoeconomic methods to the evaluation process may help streamline formulary decisions.

An interest in defining the "value" of medicine is a common thread joining today's health care professionals, especially, pharmacists. With serious concerns about rising medication costs and consistent pressure to decrease pharmacy expenditures and budgets, pharmacists must answer the question. "What is the value of the pharmaceutical goods and services I provide?" *Pharmacoeconomics,* or the discipline of placing a value on drug therapy, has evolved to provide an answer to this question.

Challenged to provide high-quality patient care in the least expensive way, pharmacists have developed strategies aimed at containing costs. However, most of these strategies focus solely on determining the least expensive alternative rather than the alternative that possesses the best value for the money. The "cheapest" alternative – with respect to drug acquisition cost – is not always the best value for patients, departments, institutions, and health care systems.

Quality patient care must not be compromised while attempting to contain costs. The products and services delivered by today's pharmacists should demonstrate "Pharmacoeconomic value", that is, a balance of both economic and clinical outcomes. Pharmacoeconomics can provide the systematic means for this quantification.

The field of pharmacoeconomics is rapidly expanding for a variety of reasons (e.g., regulations, competition). The economics of medicines can be viewed at three levels ;

Industry level: This level focuses on financial aspects of the many companies that make up the pharmaceutical industry. This level describes the financial forecasts, financial performances and related fiscal aspects of a company. This area is not part of the field of pharmacoeconomics, but economics.

Specific medicine level: This level is the primary one referred to as pharmacoeconomics and includes studies to evaluate costs and benefits of specific medicines. Studies usually compare a medicine with others or to other modalities but may evaluate a single treatment. The field of pharmacoeconomics identifies, measures, and compares the costs and outcomes of using treatments.

Individual patient level: While assessments of individual patient costs and benefits are quantitatively evaluated as part of pharmacoeconomic studies at the medicine level, another economic aspect can be studied in clinical trials. This involves the attitudes of a person toward work related functions to be productive.

18.2 Principles of Pharmacoeconomics

Definition: Pharmacoeconomics has been defined as "*the description and analysis of the costs of drug therapy to health care systems and society.*" More specifically, pharmacoeconomic research is the process of identifying, measuring, and comparing the costs, risks, and benefits of programs, services, or therapies and determining which alternative produces the best health outcome for the resource invested. For most pharmacists this translates into weighing the cost of providing a pharmacy product or service against the consequences (outcomes) realized by using the product or service, to determine which alternative yields the optimal outcome per rupee spent. This information can assist clinical decision makers in choosing the most cost-effective treatment options. Pharmacoeconomic analysis employs tools for examining the impact (desirable and undesirable) of alternative drug therapies and other medical interventions.

The Pharmacoeconomic equation

Costs → Rx → Outcomes

The center of the equation, the drug product is symbolized by the symbol Rx. If just the left hand side of the equation is measured without regard for outcomes, this is a cost analysis (or a partial economic analysis). If just the right hand side of the equation is measured without regard to costs, this is a clinical or outcome study (not an economic analysis). To be a true pharmacoeconomic analysis, both sides of the equation must be considered and compared.

Pharmacoeconomics is not synonymous with outcomes research. Although pharmacoeconomics is a division of outcomes research, not all outcomes research is pharmacoeconomic research. Outcomes research is defined more broadly as studies that attempt to identify, measure, and evaluate the results of health care services in general.

18.3 Cost Determination

Cost is defined as the value of the resources consumed by a program or drug therapy of interest. *Consequence* is defined as the effects, outputs, or outcomes of the program of drug therapy of interest. Consideration of both costs and consequences differentiates most pharmacoeconomic evaluation methods from traditional cost-containment strategies and drug-use evaluations.

Assessing costs and consequences – the value of a pharmaceutical product or service- depends heavily on the perspective of the evaluation. Treatment of an illness may include all four types (Direct medical, Direct non medical, Indirect non medical, Intangible), of costs. To determine what costs are important to measure, the perspective of the study must be determined. Perspective is a pharmacoeconomic term that describes whose costs are relevant based on the purpose of the study. Economic theory suggests that the most appropriate perspective is that of society. Societal costs include costs to the insurance company, costs to the patient, and indirect costs due to the loss of productivity. The most common perspectives used in the pharmacoeconomic studies are the perspective of the institution (hospital or clinic) or the perspective of the payer. Perspectives include the following:

- Patient
- Provider
- Hospital or health system
- Third-party payer or managed-care-organization
- Government
- Society

A pharmacoeconomic evaluation can assess the value of a product or service from single or multiple perspectives. However, clarification of the perspective is critical since the results of a pharmacoeconomic evaluation depend heavily on the perspective taken.

The economic effects of a medical care treatment may be viewed as the sum of its costs and benefits. The costs include:

- the cost of the treatment itself
- the cost of treating adverse effects
- the medical costs incurred during extended life years (if mortality is postponed).

These are the direct, medical costs of treatment.

Two other costs may also be involved:

- expenses incurred for nonmedical services (e.g., transportation)
- earnings lost by the patient or family members as a result of receiving the treatment (i.e., indirect costs).

The benefits of the treatment relate to its impact on the costs of illness. The items are similar conceptually to those above and include the medical costs, non-medical expenses and lost earnings associated with the illness that are avoided or saved because of treatment.

Once the perspective is clear, a full evaluation of the relevant costs and consequences can begin.

Health care costs or economic outcomes can be grouped into several categories.

- Direct medical
- Direct nonmedical
- Indirect nonmedical
- Intangible costs

Direct medical costs, are those incurred for medical products and services used to prevent, and/or treat a disease (e.g. drugs, labs, hospitalizations).

Direct nonmedical costs are any costs for nonmedical services that are results of illness but do not involve purchasing medical services (e.g., costs of transportation and hotel rooms near a treatment center).

Indirect nonmedical costs are the costs of reduced productivity (e.g. morbidity and morality costs).

Intangible costs are those costs incurred that represent other nonfinancial outcomes of disease and medical care, which are not appropriately expressed in a rupee / dollar value (e.g., pain, suffering, grief).

Costs can also be measured as "opportunity costs". Opportunity costs represent the economic benefit forgone when using one therapy instead of the next best alternative therapy, that is, the greatest possible benefit that might have been obtained by using the resources elsewhere. Table 18.1 contains examples of these costs.

Consequences (or outcomes) can also be categorized. Types of outcomes include economic (discussed previously), clinical and humanistic outcomes. Clinical outcomes are the medical events that occur as a result of disease or treatment. Humanistic outcomes are the consequences of disease or treatment on patient functional status or quality of life along several dimensions (e.g., physical function, social function, general health and well-being, life satisfaction). These consequences (outcomes) can also be categorized as positive or negative. An example of a positive outcome is a desired effect of a drug, possibly manifested as an efficacy or effectiveness measure of a drug. A negative outcome is an undesired or adverse effect of a drug, possibly manifested as a treatment failure or an adverse drug reaction (ADR). Pharmacoeconomic evaluations should include assessments of both positive and negative outcomes. Evaluating only positive outcomes may be misleading because of the detriment and expense associated with negative outcomes.

Table 18.1 Example of Health Care Cost Categories

Cost Category	**Costs**
Direct Medical costs	Drugs
	Supplies
	Laboratory tests
	Health care professionals' time
	Hospitalization
Direct nonmedical costs	Transportation
	Food
	Family care
	Home aides
Indirect nonmedical costs	Patient lost wages (morbidity)
	Spouse, family, or friend lost wages
	Income forgone due to premature death (mortality)
Intangible costs	Pain
	Suffering
	Grief
Opportunity costs	Lost opportunity
	Revenue forgone

18.4 Scope of Pharmacoeconomics

Pharmacoeconomics helps us to address the following issues -

What drugs should be included on the hospital formulary?

Which is the best drug for a particular patient?

Which is the best drug for a pharmaceutical manufacturer to develop?

Which drug delivery system is the best for this hospital?

How do these two clinical pharmacy services compare?

What is the cost per quality year of life extended by this drug?

Will patient's Quality of Life (QOL) be improved by a particular drug therapy decision?

Which is the best drug for this particular disease?

What are the patient outcomes or various treatment modalities?

18.5 Pharmacoeconomic Models

The pharmacoeconomic methods of evaluation are listed in Fig 18.1 These methods or tools can be separated into two distinct categories, economic and humanistic evaluation techniques. These methods have been used in a variety of fields and are being applied increasingly to health care, Those most commonly used by pharmacists are discussed in the following.

Economic Evaluations ↓

Cost of illness

Cost minimization

Cost benefit

Cost utility

Humanistic Evaluations ↓

Quality of life

Patient preferences

Patient satisfaction

Fig. 18.1

(i) Economic Evaluation Methods:

The methods associated with measuring the outcomes i.e., the right hand side of the equation are of four types. They can be also called as Pharmacoeconomic models and they are of four types.

- Cost Minimization analysis
- Cost Benefit analysis

- Cost Effectiveness analysis
- Cost Utility analysis

Cost Minimization Analysis (CMA)

CMA is not a true pharmacoeconomic study, because although costs are measured, outcomes are not. For cost-minimization analysis, costs are measured in terms of monetary value and outcomes are assumed to be equivalent.

When two or more interventions are examined and demonstrated or assumed to be equivalent in terms of given outcome or consequence, costs associated with each intervention may be examined and compared. For example, measurement and comparison of costs for drug therapy of two generically equivalent drugs in which the outcome has been proven to be equal.

The advantage of this type of study is that it is relatively simple compared to the other types of analysis because outcomes need not be measured. The disadvantage of this type of analysis is that it can only be used where outcomes are assumed to be identical.

Cost-Benefit Analysis (CBA)

A cost-benefit analysis measures both inputs and outputs in monetary terms. One advantage in using CBA is, alternatives with different outcomes can be compared, because each outcome is converted to the same unit (rupee / dollar). For example, the costs (inputs) of providing a pharmacokinetic service versus a diabetes clinic can be compared with the cost savings (outcomes) associated with each service, even though different types of outcomes are expected for each alternative.

The first step in conducting a CBA is to identify clearly the intervention(s), program(s), or therapeutic regimen(s) to be evaluated. The second step is to identify and value all the resources consumed, or costs of providing each intervention, program, or regimen. Different types of resources should be recognized. In the third step the benefits are identified and valued. The fourth step in CBA is to sum the values of all costs and of all the benefits of each program, intervention, or regimen. Total costs then may be subtracted from the total benefits to determine net benefits. The benefit (yield) of an investment in a program (cost) must exceed a minimum value before it is implemented. By comparing benefit-to-cost ratios of multiple programs, one can identify the program that produces greatest yield relative to the investment.

CBA consists of identifying all the benefits that accrue from the program or intervention and converting them into monetary value in the year in which they occur. This stream of benefit amount is then discounted to its equivalent present value at the selected interest rate. On the other side of the equation, all program costs are identified and allocated through a specific year and, again, the costs are discounted to their present value at the same interest rate. If all the relevant factors remain constant, the program with the largest present value of benefits minus costs is the best in terms of its economic value.

Comparing costs and benefits (outcomes in monetary terms) is accomplished by either of the two methods. One method divides the estimated benefits by the estimated costs to produce a benefit-to-cost ratio. If this ratio is more than 1.0, the choice is cost beneficial. The other method is to subtract the costs from the benefits to produce a net benefit calculation. If this difference is positive, the choice is cost beneficial.

Cost-Effectiveness Analysis (CEA)

Cost effectiveness is defined as a *series of analytical and mathematical procedures which aid in the selection of a course of action from various alternative approaches*. Cost effectiveness is a technique designed to assist a decision maker in identifying a preferred choice among possible alternatives. A cost effectiveness analysis measures costs in monetary value and outcomes in natural health units such as cures, lives saved, or blood pressure. This is the most common type of pharmacoeconomic analysis found in pharmacy literature. An advantage of using CEA is, health units are common outcomes practitioners can readily understand and these outcomes do not need to be converted to monetary values. On the other hand, the alternatives used in the comparison must have outcomes that are measured in the same units. If more than one natural outcome is important when conducting the comparison, a cost-effectiveness ratio should be calculated for each type of outcome. Outcomes cannot be collapsed into one unit measure in CEAs as they can with CBAs (outcome = Rupee value) or CUAs (outcome = quality adjusted life years).

The basic framework of CEA involves the comparison of the net resource effects (costs) of an intervention with some non monetary measures of its net effect on health outcome (effectiveness). This frequently is expressed as the ratio of the two and is called as a cost-effectiveness ratio. The resulting ratio takes the form of rupee unit of effectiveness.

One of the most controversial aspects of CEA is the issue of whether to include healthcare costs occurring in the added years of life. Some feel that these costs, which include the costs of treating diseases that would have occurred if the patient had not lived longer as a result of the original intervention, should be incorporated. Others feel that these should not be included, since this over estimates the costs associated with life saving interventions. Furthermore, it seems inconsistent to include consumption of healthcare resources in added years without productivity and other types of consumption that also come with prolonged life.

Cost effectiveness methodology requires that clear, articulate objectives be set. Following this process, it is recommended that five types of measurements be made for each alternative:

- outcome/impact
- operation use
- personnel and equipment needed
- cost factors and discount rates, and
- costs

Cost-Utility Analysis (CUA)

A cost utility analysis takes patient preferences, also referred to as "utilities", into account when measuring health consequences. This is an economic tool in which the intervention consequence is measured in terms of patient preference or quality of the health care outcome. It is much the same as cost-effectiveness analysis with the added dimension of a particular point of view – most often that of the patient. The most common unit used in conducting CUAs is QALYs (quality adjusted life years), which incorporates both the quality and quantity of life. The advantage of using this method is that different types of health outcomes can be compared using one common unit (QALYs) without placing monetary value on these health outcomes (like CBA). The disadvantage of this method is that it is difficult to determine an accurate QALY value. This is a relatively new type of outcome measure and is not understood or embraced by many providers or decision makers.

There are different techniques for determining scales of measurement for QALY. The three common methods for determining these scores are : rating scales, standard gamble, and time-trade off.

(ii) Humanistic evaluation Methods

Pharmacoeconomic evaluations may also focus on humanistic concerns. Methods for evaluating the impact of disease and treatment of disease on patient's health-related QOL, patient preferences and patient satisfaction are all growing in popularity and application to pharmacotherapy decisions. These methods can also assist clinicians in quantifying the value of pharmaceuticals.

QOL has been defined as the assessment of the functional effects of illness and its consequent therapy as perceived by the patient. These effects are often displayed as physical, emotional, and social effects on the patient. Measurement of health-related QOL is usually achieved through the use of patient-completed questionnaires.

18.6 Pharmacoeconomics and Drug Development

There are several stages in the process of a new drug development starting from Phase I trials to Phase IV trials. Pharmacoeconomic studies may be planned and conducted at the clinical development stage and at the Phase IV stage of post marketing. Another thought is that basic research and development activities may be partially guided by preliminary pharmacoeconomic analysis. Therefore, studies may need to be conducted at several stages of pharmaceutical research. The following is the summary of the research activity of each phase.

Phase I Trials: The objective of the initial clinical trials (Phase I) is to determine the toxicity profile of the drug in humans. The Phase I trials usually consist of administration of single, conservative doses to a small number of healthy volunteers. The effects of increasing the size and number of daily doses are evaluated until toxic effects occur or the likely therapeutic dosage is substantially exceeded. It is during this stage cost-of-illness studies should be accomplished to aid in the decision to further develop the drug and to gather background data for future pharmacoeconomic evaluations.

Phase II Trials: In Phase II trials, the drug is administered to a limited number of patients with the target disease. Patients without complications, coexisting medical conditions are preferred for these trials. This reduces the number of variables that could confound analysis of the drug's activity and permits the potential therapeutic benefit of the new drug to be more clearly demonstrated.

Phase III trials: In Phase III trials, larger numbers of patients are given the new drug in the established dosage range and the final dosage form. This larger sample size refines the knowledge gained during Phase II and helps identify patients who might have rare reactions to the drug. Patient selection is still closely supervised and some patients with coexisting medical problems are intentionally included to assess complications in the drug's use. If appropriate, patients with varying severity of the target disease are included to determine the new drug's scope of action. The drug's pharmacokinetic profile – how much of it gets into the body and how quickly, how it is metabolized and eliminated, the effects of multiple doses on drug concentrations, and the relationship between drug concentration and therapeutic activity – is extensively evaluated in patients and healthy volunteers.

Discussion, planning, and implementation of pharmacoeconomic studies during this level of research are important. The prospective clinical study that has incorporated a pharmacoeconomic study is close to the ideal situation. Critics of these studies claim that pharmacoeconomic evaluations will hinder the new drug application process. Advocates of pharmacoeconomic evaluation correctly note that, unless a new drug treatment has no alternatives and are truly a breakthrough; the value of using it must be scientifically studied.

Phase IV trials: During the post marketing phase (Phase IV), prospective and retrospective pharmacoeconomic studies can be designed and conducted to support the use of the drug. Post marketing pharmacoeconomic studies are extremely important in that they allow one to study the costs and consequences of drug therapy without altered interventions that occur in strictly controlled clinical trials.

18.7 Relationship between Economic Evaluations and Clinical Trials

Clinical Trials are used to evaluate the efficacy and safety of therapies. The relationship between economic evaluations and clinical trials are threefold.

- The pharmacoeconomic evaluation may be a secondary objective of a trial designed for safety and efficacy.
- The pharmacoeconomic evaluation may be the principal purpose of a clinical trial.
- A pharmacoeconomic evaluation may be done retrospectively on clinical data obtained in previous trials.

A pharmacoeconomic evaluation has a different focus than the traditional clinical trial in two respects. First, the economic evaluation is more concerned about extrapolating to what happens in "real life" than under controlled conditions. In other words, the economic study is more interested in effectiveness (what happens under actual conditions of use) rather than efficacy (what occurs in ideal conditions).

Second, the economic study attempts to measure different outcomes. While the clinical trial focuses on medical indicators (e.g., blood pressure), the economic study is designed to measure the effects on resource consumption, productivity, and / or quality of life.

As pharmacoeconomic data are becoming increasingly important to practitioners making drug formulary decisions, it is important to have these data as swiftly as possible after the drug receives FDA approval. For doing this, discussion and planning for pharmacoeconomic evaluation should begin during the early stages of drug development. Studies designed to evaluate the costs of disease and current treatments can begin early in stages I and II. QOL instrument development and validation can also be conducted simultaneously with the clinical trials. Cost-effectiveness and costs associated with toxicities and treatment failures can initially begin in Phase II or III, because Phase II trials are rigidly controlled, often much of the pharmacoeconomic data profile of a drug is generated after the drug is marketed. Once a drug is marketed (Phase IV), either prospective or retrospective pharmacoeconomic studies may be designed and conducted utilizing pharmacoepidemiological and pharmacoeconomic methodologies.

In short, an economic evaluation may be added as a component to a clinical trial with the goal to monitor or estimate:

- Resource consumption: health services and other (direct costs and benefits)
- Lost productivity through morbidity and /or premature death (indirect costs and benefits)
- QOL or willingness to pay.

18.8 Relationship of Pharmacoeconomics and Quality of Life

The types of outcomes of a medical treatment for a specific patient include three broad areas:

- ***Clinical:*** The changes in an individual patient's signs and symptoms of disease, as well as other directly measurable benefits. Health outcomes in medicine (as opposes to clinical trials) are assessed under the subject of outcomes research.
- ***Economic:*** The costs of the patient's treatment, who is paying, and what limitations are being placed on the system because of economic factors. Health care costs are assessed under the subject of health outcomes.
- ***Personal:*** The quality of life benefits, the patient assesses himself/herself in terms of how treatment affects the broad domains and their components.

There is an overlap between pharmacoeconomic and quality of life assessments, depending on the specific situation. In the clinical area, certain measures are essential for assessing cost effectiveness. Although cost/benefit analysis express clinical benefits in monetary terms, the clinical parameters must be measured. Cost/utility analysis usually require patient judgments though these may be estimated, based on clinician or investigator judgments. Although quality of life may change as a result of an individual's clinical changes, these changes are often an indirect result of the clinical effect. Economic parameters are clearly of paramount importance in pharmacoeconomics. Economics is also considered an independent domain in quality of life and usually focuses on vocational and work performance, although direct costs of treatment and its side effects are also critical in many cases for their impact on patients. Economics related to quality of life may overlap with, but generally differs greatly from, economic aspects of most pharmacoeconomic areas.

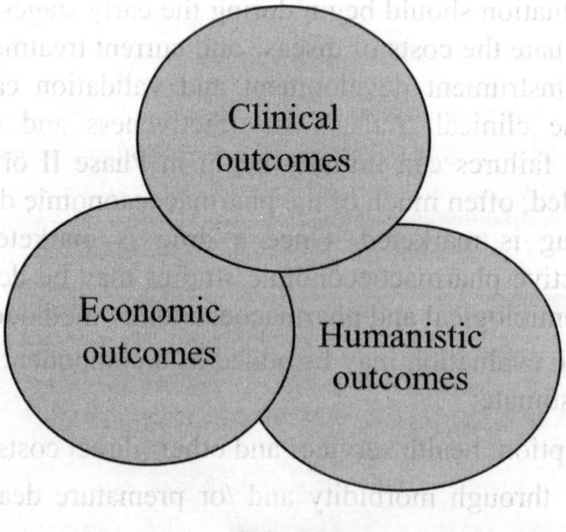

Fig. 18.2

18.9 General Steps in Designing an Economic Evaluation

There are several steps in designing the pharmacoeconomic study that should be addressed for the specific economic methodology (e.g., cost-effectiveness versus cost-benefit).

- *Define the problem* – This step is self explanatory. What is the question that is the focus of the analysis? The important thing to remember in this step is to be specific.
- *Determine the Study's perspective* - It is important to identify from whose perspective the analysis will be conducted. Is the analysis being conducted from the perspective of the patient or from that of the hospital, clinic, insurance company or society? Depending on the perspective assigned to the analysis, different results and recommendations based on these results may be identified.
- *Determine specific treatment alternatives and outcomes* - In this step, all the treatment alternatives to be compared in the analysis should be identified. This selection should include the best clinical options and / or options that are used most often in that setting at the time of the study. If a new treatment option is being considered, comparing it with an outdated treatment or a treatment with low efficacy rates is a waste of time and money. This new treatment should be compared with the next best alternative or the alternative it may replace. The alternatives may be drug treatments or nondrug treatments.
- *Select the appropriate pharmacoeconomic model* – The pharmacoeconomic model selected will depend on how the outcomes are measured. Costs (inputs) for all four types of analysis are measured in monetary value. When all outcomes for each alternative are expected to be the same, CMA is used. If all the outcomes for each alternative considered are measured in monetary units, CBA is used. When outcomes of each treatment alternative are measured in the same nonmonetary units, CEA is used. When patient preferences for alternative treatments are being considered, a CUA is used.
- *Measure inputs and outcomes* - All resources consumed by each alternative should be identified and measured in monetary value. The cost for each alternative should be listed and estimated. When evaluating alternatives over a long period of time (e.g., greater than 1 year) the concept of discounting should

be applied. Measuring outcomes can be relatively simple (e.g., cure rates) or relatively difficult (e.g., QALYs). Outcomes may be measured prospectively or retrospectively. Prospective measurements tend to be more accurate and complete, but may take considerably more time and resources than retrospective data retrieval.

- *Identify the resources necessary to conduct the analysis* - The availability of resources to conduct the study is an important consideration. Data may be obtained from a variety of sources, including clinical trials, medical literature, medical records, prescription profiles or computer databases.
- *Establish the probabilities for the outcomes of the treatment alternatives* – Probabilities for the outcomes identified should be determined. This may include the probability of treatment failures or success or adverse reactions to a given treatment or alternative.
- *Construct a decision tree* – Decision analysis can be a very useful tool when conducting pharmacoeconomic analysis. Constructing a decision tree creates a graphic display of the outcomes of each treatment alternative and the probability of their occurrence. Decision analysis is a tool that can help visualize pharmacoeconomic analysis. Decision analysis is the application of an analytical method for systematically comparing different decision options. Decision analysis graphically displays choices and performs the calculations needed to compare these options. It assists with selecting the best or most cost effective alternative. This method of analysis assists in making decisions when the decision is complex and there is uncertainty about some of the information.
- *Conduct a sensitivity analysis* – Whenever estimates are used, there is a possibility that these estimates are not precise. These estimates may be referred to as "assumptions". A sensitivity analysis allows one to determine how the results of an analysis would change when these assumptions are varied over a relevant range of values.
- *Present the results* – The results of the analysis should be presented to the appropriate audience, such as P & T committees, medical staff, or third party payers. The steps outlined in this section should be employed when presenting the results. State the problem, identify the perspective, and so on. It is imperative to acknowledge or clarify any assumptions.

Table 18.3 Steps in designing a Pharmacoeconomic evaluation in managed care hospital settings.

- Define the pharmacoeconomic problem
- Create a cross-functional project team
- Determine the study's perspective
- Determine the treatment alternatives and outcomes
- Select the appropriate pharmacoeconomic method
- Place monetary values on the outcomes
- Identify resources
- Establish the probabilities of outcome events
- Use decision analysis
- Discount costs or perform a sensitivity or incremental cost analysis
- Present the results
- Develop an intervention or policy
- Implement invention or policy and educate key professionals
- Document quality of care and potential cost savings through follow-up.

18.10 Applications of Pharmacoeconomics for Drug Therapy Decisions

To Pharmaceutical manufacturers

The Pharmacoeconomic research may be applied at many stages during the drug therapy decision process. It can be a very useful tool long before a drug is approved for use by the FDA. Pharmaceutical manufacturers need to spend enormous resources in the drug development process. If proper pharmacoeconomic research is conducted the manufacturers can avoid spending vast resources to the development of a drug that does not provide competitive advantage. Competitive advantage in the present health care environment may be defined as a drug that is cost-effective. Cost effective can mean a drug that is less costly and at least as effective as an alternative; more effective and more costly than an alternative, but improved health outcomes justify additional expenditures; or less effective and less costly than an existing alternative, but a viable alternative for some patients.

The potential for an investigational new drug to leave the laboratory is a function of its expected safety and efficacy, which are both factors comprised of several specific measures or evaluations (e.g., toxicology, adverse reactions, teratogenecity, and pharmacology). An additional factor worth considering is the expected pharmacoeconomics of the investigational drug. That factor also would be comprised of specific evaluations such as the societal and individual costs of the illness for which the drug is indicated, the costs and consequences of existing treatment methods, and the impact of the disease and existing treatments on patient quality of life (QOL). Having such information very early in the development of a drug would help reduce uncertainties and contribute to the knowledge base used to decide whether to further evaluate a treatment via prospective clinical trials. Cost efficacy and QOL components can be incorporated into appropriate Phase III studies to provide additional information regarding a drug's impact on patient outcome. If such parameters are applied systematically to all new treatment candidates, the scientific basis of drug therapy decision making will increase substantially.

To Healthcare Practitioners

One of the primary uses of pharmacoeconomics in clinical practice is to aid clinical and policy decision making. Complete pharmacotherapy decisions should contain three basic evaluation components: clinical, economic, and humanistic outcomes; that is, pharmacoeconomics value of a drug or service as illustrated in Fig. 2. No longer can drug selection decisions be based solely on acquisition costs. This strategy is misleading because of the inability to capture potential costs associated with diminished safety and efficacy profiles. Through the appropriate application of pharmacoeconomic principles and methods, incorporating these three critical components into clinical decisions can be accomplished.

Pharmacoeconomic data can be a powerful tool supports various clinical decisions, including effective formulary management, individual patient treatment, medication policy, and resource allocation. For example, pharmacoeconomics can provide critical cost-effectiveness data to support formulary addition or removal. In fact, the pharmacoeconomic assessment of formulary actions is becoming a standardized part of many pharmacy and therapeutic (P&T) committee decision making process, if based on sound pharmacoeconomic data. When competing for hospital resources, pharmacoeconomics can provide the data necessary to justify that a pharmacy service maximizes the resources allocated to it by hospital administration. Evaluating the impact a drug has on a patient's health-related quality of life can be useful when deciding between two agents for an individual patient treatment decision.

In the past, inclusion of economic outcomes (costs) in clinical decisions seemed to necessitate a compromise in the quality of care delivered. However, when used appropriately, pharmacoeconomics can assist in balancing cost with patient outcome (quality of care), often resulting in maintaining or improving quality of care, with potential cost savings. Best valued drugs will be those with optimal patient outcome per rupee/ dollar spent compared to competitors.

In the cost conscious environment, pharmacoeconomic research is important to the healthcare practitioner.

Table 18.4 Benefits of pharmacoeconomics for clinicians.

- Pharmacoeconomics can assess the value of the products and services that pharmacists provide.
- Pharmacoeconomics can assist in choosing between competing treatment alternatives.
- Pharmacoeconomics can provide data necessary to make better medication use decisions.
- Pharmacoeconomics can assist pharmacists in balancing cost with quality and patient outcome

To Pharmacists

Drug use evaluation is one of the important services provided by pharmacists. Ideally, that value should be translated into patient and financial outcomes. Apart from concentrating on inappropriately prescribed therapy and overprescribing, drug use evaluation focuses on the most cost-effective therapy. A high degree of sophistication is required in order to make such a determination fairly, considering patient factors, disease factors, and other issues.

Drug formulary services, pharmacy and therapeutics committees are viewed as a means of reducing drug budgets and have had some value in encouraging drug therapy cost considerations, but they do not provide incentives to take into account overall medical costs, nor do they necessarily consider all consequences such as potential drug interactions, adverse reactions, and treatment response rates. Conducting cost-effectiveness studies allows an evaluation of total costs and consequences from various perspectives.

Conclusion

The principles and methods of pharmacoeconomic provide the means to quantify the value of pharmacotherapy through balancing costs and outcomes. Providing quality care with minimal resources is the future and the future is here. By understanding the principles, methods and application of pharmacoeconomics, pharmacists will be prepared to determine and quantify the value of pharmacotherapy to the health care system and society.

Study Outline

Pharmacoeconomics is defined as "The description and analysis of the costs of drug therapy to health care systems and society". It is the process of identifying, measuring and comparing the costs, risks, and benefits of programs, services or therapies and determining which alteranative produces the best health out come for the resource invested.

Health care costs can be grouped into several categories:

- Direct Medical
- Direct Non medical
- Indirect Non medical
- Intangible costs

The pharmacoeconomic methods of evaluation can be broadly categorized into two distinct categories

- Economic evaluations
- Humanistic evaluations

The methods associated with measuring the outcomes i.e., the right hand side of the equation is of four types:

- cost minimization analysis
- cost benefit analysis
- cost effectiveness analysis
- cost utility analysis

The principles of Pharmacoeconomics can be applied in making drug therapy decisions by pharmaceutical manufacturers, healthcare practitioners, pharmacists.

CHAPTER 19

Pharmacoepidemiology

Objectives

After reading this chapter, the student should be able to:

- Understand the terms Epidemiology and Pharmacoepidemiology.
- Discuss the importance of Pharmacoepidemiology and its contribution to medicine.
- Explain various study designs used for Pharmacoepidemiology studies.
- Understand the need for Pharmacoepidemiological studies.

19.1 Introduction

Modern medicine has been blessed with a pharmaceutical armamentarium that is much more powerful than what it had before. Although this has given us the ability to provide much better medical care for our patients, it has also resulted in the ability to do much greater harm. The history of pharmaceutical regulation parallels the history of major adverse drug reaction disasters. The harm that drugs can cause has led to the development of the field of pharmacoepidemiology.

Pharmacoepidemiology is the science concerned with the benefit and risk of drugs used in populations and the analysis of the outcomes of drug therapies. Pharmacoepidemiologic data comes from both clinical trials and epidemiological studies with emphasis on methods for the detection and evaluation of drug-related adverse effects, assessment of risk vs benefit ratios in drug therapy, patterns of drug utilization, the cost-effectiveness of specific drugs, methodology of post marketing surveillance, and the relation between pharmacoepidemiology and the formulation and interpretation of regulatory guidelines.

19.2 Definition

***Pharmacoepidemiology** is the study of the use of and the effects of drugs in large number of people.* The term pharmacoepidemiology obviously contains two components: "Pharmaco" and "epidemiology". Therefore, Pharmacoepidemiology can be considered, a combination of clinical pharmacology and epidemiology.

***Pharmacoepidemiology** may be defined as the study of utilization and effects of drugs in large number of people.* To accomplish this study, pharmacoepidemiology borrows from both pharmacology and epidemiology. Thus, *Pharmacoepidemiology can be called a bridge science spanning both pharmacology and epidemiology.* Pharmacology is the study of the effect of drugs and clinical pharmacology is the study of effect of drugs in humans. Part of the task of clinical pharmacology is to provide a risk benefit assessment for the effect of drugs in patients. Doing the studies needed to provide an estimate of the probability of beneficial effects in populations, or the probability of adverse effects in populations and other parameters relating to drug use may benefit from using epidemiological methodology. ***Pharmacoepidemiology** then can also be defined as the application of epidemiological methods to pharmacological issues.*

***Epidemiology** can be defined as the study of the distribution and determinants of diseases in populations.* Epidemiological studies can be divided into two main types:

- *Descriptive epidemiology* describes disease and/or exposure and may consist of calculating rates, e.g., incidence and prevalence. Such descriptive studies do not use control groups and can only generate hypothesis, not test them. Studies of drug utilization would generally fall under descriptive studies.
- *Analytic epidemiology* includes two types of studies: observational studies, such as case-control and cohort studies, and experimental studies which would include clinical trials such as randomized clinical trials. The analytic studies compare an exposed group with a control group and are usually designed as hypothesis testing studies.

Epidemiology is also subdivided into two areas. The field began as the study of infectious diseases in large populations that is epidemics. More recently, it has also been concerned with the study of chronic diseases. The field of pharmacoepidemiology uses the techniques of chronic disease epidemiology to study the use and effects of drugs. The major application of the principles of pharmacoepidemiology is after a drug is marketed, though it can be applied even at the stage of clinical trials before a drug is marketed.

Clinical pharmacology is divided into two basic areas: pharmacokinetics and pharmacodynamics. *Pharmacokinetics* is the study of the relationship between the dose administered and the serum or blood level achieved. It deals with the absorption, distribution, metabolism, and excretion. *Pharmacodynamics* is the study of the relationship between drug level and the drug effect. Together, these two fields allow us to predict the effect one might observe in patient from administering a certain drug regimen. Pharmacoepidemiology encompasses elements of both these fields, exploring the effects achieved by administering a drug regimen. It does not normally involve or require the measurement of drug levels.

One central principle of clinical pharmacology is that therapy should be individualized, or tailored to the needs of the specific patient at hand. This individualization of therapy requires determination of a risk/benefit ratio specific to the patient at hand. Doing so requires a prescriber to be aware of the potential beneficial and harmful effects of the drug in question and to know how elements of the patient's clinical status might modify the probability of a good therapeutic outcome.

Pharmacoepidemiology benefits from the methodology developed in general epidemiology and may further develop them for applications of such methodology unique to pharmacoepidemiology. There are also some areas that are altogether unique to pharmacoepidemiology, e.g., pharmacovigilance. Pharmacovigilance is a type of continual monitoring for unwanted effects and other safety-related aspects of drugs that are already on the market. In practice, pharmacovigilance refers almost exclusively to the spontaneous reporting systems which allow health care professionals and others to report adverse drug reactions to a central agency. The central agency can then combine reports from many sources to produce a more informative safety profile for the drug product that could be done based on one or a few reports from one or a few health care professionals.

Specifically, the field of pharmacoepidemiology has primarily concerned itself with the study of adverse drug effects. Adverse reactions have traditionally been separated into those which are the result of an exaggerated but otherwise usual pharmacological effect of the drug, sometimes called *Type A reactions*, versus those which are aberrant effects, called as *Type B reactions.* Type A reactions tend to be common, dose related, predicatble and less serious. They can usually be treated by simply reducing the dose of the drug. In contrast , Type B reactions tend to be uncommon, not related to dose, unpredictable, and potentially more serious. They usually require cessation of the drug. They may be due to what are known as hypersensitivity reactions or immunologic reactions. Alternatively, Type B reactions may be some other idiosyncratic reaction to the drug, either due to some inherited susceptibility or due to some other mechanism. Regardless, Type B reactions are the most difficult to predict or even detect, and represent the major focus of pharmacoepidemiologic studies of adverse drug reactions.

The usual approach to study adverse drug reactions has been the collection of spontaneous reports of drug related morbidity and mortality. However, determining causation in case reports of adverse reactions can be problematic, as can attempts to compare the effects of drugs in the same class. This has led the academic investigators, industry personnel, and the legal community turns to the field of epidemiology. Specifically, studies of adverse effects have been supplemented with studies of adverse events. In the former, investigators examine case reports of purported adverse drug reactions and attempt to make a subjective clinical judgment on an individual basis about whether the adverse outcome was actually caused by the antecedent drug exposure. In the latter, controlled studies are performed examining whether the adverse outcome under study occurs more often in an exposed population than in an unexposed population. *This union of the fields of clinical pharmacology and epidemiology has resulted in the development of a new field* ***Pharmacoepidemiology.***

19.3 Importance of Pharmacoepidemiology and its Contributions

The potential contributions of pharmacoepidemiology are significant although the field is still new. The contributions made by pharmacoepidemiology are

- Information which supplements that are available from premarketing studies – better quantitation of the incidence of known adverse and beneficial effects
    - Higher precision
    - In patients not studied prior to marketing, e.g., the elderly, children, in pregnant women
    - As modified by other drugs and other illnesses
    - Relative to other drugs used for the same indication.
- New types of information not available from premarketing studies
    - Discovery of previously undetected adverse and beneficial effects.
        - Uncommon effects
        - Delayed effects
    - Patterns of drug utilization
    - The effects of drug overdoses
    - The economic implication of drug use.
- General contributions of pharmacoepidemiology
    - Reassurances about drug safety
    - Fulfillment of ethical and legal obligations.

Pharmacoepidemiology in Practice

The basic idea of pharmacoepidemiology is to measure the source, diffusion, use and effects of drugs in a population and to determine the frequency and distribution of drug outcomes in that population.

The focus of this type of research includes –

- What is being used (an assessment of specific drugs being used in certain situations)
- How it is being used (an assessment of the patterns of use, including how much, where and when, and by whom) and
- Why it is being used (an assessment of the reasons for drug-taking behaviors and the functions that drugs serve in society).

The World Health Organization focuses its pharmacoepidemiological efforts in ensuring the quality, safety, and efficacy of drugs and their use in specific populations. The organization's pharmacoepidemiological studies are performed to

- describe current patterns of drug use in specific patient populations
- determine changes in drug use over time
- measure the effects of information, education, promotional activities, media accounts and price on drug use
- detect inappropriate drug use and associated problems
- estimate drug needs in terms of disease patterns and outbreaks and
- Plan the selection, supply and distribution of drugs.

The research methods used most often by pharmacoepidemiologists are:

- the *cross sectional study* a prevalence survey of health and illness in the population at one point in time;
- *the case control study*, a retrospective analysis comparing subjects with the condition (cases) to those without it (controls) with respect to possible risk or causative factors; and
- *the cohort study*, an incidence study that follows a population free of health problems over time, examining subsequent development of problems and factors associated with them.
- *clinical trials*, an experimental approach that tests the value of a new treatment or intervention compared with a standard treatment or a placebo, are also considered to be an epidemiological method.

Many sources of data and information about drug taking behavior exist (Table19.1). Each source of data has its own unique advantages and limitations. Many studies report only frequencies of use without any basis in the population from which they are derived. Epidemiological measures are based on rates, with a numerator divided by a denominator. Reporting that 100 patients are experiencing an adverse reaction to a new drug (the numerator), without giving a sense of whether this effect is occurring in a population of 10000 or 1000000 users of that drug (the denominator) provides only marginally useful information. Denominator data are very important because, without them, comparisons are impossible.

Table 19.1 Sources of Data on Drug Use

Sources of Data on Drug Use
Institutional record systems and databases
Drug utilization studies
Hospital based medical audits (inpatient)
System wide databases
Institutionally based reviews (outpatient)
Health insurance groups and third party payers
Pharmaceutical organizations
Commercial vendors of marketing studies and sales data
National Databases
Government sponsored studies
Essential drug lists and inventory data
Pharmacoepidemiological surveillance systems
Field Data
Records of drug dispensers, sellers and distributors
Drug-taking behaviors of individuals and small groups
Experimental Data
Clinical trial results

Drug development and approval process are greatly dependent on data and information generated through epidemiological studies. Clinical trials test the value of drugs, such as the benefits of using propranolol to treat hypertension and other cardiovascular conditions. Post marketing surveillance detects and measures adverse drug reactions and other unintended effects after a drug product has been released to the market place. Relatively new efforts have been studying the benefits and costs of drug use in economic terms (pharmacoeconomics) and in terms of patient-centered care employing quality-of-life indicators.

The future of pharmacoepidemiological studies has unlimited potential. This field represents the primary scientific approach for the pharmacy profession's new mission in patient care. Its approaches and techniques for assessing the nature and extent of drug use and the reasons behind unsafe or irrational use allow the development of strategies to prevent or limit drug use problems (Table 19.2). With these tools, the products of drug development can be used more effectively, while minimizing problems, for the benefit of both individual patients and society.

Table 19.2 Problem solving with pharmacoepidemiology

Problem areas
Medical drug use
Beneficial effects of drug therapy
Risks (e.g., adverse reactions, side effects) of drug therapy
Inappropriate prescribing behaviors
Patient noncompliance
Irrational self medication practices
Poor drug use outcomes
Cost-effectiveness of drug therapy
Nonmedical drug use
Social – recreational drug use and associated problems
Acute incidents of drug toxicities (e.g., overdoses)
Chemical dependencies
Outbreaks and sources of drug epidemics

19.4 Study Designs Available for Pharmacoepidemiology Studies

Pharmacoepidemiology applies the methods of epidemiology to the content area of clinical pharmacology. To understand the methodologies and approaches specific to the field of pharmacoepidemiology, the basic principles of the field of epidemiology should be understood.

Overview of scientific method

The scientific method is a three stage process.

- In the first stage one studies a sample of study subjects.
- Second, one generalizes the information obtained in this sample of study subjects, drawing a conclusion about a population in general. This conclusion is referred to as an association.
- Third, one generalizes again, drawing a conclusion about scientific theory or causation.

Any given study is performed on a selection of individuals, who represent the study subjects. These study subjects should theoretically represent a random sample of defined population. For example, one might perform a randomized clinical trial of the efficacy of enalapril in lowering blood pressure, randomly allocating a total of 40 middle aged hypertensive men to receive either enalapril or placebo and observing their blood pressure six weeks later. One might expect to see the blood pressure of the 20 men treated with the active drug decrease more than the blood pressure of the 20 men treated with placebo. In this example, the 40 study subjects would represent the study sample, theoretically a random sample of middle aged hypertensive men. In reality, the study sample is almost never a true random sample of the underlying target population, because it is logically impossible to identify every individual who belongs in the target population and then randomly choose from among them. However, the study sample is usually treated as if it were a random sample of the target population.

At this point, one would be tempted to make a generalization that enalapril lowers blood pressure in middle aged hypertensive men. However, one must explore whether this observation could have occurred simply by chance that is due to random variation. If this were true, then the observation might not have been made if one had chosen a sample of 40 different study subjects. Perhaps more importantly, it might not exist if one were able to study the entire theoretical population of all middle aged hypertensive men. In order to evaluate this possibility, one can perform a statistical test, which allows an investigator to quantitate the probability that the difference seen between the two study groups could have happened simply by chance. There are explicit rules and procedures for how one should properly make this determination; the science of statistics. If the results of any study under consideration demonstrate a significant difference, then one is said to have an *association.* The process of assessing whether random variation could have led to study's findings is referred to as *statistical inference,* and represents the major role for statistical testing in the scientific method.

If there is no statistically significant difference then the process in figure 19.1 stops.

Study sample

↓ Statistical inference

Conclusion about a population

(association)

↓ Biological inference

Conclusion about scientific theory

(causation)

Fig. 19.1 Overview of the scientific method

If there is an association, then one is tempted to generalize the results of the study even further, to state that enalapril is an antihypertensive drug, in general. This is referred as *scientific or biological inference,* and the result is a conclusion about *causation,* that the drug really does lower blood pressure in a population of treated patients. To draw this type of conclusion, however, requires one to generalize to populations other than that included in the study, including types of people who were not represented in the study sample, such as women, children and the elderly. Although it may be obvious in this example that this in fact is appropriate, that may not always be the case. Unlike statistical inference, there are no precise quantitative rules for biological inference. Rather, one needs to examine the data at hand in light of all relevant data in the rest of the scientific literature, and make a subjective judgment. To assist in making that judgment, however, one can use the "Criteria for the casual nature of an association".

19.5 Types of Error in Performing a Study

There are four basic types of association that can be observed in a study. The basic purpose of research is to differentiate among them.

They are

- None (independent)
- Artifactual (spurious or false)
  - Chance (unsystematic variation)
  - Bias (systematic variation)
- Indirect (confounded)
- Casual (direct or true)

First, of course, one could have no association.

Second, one could have an artifactual association that is a spurious or false association. This can occur by either of two mechanisms: chance or bias. Chance is systematic or random variation. The other possible mechanism for creating an artifactual association is bias. Bias, here means a systematic variation, a consistent manner in which two study groups are treated or evaluated differently. This consistent difference can create an apparent association where one actually does not exist.

Third, one can have an indirect or confounded association. A *confounding variable, or confounder,* is a variable other than the risk factor and outcome under study which is related independently to both the risk factor and the outcome variable and which may create an apparent association or mask a real one. In designing a study, one must consider every variable which can be associated with the risk factor under study and the outcome variable under study, in order to plan to deal with it as a potential confounding variable. Preferably, one will be able to specifically control for the variable, using one of the following techniques –

- Random allocation
- Subject selection
  - Exclusion
  - Matching

- Data analysis
  - Stratification
  - Mathematical modeling

Fourth, and finally, there are true, casual associations.

Thus, there are three possible types of error that can be produced in a study:

- random error
- bias and
- confounding.

The probability of random error can be quantitated using statistics. Bias needs to be prevented by designing the study properly. Confounding can be controlled in either the design of the study or in its analysis. If all three types of error can be excluded, then one is left with a true, casual association.

19.6 Criteria for the Casual Nature of an Association

The criteria for casual nature of an association are mentioned below, in particular order. No one of them is absolutely necessary for an association to be a casual association. Analogously, no one of them is sufficient for an association to be considered a casual association. Essentially, the more criteria that are present, the more likely it is a casual association. The fewer criteria that are met, the less likely it is a casual association.

- *Coherence with existing information or biological plausibility*: This refers to whether the association makes sense, in light of other types of information available in the literature. These other types of information could include data from other human studies, data from studies of other related questions, data from animal studies, or data from *in vitro* studies, as well as scientific or pathophysiologic theory. For example, the association between cigarettes and lung cancer, cigarette smoking is a known carcinogen, based on animal data. In humans it is known to cause cancers of head, neck, pancreas, and the bladder. Cigarette smoke also goes down into the lungs, directly exposing the tissues in question. Thus, it certainly is biologically plausible that cigarettes could cause lung cancer. It is much more reassuring if an association found in a particular study makes sense, based on previously available information, and this makes one more comfortable that it might be a casual association.

- *Consistency of the association:* If a finding is real, we should be able to reproduce it in a different setting. This could include different geographical settings, different study designs, different populations, etc. The need for reproducibility is such that one should never believe a finding reported only once; there may have an error committed in the study which is not apparent to either the investigator or the reader.

- *Time sequence:* Time sequence says that a cause must precede an effect.
- *Specificity:* This refers to the question whether the cause ever occurs without the presumed effect and whether the effect ever occurs without the presumed cause. This criteria is almost never met in biology, with the occasional exception of infectious diseases. Measles never occurs without the measles virus, but even in this example not everyone who gets infected with the measles virus develops clinical measles. Certainly not everyone who smokes develops lung cancer, and not everyone who develops lung cancer was a smoker.
- *Strength of association:* This includes three concepts – quantitative strength, dose-response and the study design. The quantitative strength of an association refers to its size. A dose-response relationship is an extremely important and commonly used concept in clinical pharmacology and is used similarly in epidemiology. A dose response relationship exists when an increase in the intensity of an exposure results in an increased risk of the disease under study. Finally, study design refers to two concepts, whether the study was well designed and which study design was used in the studies in question.

19.7 Epidemiologic Study Designs

The epidemiologic study designs are of 6 types. They are

- Case reports
- Case series
- Analyses of secular trends
- Case-control study
- Cohort study
- Randomized clinical trial (experimental study)

Case reports: Case reports are simply reports of individual patients, as used in pharmacoepidemiology, a case report describes a patient who was exposed to a drug and experiences a particular, usually adverse, outcome. For example, one might see a published case report about a young woman who was taking oral contraceptives and who suffered a pulmonary embolism. Case reports are useful for raising hypothesis about drug effects, to be tested with more rigorous study designs. However, in a case report one cannot know if the patient reported is either typical of those with the exposure or typical of those with the disease. Certainly, one cannot usually determine whether the adverse outcome was due to the drug exposure or would have happened anyway. As such, it is very rare that a case report can be used to make a statement about causation. One exception to this would be when the outcome is so rare and so characteristic of the exposure that one knows that it was likely to be due to the drug exposure, even if the history of exposure were unclear. Another exception would be when the disease course is very predictable and the treatment causes a clearly apparent change in this disease course. Case reports can be particularly useful to document causation when the treatment causes a change in disease course which is reversible, such that the patient returns to his or her untreated state when the exposure is withdrawn, can be treated again, and when the change returns upon repeat treatment.

Case Series: Case series are collections of patients, all of whom have a single exposure, whose clinical outcomes are then evaluated and described. Often they are from a single hospital or medical practice. Alternatively, case series can be collection of patients with a single outcome, looking at their antecedent exposures. For example, one might observe 100 consecutive women under the age of 50 who suffer from a pulmonary embolism, and note that 30 of them had been taking oral contraceptives.

After drug marketing, case series are most useful for two related purposes. First, they can be useful for quantifying the incidence of an adverse reaction. Second, they can be useful for being certain that any particular adverse effect of concern does not occur in a population which is larger than that studied prior to drug marketing. In this type of study, one can be more certain that the patients are probably typical of those with the exposure or with the disease, depending on the focus of the study. However, in the absence of a control group, one cannot be certain which features in the description of the patients are unique to the exposure, or outcome.

Analyses of secular trends: Analysis of secular trends, also called "ecological studies", examine trends in an exposure that is a presumed cause and trends in a disease that is a presumed effect and test whether the trends coincide. These trends can be examined over time or across geographic boundaries. In other words, one could analyze data from a single region and examine how it changes over time, or one could analyze data from a single time period and compare how the data differ from region to region or country to country. Vital statistics are often used for these studies. As an example, one might look at sales data for oral contraceptives and compare them to death rates from venous thromboembolism, using recorded vital statistics. Analysis of secular trends is useful for rapidly providing evidence for or against an hypothesis. However, these studies lack data on individuals; they only study groups. As such, they are unable to control for confounding variables. Thus, among exposures whose trends coincide with that of the disease, analysis of secular trends is unable to differentiate which factor is likely to be the true cause.

Case- control studies: Case control studies are studies which compare cases with a disease with control, looking for differences in antecedent exposures. As an example, one could select cases of young women with venous thromboembolism and compare them with controls, looking for differences in antecedent oral contraceptive use. Case-control studies can be particularly useful when one wants to study multiple possible causes of a single disease, as one can study any number of exposures as potential risk factors using the same cases and controls. This design is also particularly useful when one is studying a relatively rare disease, as it guarantees a sufficient number of cases with the disease. Using case-control studies, one can study rare diseases with markedly smaller sample sizes than those needed for cohort studies. Case –control studies generally obtain their information on exposures retrospectively, that is recreating events that happened in the past. Information is generally obtained by abstracting medical records or by administering questionnaires or interviews. As such, they are subject to limitations in the validity of retrospectively collected exposure information. Also the proper selection of controls can be a challenging task, and inappropriate control selection can lead to selection bias, which may lead to incorrect conclusions. Nevertheless, when case-control studies are well done, subsequent well done cohort or randomized clinical trials, if any, will generally confirm their results. As such, the case-control design is a very useful one for pharmacoepidemiology studies.

Cohort studies: Cohort studies are studies which identify subsets of a defined population and follow them over time, looking for differences in their outcome. Cohort studies are generally used to compare exposed patients to unexposed patients, although they can also be used to compare one exposure to another. For example, one could compare women of reproductive age who use oral contraceptives to users of other contraceptive models, looking for the differences in the frequency of venous thromboembolism. Cohort studies can be performed either prospectively, that is simultaneous with the vents under study, or retrospectively, that is after the vents under study, by recreating those past events using medical records, questionnaires, or interviews. The major difference between the cohort and case control studies is the basis upon which patients are recruited into the study. Patients are recruited into case control studies on the basis of the presence or absence of a disease, and their antecedent exposures are then studied. Patients are recruited into cohort studies on the basis of the presence or absence of an exposure, and their subsequent disease course is then studied.

Cohort studies have the major advantage of being free of the major problem that plagues case control studies: the difficult process of selecting an undiseased control group. In addition, prospective cohort studies are free of the problem of the questionable validity of retrospectively collected data. For these reasons, an association demonstrated by a cohort study is more likely to be a casual association than one demonstrated by a case-control study. Furthermore, cohort studies are particularly useful when one is studying multiple possible outcomes from a single exposure, especially a relatively common unexposure. Thus, they are particularly useful in post-marketing surveillance studies which are looking at any possible effect of a newly marketed drug. However, cohort studies require extremely large sample sizes to study relatively uncommon outcomes. In addition, prospective cohort studies require a prolonged time period to study delayed drug effects.

Randomized Clinical Trials: Randomized clinical trials are experimental studies in which the investigator controls the therapy that is to be received by each participant. Generally an investigator uses that control to randomly allocate patients between or among the study groups, performing a randomized clinical trial. The major strength of this approach is random assignment, which is the only way to make it likely that the study groups are comparable in potential confounding variables that are either unknown or immeasurable. For theses reasons, associations demonstrated in randomized clinical trials are more likely to be casual associations than those demonstrated using one of the other techniques. Randomized clinical trials are expensive and artificial.

19.8 Reasons to Perform Pharmacoepidemiology Studies

The decision to conduct a pharmacoepidemiology study can be viewed as similar to the regulatory decision about whether to approve a drug for marketing or the clinical decision whether to prescribe a drug. In each case, decision making involves weighing the costs and risks of a therapy against its benefits.

The main costs of a pharmacoepidemiology study are obviously the costs of conducting the study itself. They clearly will vary, depending on the questions posed and the approach chosen to answer them. Regardless, with the exception of post marketing randomized clinical trials, the cost per patient is likely to be at least an order of magnitude less than the cost of a premarketing study. Other costs to consider are the opportunity costs of other research that might be left undone if this research is performed.

One risk of conducting a pharmacoepidemiology study is the possibility that it could identify an adverse outcome as associated with the drug under investigation when in fact the drug does not cause this adverse outcome. Another risk is that it could provide false reassurances about a drug's safety. Both of these can be minimized by appropriate study designs, skilled researchers, and appropriate and responsible interpretation of the results obtained.

The benefits of pharmacoepidemiology studies could be conceptualized in four different categories: regulatory, marketing, clinical and legal. Any given study will usually be performed for several of these reasons.

- Regulatory
  - Required
  - To obtain earlier approval for marketing
  - As a response to question by regulatory agency
  - To assist application for approval for marketing elsewhere.
- Marketing
  - To assist market penetration by documenting the safety of a drug.
  - To increase name recognition
  - To assist in repositioning the drug
    (i) Different outcomes, e.g., quality of life and economic
    (ii) Different types of patient, e.g., elderly
    (iii) New indications
    (iv) Less restrictive labeling
  - To protect the drug from accusations about adverse effects
- Legal
  - In anticipation of future liability litigation
- Clinical
  1. Hypothesis testing
     - Problem hypothesized on the basis of drug structure
     - Problem suspected on the basis of preclinical or premarketing human data
     - Problem suspected on the basis of spontaneous reports
     - Need to better quantitate the frequency of adverse reactions
  2. Hypothesis generating – need depends on whether
     - it is a new chemical entity
     - the safety profile of the class
     - the relative safety of the drug within its class
     - the formulation
     - the disease to be treated, including
       (i) its duration
       (ii) its prevalence
       (iii) its severity
       (iv) whether alternative therapies are available

Regulatory: The most clearest and compelling reason to perform a post marketing pharmacoepidemiology study is regulatory. A plan for a post marketing pharmacoepidemiology study is required before the drug will be approved for marketing.

Some post marketing studies of drugs arise in response to case reports of adverse reactions reported to the regulatory agency. One response to such a report might be to suggest a labeling change. Often a more appropriate response, clinically and commercially, would be to propose a pharmacoepidemiology study. This study would explore whether this adverse event in fact occurs more often in those exposed to the drug than would have been expected in the absence of the drug and, if so, how large the increased risk of the disease is. Finally, drugs are obviously marketed at different times in different countries. A post marketing pharmacoepidemiology study conducted in a country that marketed a drug relatively early could be useful in demonstrating the safety of the drug to regulatory agencies in countries that have not yet permitted the marketing of the drug. This is becoming increasingly feasible, as both the industry and the field of pharmacoepidemiology are becoming more international, and regulators are collaborating more.

Marketing: Generally pharmacoepidemiology studies are performed primarily to obtain the answers to clinical questions. However, it is clear that a major underlying reason for some pharmacoepidemiology studies is the potential marketing impact of those answers. Because of the known limitations in the information available about the effects of a drug at the time of its initial marketing, many physicians are appropriately hesitant to prescribe a drug until a substantial amount of experience in its use has been gathered. A formal post marketing surveillance study can speed that process, as well as clarify any advantages or disadvantages a drug has compared to its competitors.

A pharmacoepidemiology study can also be useful to improve product name recognition. The fact that a study is underway will often be known to prescribers, as will its results once it is publicly presented and published. This increased name recognition will presumably help sales. Pharmacoepidemiology studies can also be useful to re-position a drug that is already on the market, i.e., to develop new markets for the drug. Finally, and perhaps most importantly, pharmacoepidemiology studies can be useful to protect the major investment made in developing and testing a new drug. When a question arises about a drug's toxicity, it often needs an immediate answer, or else the drug may lose market share or even be removed from the market. Immediate answers are often unavailable, unless the manufacturer had the foresight to perform pharmacoepidemiology studies in anticipation of the problem.

Legal: Post-marketing surveillance studies can theoretically be useful as legal prophylaxis, in anticipation of eventually having to defend against product liability suits. All drugs cause adverse effects; the regulatory decision to approve a drug and the clinical decision to prescribe a drug both depend on a judgment about the relative balance between the benefits of a drug and its risks. From a legal perspective, to win a product liability suit using legal theory of negligence, a plaintiff must prove causation, damages, and negligence. However, when a manufacturer conducts pharmacoepidemiology studies and document that it was performing state-of-the-art studies to attempt to detect whatever toxic effects the drug had. In addition, such studies could make easier the defense of totally groundless suits, in which a drug is blamed for producing adverse reactions it does not cause.

Clinical

- Hypothesis testing- The major reason for most pharmacoepidemiology studies is hypothesis testing. The hypothesis to be tested can be based on the structure or the chemical class of a drug. Alternatively, hypothesis can also be based on premarketing or post marketing animal or clinical findings. For example, the hypothesis can come from spontaneous reports of adverse events experienced by patients taking the drug in question. Finally, an adverse event may clearly be due to a drug, but a study may be needed to quantitate its frequency.
- Hypothesis Generating- Hypothesis generating studies are intended to screen for previously unknown and unsuspected drug effects. In principle, all drugs could, and perhaps should, be subjected to such studies. However, some drugs may require these studies more than others. For example, it is generally agreed that new chemical entities are more in need of study than so called "me too" drugs. This is because the lack of experience with related drugs makes it more likely that the drug has possibly important unsuspected effects.

The safety profile of the drugs should also be important to the decision about whether to conduct a formal screening post marketing surveillance study. Previous experience with other drugs in the same class can be a useful predictor of what the experience with the drug in question is likely to be.

The relative safety of the drug within its class can also be helpful. A drug that has been studied in large numbers of patients before marketing and appears safe is less likely to need supplementary post marketing surveillance studies.

The disease to be treated is an important determinant of whether a drug needs additional post marketing surveillance studies. Drugs used to treat chronic illnesses are likely to be used for along period of time. As such, it is important to know their long term effects. This cannot be addressed adequately in the relatively brief time available for each pre-marketing study. Drugs used to treat common diseases are important to study, as many patients are likely to be exposed to them. Drugs used to treat mild or self-limited diseases also need careful study, because serious toxicity is less acceptable.

Conclusion

Pharmacoepidemiology is a rapidly expanding field of practice. Pharmacists can apply pharmacoepidemiological methods to their practice to measure the use and effects of drugs. Adverse drug reaction surveillance can be expanded to include not only spontaneous reports but also case-control studies using medical record review or computerized databases to quantify the relationship between drugs and adverse events. Clinical pharmacists collecting information about individual patients can systematically collect information about groups or populations of patients and then analyze the data for trends. Pharmacoeconomic analyses can be included in formulary decision making and disease-state management to determine the value of drug therapies.

Study Outline

Pharmacoepidemiology may be defined as the study of the utilization and effects of drugs in large number of people. The term pharmacoepidemiology contains two components. "Pharmaco" and "epidemiology". It is a combination of clinical pharmacology and epidemiology.

The potential contributions of pharmacoepidemiology are significant. The contributions made by pharmacoepidemiology are:

- Information which supplements that is available from premarketing studies – better quantitation of the incidence of known adverse and beneficial effects.
- New types of information not available from premarketing studies

Various types of study designs that are useful for pharmacoepidemiological studies are

- Case reports
- Case series
- Analysis of secular trends
- Case-control study
- Cohort study
- Randomized clinical trial

The pharmacoepidemiology studies are conducted for the following reasons

- Regulatory requirements
- Marketing needs
- Legal
- Clinical

CHAPTER 20

Clinical Laboratory Tests and Their Significance

Objectives

After completing this chapter, the reader should be able to understand the:

- Need for the laboratory tests
- Different tests performed on blood, urine, CSF, feces or other tests
- Normal values of different components
- Interpretation of different biochemical constituents
- Various tests used to assess the function of Liver, Kidney, Lungs and Thyroid gland

20.1 Introduction

Laboratory tests play a significant role in the total therapy of the patient. The physician bases his diagnosis, prognosis and treatment on data collected from the history of the patient, from the physical examination and from laboratory procedures. Common laboratory tests performed in a hospital are discussed in this chapter which can assist a pharmacist practicing in a hospital. When a pharmacist has an understanding of the significance of the various laboratory procedures he can adequately relate drug therapy to laboratory test results. In this chapter we discuss the significance of common laboratory tests and also various tests that are commonly employed to assess the function of Liver, Kidney, Lungs, and Thyroid gland.

20.2 Common Laboratory Tests

Common laboratory tests that are normally performed are discussed here in the following order.

- Tests performed on blood
- Tests performed on urine
- Tests performed on feces
- Miscellaneous tests

Normal values and their interpretations are presented in appendix. The normal value range will vary from one institution to another depending upon the individual differences of the laboratory personnel and the laboratory equipment.

20.3 Tests Performed on Blood

Blood is a fluid which is representative of the whole body and is composed of a fluid portion, the plasma, in which are suspended the formed elements (red cells, platelets, and white cells). The type and number of circulating cells in blood uniquely changes in response to various stimuli. Many of the changes in response to disease are nonspecific; however, there is usually some deviation from normal in one of the measurable constituents in almost all diseases. This explains why most of the diagnostic laboratory tests currently used is entitled "blood tests".

Tests performed on the blood may be divided into three general areas.

(a) Clinical chemistry tests

(b) Haematologic tests

(c) Miscellaneous tests

(a) *Clinical Chemistry Tests*

The majority of chemical determinations are done on whole blood, plasma or serum. Some of the factors that influence the chemical composition of blood in diseases are alterations of permeability of membranes of the lungs, kidneys, and liver; accumulation of nitrogenous waste products; changes in the rate of formation or metabolism of these constituents; and the administration of certain drugs. One of the most valuable instruments in the clinical laboratory is the 12-channel SMA-12 Auto Analyzer. This machine analyzes and prints on calibrated paper the levels of twelve blood constituents from a single serum specimen (*i.e.,* glucose, total bilirubin, albumin, alkaline phosphatase, urea nitrogen, uric acid, cholesterol, lactic dehydrogenase, total protein, glutamic oxaloacetic transaminase, calcium and inorganic phosphate).

- ***Albumin and Globulin; Total Protein, A/G Ratio:*** The normal range of albumin is 4-5.5 g %; for globulin, 1.5-3 g %; for total protein 6-8 g %; and the albumin-globulin (A/G) ratio is usually between 1.5:1 and 2.5:1. These tests are usually performed together. They may be useful in the diagnosis of kidney, liver, and some other diseases. The main function of the serum albumin appears to be the maintenance of osmotic pressure of the blood. One of the functions of serum globulin is to assist in maintaining the osmotic pressure of the blood. Since the globulin molecule is several times as large as the albumin molecule, it is less efficient, gram for gram, in maintaining osmotic pressure. In certain diseases, the albumin may leak out of capillary walls while the larger globulin molecules are retained within the blood stream. The body may then compensate for loss of albumin by producing more globulin so that the globulin becomes responsible for a larger share of the osmotic pressure. Despite normal or even increased total dissolved protein in the serum, osmotic pressure may be less than normal because of the lesser effectiveness of globulin and result in edema.

  In haemoconcentration due to dehydration from vomiting or diarrhea, the total protein increases and both the albumin and globulin increases in the same proportions so that the A/G ratio is unchanged. Globulins are increased in severe liver disease, multiple myeloma and certain infectious diseases.

  A low albumin level is caused by increased loss of albumin in the urine, decreased formation or decreased protein intake. Severe hemorrhage may cause low serum protein levels because following the hemorrhage, the plasma volume is restored more quickly than the protein level. Conditions in which the albumin-globulin ratio is lowered are chronic nephritis, lipid nephrosis, liver disease, amyloid nephrosis and malnutrition.

- ***Acid Phosphatase:*** This is a test to determine metastasis carcinomas of the prostate. Normally, small amounts of acid phosphatase are found in the serum. *A metastasizing prostate carcinoma releases the enzyme into the serum and increases the serum concentration markedly. Other conditions which produce elevated serum acid phosphatase levels include: Paget's disease, hyperparathyroidism, metastatic mammary carcinoma, multiple myeloma, renal insufficiency, osteogenesis imperfecta, thrombocytosis, arterial embolism, myocardial infarction, thrombophlebitis, pulmonary embolism, and sickle-cell crisis.*

- ***Alkaline Phosphatase:*** Alkaline phosphatase is present in high concentration in bone, and serum levels are elevated in growing children and in diseases associated with increased osteoblastic activity. There is normally a small amount of alkaline phosphatase in the serum. Since alkaline phosphatase is excreted into the bile, *serum levels are increased in liver diseases associated with intrahepatic or extra hepatic obstruction of the biliary passages.* Alkaline phosphatase elevation precedes bilirubin accumulation in early obstruction. *Obstruction of the common duct causes mild elevation, but obstruction of the smaller biliary ducts causes far higher levels.* The highest levels of all occur with primary biliary cirrhosis while ascending cholangitis and cholestatic hepatitis cause more moderate changes. Changes are relatively slight in infectious hepatitis and nonbiliary cirrhosis. *The levels are also elevated in hyperparathyroidism, osteitis deformans, osteomalacia, Gouch-s disease, rickets, healing fractures, hyperthyroidism (Grave's disease), leukemia, after the administration of large amounts of vitamin D and in pregnancy.*

- ***Ammonia:*** Ammonia is normally produced by bacterial action in the intestine and absorbed to the portal venous system. Most of the ammonia is removed from the portal circulation by the liver and converted into urea. As a result, *the ammonia levels rise in severe liver disease*. Blood ammonia determinations are used for evaluating the progress of severe liver damage.

- ***Bilirubin Partition (Direct and Indirect vanden Bergh Test):*** Bilirubin circulates in the blood in low concentrations. A small amount is directly excreted into the urine. The majority is excreted into the bile by the liver cells and passes into the intestines where it is bacterially reduced to urobilinogen. Urobilinogen is primarily excreted in the feces; however, some is reabsorbed into the blood and re-excreted by the liver as bilirubin or urobilinogen. The kidneys also excrete a small amount of absorbed urobilinogen into the urine. Bilirubin is formed from hemoglobin of destroyed erythrocytes by the reticuloendothelial system and is normally found enroute to the liver for excretion. When the ability of the liver to excrete bilirubin is impaired by obstruction, it is believed that the excess circulating bilirubin is free of any attached protein; However, when the increase in circulating bilirubin is due to increased destruction of red blood cells (hemolysis), it is believed that the bilirubin is bound to protein. By measuring the amount of free bilirubin (direct) and the amount bound to protein (indirect), there is some indication as to whether the patient's illness is based on obstruction or hemolysis. If most of the bilirubin is found on the direct test, the patient probably has an obstructive lesion. If most is found on the indirect test, the illness is probably hemolytic.

- ***Bilirubin Total:*** When the destruction of red blood cells becomes excessive or when the liver is unable to secrete the ordinary quantities of bilirubin produced, the concentration in the serum rises. This test enables one to discover an increased concentration of serum bilirubin before jaundice appears.

- ***Blood Sugar:*** The concentration of sugar (glucose) in the blood is maintained within a narrow range by four general mechanisms: (1) ability of the intestine to absorb glucose, (2) skeletal muscle mass, (3) ability of the liver to store and metabolize glycogen, and (4) production and release of insulin by the pancreas. Routine blood sugar determinations are performed on whole blood specimens and if plasma or serum is used, values will be higher by approximately 20 mg/100 ml than for whole blood. In evaluating a blood sugar level, it is important to consider whether venous or capillary blood was used because after a glucose load, the capillary blood levels are approximately 40 mg/100 ml higher than those of venous blood. It is also important to consider whether the patient is receiving an intravenous glucose supplement.

- ***Fasting Blood Sugar (FBS):*** The blood glucose concentration rises following a meal and it is therefore essential that this test be run on fasting blood specimens rather than random samples, the test requires that the patient has not eaten for at least eight hours so that digestion is completed. It is for this reason that the blood specimen is usually drawn in the morning before breakfast. The "fasting state" signifies that the patient has not eaten any food including cream, sugar, tea, cola drinks or drugs that affect the blood glucose level, and has not experienced emotional disturbances that may release glucose into the blood. *Blood glucose levels are elevated in diabetes mellitus; hyperactivity of the thyroid, pituitary, and adrenal glands; pancreatitis; pancreatic carcinoma; meningitis; encephalitis; hemorrhage; and following administration of anesthetics. Blood glucose levels are lowered in hypothyroidism (myxedema and cretinism), hypopituitarism, hypoadrenalism, glycogen storage disease, and overtreatment of diabetes with insulin.*

- ***Glucose Tolerance Test:*** The glucose tolerance test usually gives more information than can be derived from a fasting blood sugar. This test is intended to assist in the diagnosis of doubtful or borderline cases of diabetes, but has no quantitative significance to severity of the diabetes or insulin requirement. Blood specimens are taken fasting and half hour, 2 hours and 3 hours after ingestion of a predetermined amount of glucose. After ingestion and a lag period, the blood sugar curve rises sharply to a peak, usually in 15-60 minutes. The curve then falls steadily, but more slowly, reaching normal levels at 2 hours. It is assumed that the subsequent rise and fall of the blood sugar is due mainly to production of insulin in response to hyperglycemia and that the degree of insulin response is mirrored in the behavior of thc blood glucosc.

  The intravenous test is somewhat more sensitive than the oral since the factor of absorption from the gastrointestinal tract is not involved and is of valuc in conditions characterized by poor intestinal absorption or vomiting after glucose ingestion. *An increase in the blood level after glucose ingestion (a diminished glucose tolerance) is most commonly seen in diabetes mellitus.*

- ***Blood Urea Nitrogen (BUN):*** Urea is the chief end product of protein metabolism and is the chief component of nonprotein nitrogenous material in the blood. From its hepatic origin, urea travels through the blood to the kidneys for urinary excretion. In certain kidney disorders the ability to excrete urea may be impaired so that the concentration of urea nitrogen in the blood increases. The protein content of the diet will also influence the quantity of urea in the blood since the concentration of urea is directly related to protein metabolism. *Uremia* is the term for the condition in which urea is found in the blood in increased amounts. *The most common cause of elevated BUN values is renal disease, either acute or chronic. Other causes of elevated BUN values include urinary obstruction, intestinal obstruction, lead poisoning, cardiac failure, and conditions characterized by increased protein catabolism (i.e., burns with subsequent fluid loss, massive hemorrhage, infarction, pancreatitis, severe diabetic ketoacidosis and far-advanced carcinoma).*

- ***Calcium:*** Approximately one-half of the serum calcium is combined with proteins in the serum and the remainder is in a diffusible form. *Elevated levels of calcium are found in hyperparathyroidism, excessive administration of vitamin D, and multiple myeloma. Low values are found in hypoparathyroidism, rickets, osteomalacia, steatorrhea, and advanced renal failure.*

- ***Carbon dioxide Content and Combining Power:*** Carbon dioxide may be determined as the CO_2 content which is the actual plasma or serum content when analyzed anaerobically, or as the CO_2 combining power which is the CO_2 content of the plasma after equilibration with a gas of fixed carbon dioxide partial pressure of 40 mm. These tests estimate the plasma bicarbonate which is used to measure the acid-base balance of the body. Changes in CO_2 combining power do not always represent changes in pH of the blood since the latter depends on the ratio and not on the absolute amounts of basic and acidic substances. Measurement of the CO_2 combining power does not require anaerobic handling of blood specimens; however, the results are less accurate than measurement of total CO_2. An increase in CO_2 combining power is usually a manifestation of alkalosis while a decrease is usually a manifestation of acidosis. *High CO_2 combining power is usually found in excessive vomiting; drainage of the stomach with loss of hydrochloric acid; excessive sodium bicarbonate intake in the presence of poor kidney function; excessive administration of ACTH or cortisone; and hypoventilation. Low CO_2 combining power is usually found in diabetic acidosis, severe diarrhea or drainage of intestinal fluids, certain kidney diseases and hyperventilation.*

- ***Chloride:*** Chloride is an anion of the extra cellular fluid and is found in serum plasma, cerebrospinal fluid, tissue fluid, and urine. The test for chloride is routinely performed on plasma or serum and not on the whole blood since two-thirds of the anion is present in the plasma and only one-third in the red blood cells. Chlorides are involved in the maintenance of normal osmotic relationships, acid-base balance, and water balance of the body. There is a reciprocal relationship between the chloride and bicarbonate anions of the extra cellular fluid. *A decrease in blood chlorides (hypochloremia) is seen in diabetic acidosis, Addison's disease, heat exhaustion, excessive vomiting and diarrhea and following certain surgical procedures. An elevation in blood chlorides (hypochloremia) is seen in Cushing's syndrome, complete renal shutdown, hyperventilation and de hydration.*

- ***Cholesterol:*** The liver excretes esterified cholesterol into the plasma. Normally, one-half to three-quarters of the serum cholesterol is present in esterified form and a decline in the percentage of esters signifies hepatocellular disease, notably acute hepatitis and active cirrhosis. *Hypercholesteremia, with a normal percentage of esters accompanies obstructive jaundice, diabetes mellitus, hypothyroidism, and the nephrotic syndrome. A low level of total cholesterol, with a normal percentage of esters, accompanies hyperthyroidism and chronic malnutrition.*

- ***Creatinine:*** Creatinine is derived from muscle creatinine and phosphocreatine. Creatine in muscle is phosphorylated to phosphocreatine which is an important compound for storing muscular energy. When energy is needed for metabolic processes, phosphocreatine is broken down to creatinine. The quantity of creatine converted to creatinine is related directly to the total body muscle mass and is unaffected by variations in the rate of protein catabolism. Creatinine is exited primarily by glomerular filtration and when the filtration rate falls, the serum creatinine level rises. *An elevated blood creatinine level is usually indicative of depressed renal function.*

- ***Lactic Dehydrogenase (LDH):*** This test is used in the diagnosis of myocardial infarction. Lactic hydrogenases are enzymes found in serum and in several organs including the heart. Therefore, an increase in levels of lactic dehydrogenase is not specific but in conjunction with other tests it can help diagnose the presence of myocardial infarction. After an infarction occurs, the serum level rises in 6-12 hours and persists 1-3 weeks. *The lactic dehydrogenase is elevated in myocardial infarction, acute leukemia, malignant lymphoma, megaloblastic anemia, sickle-cell anemia, liver disease and extensive carcinomas.*

- ***Magnesium:*** *A* magnesium deficiency results in a state of tetany which in appearance is indistinguishable from the tetany of low calcium. *Serum magnesium levels are increased in acute and chronic renal disease, liver disease, and idiabetic coma. The levels are decreased in Addison's disease, malabsorption syndrome, diarrhea, chronic alcoholism and occasionally in pancreatitis.*

- ***Non-Protein Nitrogen (NPN):*** This is a kidney function test. Approximately half of the non-protein nitrogen is usually urea which is normally excreted by the kidney. The remainder consists of amino acids, ammonia, creatine, creatinine and uric acid. When kidney function is markedly diminished, the urea and therefore, the nonprotein nitrogen level in the blood rises. This measurement is less accurate than the urea nitrogen test. *Non-protein nitrogen levels are elevated in conditions of decreased kidney function, eclampsia, and hepatic failure.*

- ***P^H:*** The normal blood pH ranges from 7.35-7.45. *The blood pH is elevated in hypoventilation, severe diarrhea, Addison's disease, and diabetic acidosis. The blood pH is lowered in Cushing's syndrome, hyperventilation, and excessive vomiting.*

- ***Phosphorous, Inorganic:*** Phosphorus in the blood exists as (1) inorganic phosphorus, (2) lipid phosphorus, and (3) organic or ester phosphorus. Determinations are usually made only of inorganic phosphorus and of lipid phosphorus. The concentration of calcium in the serum and body fluids tends to vary inversely with the concentration of inorganic phosphorus. *The inorganic phosphate level is increased in severe kidney disease, hypoparathyroidism, acromegaly, and excessive vitamin D intake. Phosphorus levels are decreased in rickets and hyperparathyroidism.*

- ***Potassium:*** Potassium is essentially an intracellular cation, and the extracellular concentration is approximately the same as that in the blood. The serum potassium concentration is often not an accurate measurement of intracellular potassium and a patient may have a potassium deficiency even when the serum potassium is normal. For practical purposes, potassium depletion may be suspected from abnormally low serum potassium in combination with characteristic electrocardiogram changes or the presence of alkalosis. *A marked decrease in serum potassium may cause cardiac arrythmias and muscle weakness. A marked increase in serum potassium produces a series of electrocardiographic changes and arrythmias. There may also be depression, lethargy and coma. The only common situation of high potassium values is renal shutdown with failure to produce adequate urine quantities and, therefore, an inability to excrete enough potassium.*

  Increased serum potassium levels may be found in conditions of severe cell damage and destruction, adrenal cortical deficiency and hypoventilation. Decreased serum potassium levels occur in severe diarrhea, periodic familial paralysis, chronic kidney disease, hyper function of the adrenal cortex and following the administration of insulin and glucose in diabetes without supplementary potassium. Besides being produced by alkalosis, hypokalemia can itself lead to or cause a tendency toward alkalosis. Potassium depletion usually caused by the use of diuretic agents or electrolyte manipulations may sensitize the heart to digitalis glycosides and may produce arrythmias.

- ***Serum Transaminases:*** Transaminases are enzymes that catalyze the transfer of an amino group from an amino acid to an alpha keto acid. Organs in which transaminases are normally found are heart, liver, muscle, kidney and pancreas. In certain disease conditions in which cells are damaged, the transaminases leak from the damaged cells and the serum levels are thus elevated. The most commonly measured transaminases are the serum glutamic oxaloacetic transaminase (SGOT) and the serum glutamic pyruvic transaminase (SGPT). Elevations of serum transaminase levels are not specific. Because there are several transaminases in each type of cell, there are likely to be serum elevations of more than one type of transaminase when an organ is damaged. To be of value, the levels must be compared with the results of the physical examination and other laboratory tests.

- ***Serum Glutamic Oxaloacetic Transaminase (SGOT):*** Glutamic oxaloacetic transaminase (GOT) is present in large quantities in the liver, heart, kidneys and skeletal muscles. *Acute destruction of any of these tissues (especially heart and liver tissues) results in a rise in the serum level of this enzyme.* The test is useful in the diagnosis of myocardial infarction. The peak level is usually readied about 24 hours after infarction and returns to normal by approximately the fifth day. In acute hepatitis, SGOT levels may be elevated 10-100 times normal and remain elevated for relatively long periods of time. In extra hepatic obstruction, there is no elevation unless secondary parenchymal acute damage is present. In cirrhosis, SGOT may or may not be abnormal and depends upon the degree of hepatic decompensation of cell necrosis.

- ***Serum Glutamic Pyruvic Transaminase (SGPT):*** Glutamic pyruvic transaminase (GPT) is an enzyme found mainly in the liver. *It is elevated in liver disease but is less sensitive than the SGOT* and apparently requires somewhat more extensive or severe acute parenchymal damage to give abnormal values. It has the advantage of being relatively specific for liver cell damage. It usually returns to normal levels before the SGOT. *In cases of hepatitis, SGPT levels rise higher than SGOT levels and fall slowly reaching normal levels in about 2-3 months, unless complications occur.*

  The major clinical value of the test appears to be in the differential diagnosis of jaundice. If the jaundice is caused by disease in the liver itself, SGPT levels are likely to be considerably higher than 300 units. If the jaundice results from a condition outside the liver, the SGPT levels are likely to be less than 300 units.

  NOTE: *Cephalin Flocculation.* Both the SGOT and SGPT, if elevated, do so before the cephalin flocculation becomes abnormal but they both return to normal ranges considerably in advance of the cephalin flocculation. This explains why the cephalin flocculation sometimes will be abnormal in the presence of normal enzyme studies, due either to a minimal amount of hepatocellular damage or from obtaining the tests after the enzymes had returned to normal. In general, the cephalin flocculation is less sensitive than the SGOT, but is elevated longer and is more specific for acute hepatic cell destruction. If the SGOT is normal or only minimally elevated, the cephalin flocculation is valuable as a means to confirm acute liver cell damage. If the SGOT is elevated, there usually is little use in getting a cephalin flocculation.

- ***Sodium:*** Sodium is the chief cation of the plasma and is involved in the maintenance of osmotic pressure and acid-base balance. The sodium concentration of the plasma is maintained within a very narrow range. *Increased serum sodium levels are found in markedly restricted water intake and administration of excessive amounts of sodium. Decreased serum sodium levels are found in pregnancy, pyloric obstruction, severe nephritis, Addison's disease, diarrhea, and heat exhaustion.*
- ***Total Protein:*** *See* Albumin Globulin
- ***Urea Nitrogen:*** *See* Blood Urea Nitrogen
- ***Uric Acid:*** Uric acid is the end product of purine metabolism and is formed from the break down of cell nucleic acids. The main excretory pathway of uric acid is the kidney. Different micro puncture studies have shown that there is initially total clearance of uric acid at the glomerular level. This is followed by almost total tubular reabsorption through an active transport mechanism. The amount excreted equals the amount filtered. A second route of uric acid excretion is the gastrointestinal mucosa.

  Blood uric acid levels are usually increased in conditions characterized by excessive cell breakdown and catabolism of nucleic acids. Blood uric acid levels are elevated in gout, excessive exposure to roentgen rays, multiple myeloma, and leukemia, toxemia of pregnancy, chronic glomerulonephritis, and Fanconi syndrome.

(b) *Haematologic Tests*

Several haematologic tests are required as a part of the physical examinations performed by a physician in either his office or in the hospital. There are two primary sources of blood for laboratory tests: (1) peripheral or capillary blood and (2) venous blood. There is no significant difference between cell counts performed on venous blood or capillary blood as long as the samples are freely flowing. When several haematologic procedures are necessitated, it is more practical to collect the blood from a vein rather than a finger. If the blood sample is collected by venipuncture, an anticoagulant must be added to the specimen to prevent coagulation. Two anticoagulants which prevent coagulation by binding the calcium and which are suitable for most haematologic tests are: (1) balanced oxalate which is a mixture of ammonium and potassium oxalate and (2) Sequestrene which is disodium ethylene diamine tetra acetate or EDTA.

- ***Bleeding Time Tests:*** The Ivy bleeding time test and the Duke bleeding time test are the two commonly performed bleeding time tests. These tests measure the time necessary for active bleeding to cease from a clean, superficial wound. The main disadvantage in performing these tests is in the production of an adequate and standardized skin puncture. The bleeding time is influenced by the number and functional activity of platelets, ability of tissue constituents to initiate or accelerate clotting, elasticity of the skin and the capillary tonus. Defects in the coagulation process have little effect on the bleeding time and bleeding time is not equivalent to coagulation time. *The bleeding time is prolonged in conditions characterized by poor capillary retraction and platelet deficiency. The bleeding test is positive in thrombocytopenic purpura, thrombasthenia, von Willebrand's disease, thrombocytopathia and constitutional capillary inferiority. The bleeding time is normal in hemophilia.*
- ***Blood Counts***

  Any blood cell count is done on a small sample of whole blood (generally capillary blood). The procedures used for enumeration of the formed elements of the blood utilize microscopic techniques. The blood sample is first diluted to an appropriate volume and using either an electronic cell counter or a manual method, the various formed elements are counted to obtain the number of cells in 1 mm^3 of whole blood.

  Platelet count: Platelets are involved in coagulation of the blood and normal hemostasis. A decrease in the number of platelets may signify a generalized bleeding tendency and a prolonged bleeding time. *An increase in the number of platelets may characterize a tendency toward thrombosis. Thrombocytopenia (a decrease in platelets) occurs in thrombocytopenic purpura, aplastic anemia, Goucher's disease, and septicemia. Thrombocytosis (an increase in platelets) occurs in polycythemia, certain types of anemia, fractures, chronic myelogenous leukemia, rheumatic fever, and with some drug therapies used in the treatment of leukemia.*

  Red blood cell count: The erythrocytes contain hemoglobin which is the essential oxygen carrier of the blood. The significance of the red-cell count is limited since it may be normal in hypochromic anemias and thalassemia. The hematocrit or hemoglobin should be determined to detect the presence of anemia. If anemia is diagnosed, the red-cell count is valuable in determining the red-cell corpuscular values. *A decrease in red blood cells may result from hemorrhage or one of the anemias. (Anemia can also be caused by decreased blood cell or hemoglobin formation.) An increase in red blood cells may indicate polycythemia or hemoconcentration.*

Reticulocyte count: Reticulocytes are immature red blood cells which show basophilic reticulum under vital staining. *This test gives some indication of bone marrow activity.* If there is red cell loss through bleeding or hemolysis, erythropoiesis becomes more active and the number of circulating reticulocytes increases. In conditions of blood loss, absence of an elevated reticulocyte count indicates bone marrow hypo-function. *This test is often used to evaluate the response to anemia therapy.*

White cell differential count: There are several kinds of white blood cells (leukocytes) which can be identified microscopically. The proportions of these various types of cells in the blood may have direct attention to a particular group of diseases. The differential count consists of identification and counting of a minimum of 100 white blood cells. The number of different white cells recorded is an estimate of the approximate percentages of white cells comprising the total white blood cell count.

Neutrophils comprise approximately 60 to 70 percent of the total number of leukocytes in adults. The neutrophils (neutral staining multinucleated cells) are increased in most bacterial infections, neoplasms, drug and chemical intoxications (especially in poisonings with liver damage), and acute hemorrhage. Neutrophilia is a term designating an increase in the absolute number of neutrophils. *Decreased neutrophil counts accompany vitamin B and folic acid deficiencies, disseminated lupus erythematosus, anaphylaxis and disorders associated with splenomegaly, bone marrow damage (due to aplastic anemia, irradiation or drug idiosyncrasy).*

The ***eosinophils*** (acid staining multinucleated cells) comprise 2-4 percent of the total number of leukocytes. *The eosinophils are increased in parasitic infestations and allergic conditions, and in the Thorn test for studying the adrenal response to ACTH.*

The ***basophils*** (basic staining multinucleated cells) comprise 0-1 percent of the total leukocytes. *The basophils may be increased in some blood dyscrasias. Basophil counts are used to study allergic reactions.*

The ***lymphocytes*** comprise 22-30 percent of the total leukocytes. *The lymphocytes may be increased (lymphocytosis) in measles, whooping cough, infectious mononucleosis, infectious lymphocytosis, brucellosis, typhoid fever, syphilis, agammaglobulinemia, hepatitis, herpes zoster, herpes simplex, chickenpox, and chronic exposure to irradiation. The lymphocytes may be* *decreased (lymphopenia) in myelocytic leukemia, Hodgkin's disease, lupus erythematosus, and acute irradiation syndrome.*

The ***monocytes*** comprise 4-8 percent of the total leukocytes and are phagocytic. *The monocytes may be increased (monocytosis) during recovery from severe infections, Hodgkin's disease and lipoid storage diseases.*

- ***Clotting Time (Coagulation Time):*** This is a test which measures the length of time required for a sample of venous blood to clot. The whole blood clotting time is a measure of the time required to form intrinsic thromboplastin. Deficiencies of any factor in the intrinsic clotting scheme or in the common phase commencing with Factor X may prolong the clotting time, as may fibrinogen deficiency or presence of a circulating anticoagulant. The clotting time is difficult to standardize and demonstrates only gross abnormalities of hemostasis. *A prolonged clotting time indicates that a problem exists, but a normal clotting time does not ensure that hemostasis is normal. The whole blood clotting time is used to control heparin therapy.*

- ***Coombs' Test Direct:*** This is also known as a direct antiglobulin test. It is an immunologic procedure which reveals antigen-antibody reactions that are incomplete or weak. Coomb's serum is added to a preparation of red blood cells which is coated with antibody. Antibodies to human red cells may damage or increase the fragility of red blood cells without causing visible agglutination. This test is used early in diagnosis of erythroblastosis fetalis, autoimmune hemolytic anemia, and the cross-matching of blood for patients with a high risk of transfusion reaction. *A positive test indicates that some antibody is attached to the red cells, but does not indicate the exact nature of the antibody.*

- ***Coombs' Test, Indirect:*** This test is used in the detection of various minor blood-type factors including Rh antibodies. It is thereby possible to eliminate bloods which might cause reactions because of incompatibilities of the minor blood-type factors.

- ***Erythrocyte Sedimentation Rate (ESR):*** The erythrocyte sedimentation rate is a method of measuring the rate at which red cells settle to the bottom of a glass test tube. When blood is anticoagulated and allowed to settle, sedimentation of the erythrocytes occurs. The rate of sedimentation depends upon the number of erythrocytes, the size of the erythrocytes, and certain technical factors. Fibrinogen and globulin increases the tendency of the red cells to aggregate and to form rouleaux. *The increase in the sedimentation rate is primarily a measure of the degree of rouleaux formation.* The test is non-specific but can (1) supply objective evidence of disease at a time when other signs are lacking. This would suggest that more specific information be sought. (2) The ESR can serve as a measure of the intensity of tissue destruction or repair since the rate of sedimentation reflects the degree to which these processes are active. *The ESR is* *increased in almost all infections, in most cases of carcinoma, severe anemia, active tuberculosis, rheumatoid arthritis, and acute coronary thrombosis.* The ESR slowly returns to normal as patients recover from infectious diseases. *The ESR is decreased when the plasma fibrinogen level is decreased, i.e., severe liver diseases, polycythemia, sickle cell anemia and congestive heart failure.*

- ***Haematocrit (HCT):*** The haematocrit is the percentage of red-cell mass to original blood volume. After centrifugation of anticoagulated whole blood the percentage of packed red cells gives an indirect estimate of the number of red blood cells per 100 ml of whole blood. This in turn is an indirect estimate of the amount of hemoglobin. The hematocrit is useful in the evaluation and classification of various types of anemia. The Wintrobe test and the micro-hematocrit method are the two most commonly used procedures. *The hematocrit is decreased in anemias and after hemorrhage and is increased in polycythemia and dehydration.*
- ***Haemoglobin (HgB):*** The amount of haemoglobin, the essential oxygen carrier of the blood, per 100 ml can be used as an index of the oxygen-carrying capacity of the blood. Total blood hemoglobin depends on the number of red blood cells and on the amount of hemoglobin in each red blood cell. *The hemoglobin is decreased in polycythemia and in newborn infants. The hemoglobin is decreased in anemia and this test is useful in the differential diagnosis of certain anemias. For example, in iron deficiency anemias, the hemoglobin is decreased more than the red blood cell count whereas the red blood cell count is decreased more than the hemoglobin in pernicious anemia.*
- ***Iron-Binding Capacity (Unsaturated):*** Iron is transported in the serum from the intestines where it is absorbed to the point of use in the erythropoietic system. The iron is combined with a fraction of beta globulins and is available for formation of hemoglobin. The unsaturated iron-binding capacity is the amount of iron that the protein (transferrin) could absorb to be fully saturated. Ordinarily, the actual serum iron is approximately one-third the level of the total iron-binding capacity.

  Low values are found in iron-deficiency anemia, acute or chronic blood loss, pregnancy, and haemochromatosis. Elevated values are found in pernicious anemia, hemolytic anemia, cirrhosis, uremia, and some infections.
- ***Lupus Erythematosus (LE) Cell Test:*** The lupus erythematosus cell test is clinically important in the diagnosis of disseminated lupus erythematosus. The test depends upon the reaction of an abnormal gamma globulin factor in the serum of the patient with the nucleus of a leukocyte. This results in the formation of a swollen homogeneous mass of nuclear material which is phagocytosed by a normal granulocyte to form the LE cell.

- ***Mean Corpuscular Hemoglobin:*** *See* Red Blood Cell Indices
- ***Mean Corpuscular Hemoglobin Concentration:*** See Red Blood Cell Indices
- ***Mean Corpuscular Volume:*** *See* Red Blood Cell Indices
- ***Prothrombin Time:*** Prothrombin is formed in the liver where its production depends on an adequate intake and absorption of vitamin K. Vitamin K is produced by the normal intestinal flora so that a deficiency of the vitamin is unusual in the otherwise healthy adult. Prothrombin is converted to thrombin in the clotting process. *A low prothrombin level is usually indicative that the clotting tendency of the blood is diminished.* This test measures the time needed for citrated or oxalate plasma to clot after tissue thromboplastin and calcium chloride have been added. The prothrombin time is often done during the acute stages of myocardial infarction in order to assist the physician to determine the next dose of anticoagulant. Clotting normally occurs in 11-14 seconds depending upon the control. An abnormal result is not pathognomonic of prothrombin deficiency as any one of the factors necessary for stage II and stage III of the clotting process may be involved.

  A lowered plasma prothrombin may mean either dysfunction of the liver or a deficient supply of vitamin K. Since vitamin K is not absorbed from the intestine in the absence of bile salts, biliary obstruction of any type can result in vitamin K deficiency, a lowered prothrombin concentration and a consequent bleeding tendency in the patient. Depressed prothrombin times are also seen in premature and breast-fed infants. A prothrombin determination without preliminary parenteral administration of vitamin K can be interpreted in terms of a possible bleeding tendency due to lack of this factor in the coagulation mechanism. The plasma prothrombin activity should not be regarded as a test of liver function unless an adequate dose of vitamin K is given parenterally 24 hours before the observation is made.
- ***Red Blood Cell Indices: Mean corpuscular hemoglobin (MCH).*** The mean corpuscular hemoglobin is the amount of hemoglobin by weight in the average red blood cell.
- ***Mean corpuscular hemoglobin concentration (MCHC):*** The mean corpuscular hemoglobin concentration is an expression of the percent of the average hemoglobin concentration per cell.
- ***Mean corpuscular volume (MCV):*** The mean corpuscular volume is the volume of the average red blood cell.

(c) Miscellaneous Tests

- ***Amylase:*** The determination of serum amylase is the most useful single test in the diagnosis of pancreatic disease. The normal range of serum amylase is 60-

200 Somogyi units. *In acute pancreatitis, it is consistently elevated often to values over 500 Somogyi units. Conditions which may cause amylase elevation are mumps, perforated peptic ulcer, gallstones, intestinal obstruction, ruptured ectopic pregnancy, renal insufficiency, nonpenetrating abdominal trauma and the administration of morphine and morphine-like drugs.* The elevation in these cases is typically transient, lasting a few hours to three days. Tests for urinary amylase add little or nothing to blood amylase determination, although the elevated urinary excretion may sometimes last several days longer. *In severe destructive pancreatitis, serum amylase may go down rather than up because of the inability of the pancreas to produce enzymes.*

- ***Anti-Streptolysin O Titer:*** This is a test usually used when rheumatic fever is suspected. Since rheumatic fever is related to a recent streptococcal infection, an increase in the titer of the anti-streptolysin is usually found in rheumatic fever. The test is non-specific.

- ***Bromsulphalein Test (BSP):*** This is a test for liver function and is particularly valuable in the diagnosis of cirrhosis and other diffuse diseases not accompanied by jaundice. The BSP test is based on the ability of the liver to remove injected sulfobromophthalein sodium from the blood stream. When sulfo-bromopthalein sodium is injected intravenously, it is rapidly removed from the blood stream by the liver and excreted in the bile. The time required for its removal depends upon the size of the dose and the functional capacity of the liver. Since the dye is removed via the bile flow, it is essential that the bile flow is not obstructed in order to achieve accurate results. Doses of 5 mg/kg of body weight are normally completely removed from the blood after 45 minutes. Impairment of liver functions will show a retention of dye from 6-40 percent or more. Since sulfobromophthalein sodium may interfere with the use of phenolsulfonphthalein as a test for kidney function, at least 24 hours should elapse between the two tests.

- ***C - reactive protein (CRP):*** This is a non-specific test for inflammation and tissue breakdown. An abnormal protein (C-reactive protein) has been demonstrated in the blood during the acute phases of many inflammatory disorders. This substance forms a precipitate with the non-type-specific or somatic C polysaccharide of the pneumococcus. An animal antiserum against this protein is used as the test reagent. The test is non-specific and has the same indications, interpretations and limitations as the erythrocyte sedimentation rate (ESR). *The test is useful in following the progress of rheumatic fever.*

- ***Cephalin-Cholesterol Flocculation:*** Properly diluted serum of normal persons will not flocculate a colloidal suspension of cephalin and cholesterol. The serum of persons with damaged liver cells will flocculate the suspension. This test affords a rough quantitative measurement of liver cell function and is sometimes used to follow the course of patients with a known liver disease (i.e., cirrhosis). The test is sensitive and *frequently positive in the early stages of liver disease before jaundice appears. It is negative in acute obstruction of the biliary tract of short duration.* If the obstruction persists, secondary damage to the liver cells occurs and the cephalin flocculation test becomes positive.

- ***Congo Red Retention Test:*** In amyloidosis, deposits of amyloid tissue are laid down in the liver, kidneys and spleen and eventually interfere with proper function. The amyloid material has an affinity for congo red and the dye is removed from the blood more quickly in patients with amyloidosis. A standard dose of 10 ml of a 1 percent solution of congo red is administered intravenously. If over 80 percent of the dye is removed from the blood within one hour, there is strong presumptive evidence of amyloidosis. A negative test, however, does not rule out the disease.

- ***Icterus Index:*** Bilirubin is yellow in color. This is a simple test for measuring the approximate amount of bilirubin in the serum by measuring the degree of yellowness of the serum. *An increase in the icterus index usually parallels an increase in the serum bilirubin.* The test does not differentiate between bilirubin due to excess hemolysis or due to obstruction of the biliary tract.

- ***Latex Slide Agglutination Test:*** This is a test used in the diagnosis of rheumatoid arthritis. Serum from patients with rheumatoid arthritis will cause small biologically inert particles coated with human gamma globulin to clump together. *It is also positive in lupus erythematosus and dermatomyositis.*

- ***Protein Bound Iodine (PBI):*** This is a test of thyroid function. Thyroxine normally contains most of the serum iodine and is mainly bound to certain serum proteins. The protein-bound iodine represents the organic fraction of blood iodine that precipitates with serum proteins. The level of PBI in the serum correlates well with the thyroid status and provides an indirect estimation of thyroxine in the body. *Low serum PBI values are found in hypothyroidism and nephrosis. Serum PBI values are elevated in hyperthyroidism and pregnancy.* Since thyroxine is carried to some extent by albumin and prealbumin proteins, any condition (i.e., nephritic syndrome or severe liver disease) which leads to a marked decrease of these proteins will falsely decrease PBI. Mercurial diuretics may cause erroneously low results due to the interference of mercury, and drugs containing inorganic iodine will cause false high results. All patients should be questioned about the prior administration of these drugs before determining the protein-bound iodine. In general, all radio-opaque, iodine-containing injectable contrast media are likely to produce falsely elevated protein-bound iodine levels for six months. Some of these contrast media may exert an effect for 20 or more years.

- ***Thymol Turbidity:*** The thymol turbidity test measures the degree of turbidity produced when blood serum is mixed with a buffered thymol solution. Normal sera produce no or very little turbidity. Sera from patients with liver disease contain altered gamma globulins and phospholipids which cause pronounced turbidity. *The turbidity is usually increased in liver conditions where the liver cells are damaged.* In biliary obstruction without damage to the liver cells, the turbidity is usually normal. The thymol turbidity test is a test of liver function and roughly correlates with the results of the cephalin flocculation test, it seems less sensitive than the cephalin flocculation test and becomes positive later, but tends to remain positive longer. *The test is high in infectious hepatitis, cirrhosis, Hodgkin's disease, coccidioidomycosis, disseminated tuberculosis, lobar pneumonia, and bacterial endocarditis.*

- ***Zinc Sulfate Turbidity:*** The zinc sulfate turbidity test depends upon the amount of gamma globulins present in the sera. Since the amount of gamma globulins in the serum is elevated when the liver cells are damaged, the test is useful in evaluating the presence of liver damage. The test is not specific for liver disease because the procedure depends upon an increase in gamma globulins, and conditions in which gamma globulins are increased will give a false positive result, i.e., multiple myeloma.

20.4 Tests Performed on Urine

The urinalysis, a composite examination on a specimen of urine, is an integral part of the initial examination of patients in all branches of medicine. The urinalysis is composed of four general parts.

(a) Physical properties

(b) Chemical tests for abnormal constituents

(c) Microscopic examination of the urine sediment

(d) Special tests

(a) *Physical Properties*

- ***Urine Colour:*** Normal urine varies in color from faint yellow to amber depending upon the concentration of the urine. Color is not an adequate measurement of concentration, however, and specific gravity or osmolarity values are preferred. The three normal urinary pigments are urochrome, uroerythrin, and urobilin. Clinical conditions which affect the urine color include porphyria (red urine), alcaptonuria (brown/black urine), and extensive melanotic sarcoma (black urine). There are numerous color changes caused by some drugs and foods but these are usually of little clinical significance.

- ***Urine Odor:*** Normal urine has a characteristic, faintly *aromatic* odor due to presence of certain volatile acids. Upon standing, bacteria, in the specimen breakdown urea, ammonia is formed, and the urine acquires a strong *ammoniacal* odor. This odor is an indication that the urine specimen is too old to be worth examining and a fresh specimen should be obtained. *Urine heavily infected with bacteria is foul-smelling and in diabetic ketosis, the urine has a characteristic "fruity" or sweet odor.*

- ***Urine Transparency:*** Freshly voided normal urine is usually, but not necessarily, clear and upon standing will become cloudy. When a freshly voided specimen is cloudy, a microscopic analysis of the urinary sediment can usually ascribe the cloudiness to amorphous phosphates, amorphous urates, pus, blood, bacteria or fat.

- ***Specific Gravity:*** Specific gravity of urine is the ratio of the weight of a given volume of urine to the weight of the same volume of water at a temperature of 4°C. The normal range is 1.010 to 1.030 and the morning specimen shows the greatest concentration with a specific gravity of 1.020 or higher. The specific gravity of urine always should be reported to the third decimal point to have clinical significance and since it is a ratio, there are no units.

  The specific gravity of the urine is dependent upon the concentrating ability of the kidneys and the state of hydration of the patient. It is a reflection of the amount of dissolved substances present in the solution and varies inversely with urine volume. *The specific gravity is decreased in high fluid intake, low salt intake, diabetes insipidus and chronic nephritis. The specific gravity is increased in diabetes mellitus, acute glomerulonephritis, fever, sweating, vomiting, and diarrhea.*

- ***pH:*** The pH of urine depends greatly upon the acid-base composition of the blood. The kidney maintains the blood at constant pH range by excreting into the urine any excess ions which might alter the pH of the blood. Therefore, the urinary pH varies and changes do not necessarily indicate abnormality. Freshly voided urine usually has a pH value of 5 or 6; however, because of the presence of phosphate salts and other buffers in the glomerular filtrate and of ammonia formed by the tubular cells, the kidney is capable of producing urine ranging from pH 4.5 to 8.0. The pH of the urine influences the preservation of formed elements in the urine sediment. In renal insufficiency, the ability to excrete acid is reduced owing chiefly to impairment in ammonia excretion. It is not uncommon for urine to be alkaline following a heavy meal or after ingestion of large amounts of alkaline salts. Otherwise, the presence of constantly alkaline urine may be due to the presence of urea-splitting organisms in the urine, a potassium deficiency, primary aldosteronism, after blood transfusions, or frequent vomiting. *Strongly acidic urine occurs in acidosis, diabetes mellitus, gout, and after ingestion of ammonium chloride, ammonium mandelate, or a high protein diet.*

(b) *Chemical Tests for Abnormal Constituents*

- ***Acetoacetic Acid:*** See Ketones
- ***Acetone:*** See Ketones
- ***Albumin:*** Ordinarily the albumin in the blood does not pass through the glomerulus into the urine. Albuminuria refers to albumin that has passed from the blood into the urine and as the glomerular membrane is progressively damaged, proteins appear in the urine in the order of their molecular size. Albumin has the smallest molecular size and is released first and is followed by the globulins and rarely fibrinogen. The test for urinary protein is probably the most significant single finding in the detection and diagnosis of renal disease. Proteinuria must be correlated with the microscopic examination of the urinary sediment and treatment should be started as soon as possible in order to prevent permanent renal damage. *Slight albuminuria may occur after excessive muscular exertion, exercise, protein ingestion and in late pregnancy. Albuminuria may be caused by (1) increased permeability of the glomerulus and (2) decreased reabsorption of protein by the renal tubular cells. Albuminuria is found in all stages of nephritis, nephrosis and nephrosclerosis. Albuminuria is also common in hypertension, certain infectious processes involving the kidney, (i.e., tuberculosis, pyelonephritis, pyelitis, septic emboli), non-infectious processes (i.e., polycystic disease, hemorrhage, incompatible transfusions, amyloidosis, calculi), and diabetes mellitus. Mercurial compounds and gold salts may produce albuminuria secondary to tubular damage. If venous return from the kidneys to the heart is impaired (i.e., renal vein thrombosis, congestive heart failure, constrictive pericarditis), albuminuria may result.*
- ***Beta Hydroxybutyric Acid:*** see Ketones
- ***Bilirubin:*** This is a test of liver function. Bilirubin is formed from hemoglobin by the reticuloendothelial system and is normally excreted from the body by the liver through the intestine. Free bilirubin linked to protein is excreted by the liver rather than the kidneys because it cannot pass through the glomerular capsule. The urine normally contains no bilirubin. Bilirubin which has passed through the

liver (post hepatic) diffuses more readily than prehepatic bilirubin. Consequently, the bilirubin of obstructive jaundice is found in the urine earlier than that of hemolytic jaundice. Bilirubin may be absent in patients with hemolytic jaundice with a fairly high icterus index. In infectious or toxic hepatitis, cholangitis, and in partial obstruction of the biliary tract, bilirubin is present because the liver is unable to handle the bilirubin absorbed from the intestinal tract plus the bilirubin formed by the reticuloendothelial system. *A less common, but important cause of bilirubin in the urine is an excessive production of bilirubin associated with pathologically increased destruction of erythrocytes.*

- ***Chlorides, Quantitative:*** This test is performed to evaluate the urinary excretion of chlorides. A normal person will excrete extremely small amounts of sodium and chloride in the urine when he is fed a diet low in these elements. The ability of the body to conserve sodium and chloride depends upon the functional integrity of the adrenal cortex. *A decrease in urinary chlorides occurs when there is a decrease in blood chlorides, starvation, excessive sweating, vomiting, pneumonia, ascites, pleuritic effusion, heart failure, nephritis, nephrosis and burns. In Addison's disease, there is increased urinary excretion of chloride in spite of decreased plasma chloride.*

- ***Clearance Tests:*** Clearance is the volume of blood or plasma that contains the amount of a substance which is excreted in the urine in one minute. Clearance tests allow the physician to evaluate the extent of renal damage and to differentiate between glomerular lesions and tubular lesions.

  The three specific functions of the kidney which are commonly measured are:

  1. Renal plasma flow
  2. Glomerular filtration rate
  3. Tubular function

  The ***renal plasma flow*** is commonly determined by using sodium p-aminohippurate (PAH) which, at low blood concentrations, is almost completely removed by tubular excretion in a single circulation through the kidney.

  The ***glomerular filtration rate*** is determined by measuring the clearance of any substance that is filtered at the glomerulus but is not excreted or reabsorbed by the tubules. Inulin clearance, creatinine clearance, and urea clearance are all methods of measuring the glomerular filtration rate.

  The ***tubular function*** may be subdivided into tubular secretion and tubular absorption. Diodrast, para-aminohippuric acid, and phenol red can overload tubular secretory mechanisms and high blood levels of glucose can exceed tubular reabsorption. The clearance rate of these substances (after being corrected for that amount simultaneously filtered by the glomerulus) is an indication of average tubular function (Tm).

- ***Concentration and Dilution:*** These tests measure the ability of the kidneys to concentrate and dilute urine. The normal kidneys excrete urine that differs markedly in volume and specific gravity at different periods within a 24 hour period. These variations represent an attempt to maintain normal body fluids under conditions of varying fluid intake. Damaged kidneys lose partially or completely this ability to respond to the needs of the body with the result that the urine has almost the same specific gravity throughout the day.
- ***Diacetic Acid:*** *See* Ketones
- ***Glomerular Filtration Rate:*** *see* Clearance Tests
- ***Haemoglobin:*** Blood in the urine may appear as intact red blood cells (haematuria) or dissolved hemoglobin derived from destroyed red blood cells (haemoglobinuria). Haematuria is the result of bleeding somewhere along the urinary tract. The site of bleeding is determined by more precise methods. Haemoglobinuria usually results from conditions outside the urinary tract. *The red blood cells are haemolyzed and the dissolved hemoglobin in the plasma is excreted by the kidney. This occurs in severe burns, transfusion reactions, severe malaria, poisoning and paroxysmal haemoglobinuria.*
- ***Ketones:*** Ketone bodies are normal products of fat metabolism and include: acetone, diacetic acid, and beta-hydroxybutyric acid. They are not normally detectable in blood or urine. The ketone bodies are utilized by muscle tissue as an energy source; however, if an excessive amount of fat is metabolized, the muscles may be unable to utilize all the resulting ketone bodies. Ketosis (increased concentration of ketones in the blood) and ketonuria (increased concentration of ketones in the urine) are the clinical results.

  Acetone This test is important in the diagnosis of ketosis. In diabetes mellitus, sugar is not utilized properly and excessive fat is metabolized. The fatty acids are broken down into aceto acetic acid and beta-hydroxybutyric acid which are converted to acetone and excreted by the kidneys. There is normally no acetone in the urine of adults. Acetone in the urine indicates a severe disorder of metabolism and is present in diabetes mellitus, in a certain percentage of small children, and in starvation. It is also increased if the patient received sulfobromophthalein sodium (BSP) or phenolsulfonphthalein in the past 48 hours.

  Beta-Hydroxybutyric acid Of the three ketone bodies, beta-hydroxybutyric acid is relatively non-toxic. It is excreted in the urine in combination with a fixed base (sodium) and loss of the body cations may lead to acidosis. In uncontrolled diabetes, acetone is the first ketone body to appear, diacetic acid is later excreted and when the situation becomes severe, beta-hydroxybutyric acid appears.

Diacetic (aceto-acetic) acid The test for diacetic acid is used in the diagnosis of metabolic ketosis. Like acetone, diacetic acid is produced when glucose is not properly utilized and excessive fat is metabolized. A positive test for diacetic acid indicates a more severe degree of ketosis than a positive acetone test alone.

Myoglobin Myoglobin is a normal constituent of muscle and similar in many respects to hemoglobin. Myoglobin appears in the urine after extensive destruction of muscle *(i.e.,* crush injuries or following occlusion of a main limb artery, and in the rare disease termed acute paralytic myoglobinuria or acute recurrent rhabdomyolysis). Myoglobin has one quarter the molecular weight of hemoglobin and is more rapidly cleared by the kidney. Myoglobin is quite soluble in alkaline urine, but if the urine is acidic, the myoglobin may precipitate in the kidney tubules and cause kidney damage.

- ***Porphyrins:*** Porphyrins are pigments which are normally contained in red blood cells. Normally, there is an insignificant amount of porphyrin in the urine. In lead poisoning and toxic liver damage, some blood disorders, pellagra, and congenital porphyria, the urinary excretion of porphyrins rises.
- ***Renal Plasma Flow:*** *see* Clearance Tests
- ***Sugar:*** Traces of sugar, particularly glucose, may occur in normal urine. The occurrence of any sugar in the urine is termed glycosuria. Sugars that may be present in the urine are glucose, pentose, galactose, lactose and levulose. All tests for urine sugar may be classified as either nonspecific tests for sugars, which are based on the reducing ability of glucose, or specific tests for glucose, which are based on the enzyme of glucose oxidase.

  The renal threshold is the lowest blood glucose concentration that will result in glycosuria, and at this point (usually 170-180 mg %) any additional glucose will not be reabsorbed into the blood but will be excreted in the urine. When glucose is detected in urine, it is important to determine if the underlying cause is benign or pathologic. Benign glycosuria occurs after eating a large quantity of glucose or other carbohydrate or after emotional reactions. *Pathologic glycosuria is due chiefly to diabetes mellitus, but may also occur in pregnancy, hyperthyroidism, increased intracranial pressure, hyperpituitarism, chronic liver disease, and acidosis of anesthesia or asphyxia.*
- ***Tubular Function:*** see Clearance Tests
- ***Urobilinogen:*** When bilirubin enters the intestine, it is acted upon by bacteria which convert it to urobilinogen. This is a test used to differentiate between complete and incomplete obstruction of the biliary tract. Tests for urine urobilinogen are valuable in early detection of liver damage because one of the

first mechanisms altered in a damaged liver is the inability to remove urobilinogen from the blood and excrete it via the intestine. As a result, urobilinogen is removed by the kidney. *Increases in urinary urobilinogen occur in many conditions including hemolytic diseases, liver damage, congestive heart failure, and severe infections.* However, in complete obstructive jaundice without infection there is ordinarily no excess urobilinogen in the urine.

(c) *Microscopic Examination of the Urine Sediment*

The centrifuged sediment of the urine contains all the insoluble materials that have accumulated in the urine in the process of glomerular filtration and during passage of the fluid through tubules of the kidneys and lower urinary tract. When renal disease is present, it is often possible to surmise from examination of the urine sediment, the nature of the pathologic process in the kidney and its degree of activity. Localization of disease in the lower urinary tract may be aided by use of fractional urine collection.

- ***Significance of Cells in Urine Sediment***

  Leukocytes: The white blood cells that appear in urine are predominantly polymorphonuclear neutrophils. Pyuria is the condition in which increased numbers of white cells are found in the urine. The presence of increased numbers of leukocytes in the sediment is often indicative of urinary tract infection, especially when clumping occurs. Occasional white cells are frequently found in normal urine sediment. Increased numbers of leukocytes and epithelial cells occur in glomerulonephritis and other diseases not associated with bacterial infection.

  Erythrocytes: Erythrocytes, like leukocytes, may enter the urine from any part of the urinary tract. Haematuria is the condition in which red blood cells are found in the urine. In the urine, red blood cells act as osmometers and alter in size and appearance depending on the osmolarity of the urine. In concentrated urine, they lose their usual biconcave contour and become small and crenated. In dilute urine, they may appear large and swollen, or they may rupture leaving only a ring of stroma or "ghost cell."

  Increased numbers of red blood cells may appear in the urine during the acute febrile phase of streptococcal infections without significant disease of the kidneys or urinary tract. Haematuria occurs in glomerulonephritis; renal infarction; tuberculosis of kidneys; pyelonephritis; carcinomas of kidneys, ureters and bladder; polycystic kidneys; calculi; and hemorrhagic diseases such as purpura haemorrhagica and hemophilia. Haematuria has occurred following anticoagulant therapy of thrombophlebitis, phlebothrombosis, etc.

  Epithelial cells: Cells of the renal tubular epithelium are round, mononuclear and generally larger than leukocytes. Their presence in the urine in elevated numbers signifies degenerative exfoliation of the tubular epithelium and may appear in glomerulonephritis and other vascular nephritides following exposure to nephrotoxic substances or during acute infections involving the renal medulla. When intense degenerative changes occur, whole sheets of epithelial cells may appear in the sediment. Large numbers of renal tubular epithelial cells are usually excreted in the urine of patients with massive proteinuria from any cause.

- ***Significance of Casts in Urine Sediment***

  Casts are cylindrical structures that form in the kidney tubules by the coagulation of protein. The occurrence of casts is called cylindruria. For casts to form, protein must be present in tubular urine in sufficient concentration and under conditions favorable to coagulation. Within the coagulum may be trapped the cells, bacteria crystals and other debris present at the site of formation. Thus, the cast provides a method of examining the contents of the kidney tubule because anything present within a cast roust have been present in the tubule.

  Noncellular casts The noncellular casts are hyaline, granular, waxy and fatty in type.

  Hyaline casts result from precipitation of protein within the kidney tubule lumens and are seen in increased numbers when proteinuria is present from any cause. Hyaline casts should be carefully inspected for inclusions since the presence of formed elements within the casts indicates that these are derived from the kidney rather than the lower urinary tract.

  Granular casts are thought to represent cellular casts that have undergone degenerative changes after formation. Their presence suggests nephrosis, orthostatic proteinuria or some type of glomerulonephrosis.

  Waxy casts may represent the final degenerative end product in the evolution of cellular casts. They do not occur in normal urine and are most often seen in chronic renal disease of long duration.

  Fatty casts may appear in the nephrotic syndrome. They consist of lipid droplets in the epithelial cell or granular casts.

- ***Significance of Crystals in Urine Sediment***

  Crystals can be divided into those that appear in acid urine and those that appear in neutral or alkaline urine. Increased quantities of crystals may occur in patients who tend to form renal stones and there are certain chemicals that may crystallize in the urine *(i.e.,* cystine, leonine, tyrosine) in certain metabolic diseases.

(d) ***Special Tests***

- ***Ferric Chloride Test on Urine:*** see Phenyl-ketonuria Test

- ***17-Hydroxycorticosteroids:*** This is primarily a test of adrenal cortex function. The adrenal cortex produces corticosteroids which are altered and then excreted primarily in the urine. The urinary excretion of 17-hydroxycorticosteroids is an indication of the rate at which the adrenals are producing the corticosteroids. In Cushing's syndrome (hyperadrenalism), the urinary levels are higher than normal. However, the reverse is not necessarily true. In cases of adrenal cortical under function, the urinary levels may be within the normal range. If adrenal cortical under function is suspected, but the urinary 17-hydroxycorticosteroid levels are normal, ACTH may be administered and then the 17-hydroxycorticosteroid excretion levels retested. If adrenal cortical function is normal, the urinary excretion of 17-hydroxycorticosteroids will rise markedly after ACTH. However, if adrenal cortical function is poor, the urinary levels of 17-hydroxycorticosteroids will not rise appreciably.
- ***Immunologic Test for Pregnancy:*** The immunologic tests rely upon commercially available anti-human chorionic gonadotropin antibody (anti-HCG). After fertilization of the ovum, chorionic gonadotropin is produced. When the test is performed, the patient's serum or urine is incubated with the antibody; HCG, if present, reacts with it and thereby inactivates the antibody. The incubated antibody sample mixture is then added to an indicator. If HCG is present in the sample, the antibody is inactivated and the red cells or particles remain unagglutinated. If the sample does not contain HCG, the antibody remains active, and agglutination occurs. The test has a 95-99 percent accuracy rate.
- ***17-Ketosteroid Excretion:*** The urinary 17-ketosteroids are metabolites of adrenal cortical steroids, adrenal androgens and gonadal androgens. They represent an index of the activity of the adrenal cortex and the gonads in the male and an approximation of the activity of the adrenal cortex in the female. In normal subjects, there is a moderate variation in the 17-ketosteroid excretion in a 24-hour period. The urinary 17-ketosteroid values for normal subjects are higher in men than in women. In children, the level is normally very low.

  Normal levels are found in adrenal benign tumor, menopausal women and thyrotoxicosis. Low levels of 17-ketosteroids are found in adrenal hypofunction (*i.e.,* Addison's disease, myxedema, pituitary hypofunction, primary ovarian agenesis, eunuchoid men, and starvation. High levels of 17-ketosteroids are found in adrenal hyperplasia, adrenal malignant tumor, adreno-genital syndrome and idiopathic hirsutism. Very marked elevations, over 100 mg a day, suggest either carcinoma of the adrenal cortex or the extremely rare interstitial cell tumor of the testis.
- ***Phenolsulfonphthalein (PSP) Test:*** This test measures the secretory activity of the proximal tubules. In the plasma, phenolsulfonphthalein (PSP) is reversibly bound to the albumin fraction of plasma protein. Because of this binding, very

little of the dye is excreted by glomerular filtration and over 90 percent of an administered dose is excreted by the renal tubules.

The PSP test is an empirical measure of the rate of excretion of a standard test dose of the dye over a fixed period of time. The rate of excretion depends chiefly on the renal plasma flow since the test dose produces too low a concentration in the plasma to saturate the tubular excretory mechanism. The dye is given as a single intravenous injection and is most rapidly excreted during the first few minutes after injection when the plasma concentration is high. After the plasma concentration is reduced to low levels, the remainder of the dose is excreted more slowly. In normal kidney function, 30 percent of the dye is excreted after 15 minutes, an additional 15 percent after 30 minutes, and another additional 10 percent after 60 minutes.

In the presence of reduced renal blood flow or inactive renal tubules, the blood must be recirculated through the kidney over a longer period of time to excrete the same amount of dye. If allowed sufficient time, the damaged kidney will excrete the same amount of PSP as the normal kidney and abnormally low excretion may be apparent only during the first 15 or 20 minutes after injection. The cumulative excretion over a period of 2 hours may be the same for normal and damaged kidneys and is usually 70-80 percent of the test dose. Approximately 15-25 percent of the test dose is excreted by the liver and is not recovered in the urine. The test is not reliable in hepatorenal disease. In summary, this test is a crude measure of the integrity of the renal tubules and their rate of perfusion with plasma,

- ***Phenylketonuria Test (Ferric Chloride Test):*** This test is designed to uncover early cases of phenylketonuria. In this condition, the patient— an infant—is unable to metabolize phenylalanine properly. As a result, pathologic metabolic end products are formed which lead to permanent mental deficiency. If the disorder is recognized early, a phenylalanine deficient diet can be prescribed and the mental deficiency avoided.

20.5 Tests Performed on Feces

- ***Blood:*** In bleeding lesions of the upper intestinal tract, gross blood is not detected macroscopically in the stool because of the effect of digestion. In such cases it is necessary to do a test for occult blood (guaiac test). The test for occult blood may be positive for ruptured varicose veins of the esophagus or stomach; swallowed blood from pulmonary hemorrhage; rupture of aortic aneurysm into the esophagus; carcinoma of the esophagus, stomach or intestine; ulcer of stomach or duodenum; intestinal ulcers due to typhoid fever or tuberculosis; embolism of the superior mesenteric artery; venous thrombosis of mesenteric veins; ulcerative colitis; bacillary and amebic dysentery; hemophilia; hemolytic jaundice; and purpura.

In general, blood originating from a lesion in the lower colon is bright red and hemorrhage from the upper gastrointestinal tract results in a tarry stool. The presence of blood in any tarry or red stool should be confirmed by a chemical test for occult blood. *Any degree of positiveness of the guaiac test for occult blood usually signifies bleeding in the gastrointestinal tract and a thorough investigation for the source of bleeding is indicated.*

- ***Fat Determination:*** Very few neutral fat globules are found in the normal stool. The presence of large amounts of neutral fat may suggest that the patient has been taking an oily laxative. This test is used to study any patients with symptoms suggesting intestinal malabsorption and to confirm a diagnosis of steatorrhea (excess fat in the stools). Total fat is increased in the feces in ileitis, extrahepatic obstructive jaundice, and pancreatitis, obstruction of the pancreatic duct, sprue, and celiac disease. Some patients with pancreatic insufficiency may have an increase in neutral fat content of the stools. An increase of fat content of the stool does not, however, permit a specific diagnosis of pancreatic deficiency to be made since pancreatic enzymes may be normal in certain instances of itorrhea.
- ***Cuaiac Test* - see *Blood Parasites:*** Examinations of feces for parasites performed in order to identify the parasites their eggs. The therapy will usually depend the type of parasite found so that precise identification is important.

20.6 Miscellaneous Tests

- ***Basal Metabolic Rate (BMR):*** The oldest and least specific test of thyroid function is the basal metabolic rate (BMR). This measurement of oxygen consumption is expressed as kilocalories vended per square meter of body surface per hour, with the fasted patient in a condition of steal and mental repose.

  The BMR may be elevated in hyperthyroid, anxiety, infection, leukemia, cardiovascular disease, acidosis, polycythemia, severe anemia, acromegaly, diabetes insipidus, and Cushing's disease. The BMR may be decreased in hypothyroidism, hypopituitarism, malnutrition, Addison's disease, anorexia nervosa and nephrotic syndrome. This test is often replaced by more specific tests of thyroid function.
- ***Chloride in Sweat:*** This is a test for cystic fibrosis of the pancreas. Children with cystic fibrosis excrete greater quantities of chloride in their perspiration than do normal children.

- ***Radioiodine Uptake*:** The radioiodine uptake is used in the diagnosis of certain thyroid conditions. It is based on the fact that the radioactive isotope of iodine, I^{131}, is taken up the thyroid in the same manner as ordinary line. The breakdown of I^{131} to more stable elements results in the release of gamma rays which can be detected and counted by a scintillation counter. The degree of radioactivity is a measure of the degree of iodine uptake. Uptake below normal suggests hypothyroidism and uptake above normal suggests hyperthyroidism.
- ***Thorn Test:*** The thorn test is a test of adrenal function. It is based on the fact that ACTH produces a decrease of at least 50 percent in four hours in persons with a normally functioning adrenal cortex. Patients with normal adrenal function respond to ACTH injections by a decrease in the circulating eosinphils and an increase in the excretion of uric acid as compared to creatinine. Patients with Addison's disease do not respond to ACTH injections. The thorn test is also a test of adrenal cortical reserve before surgery and a test to differentiate functional hypopituitarism from organic disease of the adrenal cortex.

20.7 Liver Function Tests

Liver function tests represent a broad range of normal functions performed by the liver. The diagnosis of liver disease depends upon a complete history, complete physical examination, and evaluation of liver function tests and further invasive and noninvasive tests.

The hepatobiliary tree represents hepatic cells and biliary tract cells. Inflammation of the hepatic cells results in elevation in the alanine aminotransferase (ALT), aspartate aminotransferase (AST) and possibly the bilirubin. Inflammation of the biliary tract cells results predominantly in an elevation of the alkaline phosphatase. In liver disease there are crossovers between purely biliary disease and hepatocellular disease.

- ***Alanine Aminotransferase (ALT) or Serum Glutamic Pyruvate Transaminase (SGPT):*** ALT is the enzyme produced within the cells of the liver. The level of ALT abnormality is increased in conditions where cells of the liver have been inflamed or undergone cell death. As the cells are damaged, the ALT leaks into the bloodstream leading to a rise in the serum levels. Any form of hepatic cell damage can result in an elevation in the ALT. The ALT level may or may not correlate with the degree of cell death or inflammation. ALT is the most sensitive marker for liver cell damage.
- ***Aspartate Aminotransferase (AST) or Serum Glutamic Oxoloacetic Transaminase (SGOT):*** This enzyme also reflects damage to the hepatic cell. It is less specific for liver disease. It may be elevated and other conditions such as a myocardial infarct (heart attack). Although AST is not a specific for liver as the

ALT, ratios between ALT and AST are useful in assessing the etiology of liver enzyme abnormalities.

- ***Alkaline Phosphatase:*** Alkaline phosphatase is an enzyme, which is associated with the biliary tract. It is not specific to the biliary tract. It is also found in bone and the placenta. Renal or intestinal damage can also cause the alkaline phosphatase to rise. If the alkaline phosphatase is elevated, biliary tract damage and inflammation should be considered. However, considering the above other etiologies must also be entertained. One way to assess the etiology of the alkaline phosphatase is to perform a serologic evaluation called isoenzymes. Another more common method to asses the etiology of the elevated alkaline phosphatase is to determine whether the GGT is elevated or whether other function tests are abnormal (such as bilirubin). *Alkaline phosphatase may be elevated in primary biliary cirrhosis, alcoholic hepatitis, PSC, gallstones in choledocholithiasis.*

- ***Gamma Glutamic Transpeptidase (GGT):*** This enzyme is also produced by the bile ducts. However, it is not very specific to the liver or bile ducts. It is used often times to confirm that the alkaline phosphatase is of the hepatic etiology. Certain GGT levels, as an isolated finding, reflect rare forms of liver disease. *Medications commonly cause GGT to be elevated. Liver toxins such as alcohol can cause increases in the GGT.*

- ***Bilirubin:*** Bilirubin is a major breakdown product of haemoglobin. Haemoglobin is derived from red cells that have outlived their natural life and subsequently have been removed by the spleen. During splenic degradation of red blood cells, haemoglobin (the part of the red blood cell that carries oxygen to the tissues) is separated out from iron and cell membrane components. Haemoglobin is transferred to the liver where it undergoes further metabolism in a process called conjugation. Conjugation allows haemoglobin to become more water-soluble. The water solubility of bilirubin allows the bilirubin to be excreted into bile. Bile then is used to digest food.

  As the liver becomes irritated, the total bilirubin may rise. It is then important to understand the difference between total bilirubin, which has undergone conjugation (that is hepatic cell metabolism), and at portion of bilirubin which has not been metabolized. These two components are called total bilirubin and direct bilirubin. The direct bilirubin fraction is that portion of bilirubin that has undergone metabolism by the liver. When this fraction is elevated, the cause of elevated bilirubin (hyperbilirubinemia) is usually outside the liver. These types of causes are typically gallstones. This type of abnormality is usually treated with surgery (such as a gallbladder removal or choleycystectomy).

  If the direct bilirubin is low, while the total bilirubin is high, this reflects liver cell damage or bile duct damage within the liver itself.

- ***Albumin:*** Albumin is the major protein present within the blood. Albumin is synthesized by the liver. As such, it represents a major synthetic protein and is a marker for the ability of the liver to synthesize proteins. It is only one of many proteins that are synthesized by the liver. It represents a reliable and inexpensive laboratory test to assess the degree of liver damage present in the in any particular patient. When the liver has been chronically damaged, the albumin may be low. This would indicate that the synthetic function of the liver has been markedly diminished. Such findings suggest a diagnosis of cirrhosis. *Malnutrition can also cause low albumin (hypoalbuminemia) with no associated liver disease.*

- ***Prothrombin time (PT):*** Another measure of hepatic synthetic function is the prothrombin time. Prothrombin time is affected by proteins synthesized by the liver. Particularly, these proteins are associated with the incorporation of vitamin K metabolites into a protein. This allows normal coagulation (clotting of blood). Thus, in patients who have prolonged prothrombin times, liver disease may be present. Since a prolonged PT is not a specific test for liver disease, confirmation of other abnormal liver tests is essential. This may include reviewing other liver function tests or radiology studies of the liver. Diseases such as malnutrition, in which decreased vitamin K ingestion is present, may result in a prolonged PT time. An indirect test of hepatic synthetic function includes administration of vitamin K (10mg) subcutaneously over three days. Several days later, the prothrombin time may be measured. If the prothrombin time becomes normal, then hepatic synthetic function is intact. This test does not indicate that there is no liver disease, but is suggestive that malnutrition may coexist with (or without) liver disease.

- ***Platelet count:*** Platelets are cells that form the primary mechanism in blood clots. They're also the smallest of blood cells. They are derived from the bone marrow from the larger cells known as megakaryocytes. Individuals with liver disease develop a large spleen. As this process occurs platelets are trapped with in the sinusoids (small pathways within the spleen) of the spleen. While the trapping of platelets is a normal function for the spleen, in liver disease it becomes exaggerated because of the enlarged spleen (splenomegaly). Subsequently, the platelet count may become diminished.

- ***Serum protein electrophoresis:*** This is an evaluation of the types of proteins that are present with in a patient's serum. By using an electrophoretic gel, major proteins can be separated out. This results in four major types of proteins. These are 1) albumin, 2) alpha globulins, 3) beta globulins and 4) gammaglobulins. This test is useful for evaluation of patients who have abnormal liver function tests since it allows a direct quantification of multiple different serum proteins. If the gamma globulin fraction is elevated, autoimmune hepatitis may be present. In addition a deficiency in the alpha globulin fraction can result in the diagnosis, or a clinical clue, to A. alpha-1 antitrypsin deficiency. This is a simple blood test that is commonly performed by hepatologists

Other tests

- ***5' nucleotidase (5'NTD):*** 5' *nucleotidase* is another test specific for cholestasis or damage to the intra or extra hepatic biliary system, and in some laboratories, is used as a substitute for GGT for ascertaining whether an elevated ALP is of biliary or extra-biliary origin.
- ***Coagulation tests:*** The liver is responsible for the production of coagulation factors. The *international normalized ratio* (INR) measures the speed of a particular pathway of coagulation, comparing it to normal. If the INR is increased, it means it is taking longer than usual for blood to clot. The INR will only be increased if the liver is so damaged that synthesis of *vitamin K*-dependent coagulation factors has been impaired: it is not a sensitive measure of liver function. It is very important to normalize the INR before operating on people with liver problems (usually by transfusion with blood plasma containing the deficient factors) as they could bleed excessively.
- ***Serum glucose (BG, Glu):*** The liver's ability to produce glucose (*gluconeogenesis*) is usually the last function to be lost in the setting of fulminant liver failure.
- ***Lactate dehydrogenase (LDH):*** *Lactate dehydrogenase* is an enzyme found in many body tissues, including the liver. Elevated levels of LDH may indicate liver damage

Table 20.1 Standard liver panel

Measurement	Significance	Reference range
Alanine transaminase (ALT)	*Alanine transaminase* (ALT), also called *Serum Glutamic Pyruvate Transaminase* (SGPT) or Alanine aminotransferase (ALAT) is an enzyme present in hepatocytes (liver cells). When a cell is damaged, it leaks this enzyme into the blood, where it is measured. ALT rises dramatically in acute liver damage, such as viral hepatitis or paracetamol (acetaminophen) overdose. Elevations are often measured in multiples of the upper limit of normal (ULN).	5 to 40 IU/L
Aspartate transaminase (AST)	*Aspartate transaminase* (AST) also called *Serum Glutamic Oxaloacetic Transaminase* (SGOT) or aspartate aminotransferase (ASAT) is similar to ALT in that it is another enzyme associated with liver parenchymal cells. It is raised in acute liver damage, but is also present in red cells and cardiac and skeletal muscle and is therefore not specific to the liver. The ratio of AST to ALT is sometimes useful in differentiating between causes of liver damage.	10 to 40 IU/L

Table 20.1 *Contd...*

Measurement	Significance	Reference range
Alkaline phosphatase (ALP)	*Alkaline phosphatase* (ALP) is an enzyme in the cells lining the *biliary ducts* of the liver. ALP levels in plasma will rise with large bile duct obstruction, intrahepatic cholestasis or infiltrative diseases of the liver. ALP is also present in bone and placental tissue, so it is higher in growing children (as their bones are being remodelled) and elderly patients with Paget's disease.	30 to 120 IU/L
Total bilirubin (TBIL)	Bilirubin is a breakdown product of haem (a part of haemoglobin in red blood cells). The liver is responsible for clearing the blood of bilirubin. It does this by the following mechanism: bilirubin is taken up into hepatocytes, *conjugated* (modified to make it water-soluble), and secreted into the bile, which is excreted into the intestine. Increased total bilirubin causes jaundice, and can signal a number of problems: 1. **Prehepatic**: Increased bilirubin *production*. This can be due to a number of causes, including hemolytic anemias and internal hemorrhage. 2. **Hepatic**: Problems with the liver, which are reflected as deficiencies in bilirubin *metabolism* (e.g. reduced hepatocyte uptake, impaired conjugation of bilirubin, and reduced hepatocyte secretion of bilirubin). Some examples would be cirrhosis and viral hepatitis. 3. **Post hepatic**: Obstruction of the bile ducts, reflected as deficiencies in bilirubin *excretion*. (Obstruction can be located either within the liver or outside the liver.)	2 - 14 μmol/L
Direct bilirubin	The diagnosis is narrowed down further by looking at the levels of direct bilirubin. If direct (i.e. conjugated) bilirubin is normal, then the problem is an excess of unconjugated bilirubin, and the location of the problem is upstream of bilirubin excretion. Hemolysis, viral hepatitis, or cirrhosis can be suspected. If direct bilirubin is elevated, then the liver is conjugating bilirubin normally, but is not able to excrete it. Bile duct obstruction by gallstones or cancer should be suspected.	0 – 4 μmol/L
Gamma glutamyl transpeptidase (GGT)	Although reasonably specific to the liver and a more sensitive marker for cholestatic damage than ALP, Gamma glutamyl transpeptidase (GGT) may be elevated with even minor, sub-clinical levels of liver dysfunction. It can also be helpful in identifying the cause of an isolated elevation in ALP. GGT is raised in alcohol toxicity (acute and chronic). In some laboratories, GGT is not part of the standard LFTs and must be specifically requested.	0 to 51 IU/L

20.8 Kidney Function Tests

In the diseased kidney, only one function of this complex organ may be affected while the others remain undisturbed. Since the extent of renal damage is not measured by renal function tests, the results of specific tests have meaning only when correlated with other observations and tests of the urine. Generally, information regarding the rate of glomerular filtration and tubular reabsorption and excretion is sought in specific tests, but without correlation with other tests, these tests can only approximate the kidney functional capacity.

Tests used to determine kidney function can be divided into three categories:

- ascertainment of the ability of the kidney to concentrate or dilute the urine,
- measurement of renal capacity to excrete a foreign substance or metabolic waste products, and
- determination of renal capability to clear waste products from the blood into the urine.

Impaired kidney function may be "prerenal", "renal", or "post renal".

- *Prerenal azotemia* results from under perfusion of the kidney which may be due to dehydration, hemorrhage, shock, congestive heart failure. Glomerulonephritis is likely also to be "prerenal" if mild, since it compromises renal blood flow more than tubular function.
- *Renal azotemia* has several familiar causes like acute tubular necrosis, chronic interstitial nephritis, some glomerulonephritis, etc.
- *Post renal azotemia* results from obstruction of urinary flow which may be due to prostate trouble, stones, surgical mishaps, tumors.

Indications for Renal function tests

- Newly discovered high blood pressure or diabetes
- Abnormal urinalysis (anything more than "trace protein" or "honeymoon cystitis")
- Any medical problem serious enough to admit the patient to the hospital

The kidney function tests that are commonly done are

- Serum urea ("blood urea nitrogen", "BUN") level
- Serum creatinine
- Creatinine clearance
- Urinalysis

- ***Serum Urea ("BUN"):*** Clinical chemists used to measure only the nitrogen in urea, hence the "urea nitrogen" measurement on lab reports.

  Normal blood urea nitrogen is 8-25 mg/dL (2.9-8.9 mmol/L).

  Urea is filtered by the glomerulus. If the glomerular filtrate is flowing slowly through the proximal tubule, urea tends to be passively reabsorbed and return to the bloodstream. Blood urea levels are quite sensitive indicators of renal disease, becoming elevated when renal function drops to around 25-50% of normal (remember the kidney has great functional reserve). The interpretation of the BUN is usually straightforward, though there are a few things to remember. *Increased BUN is, by definition, azotemia. It is due either to increased protein catabolism or impaired kidney function.*

Increased protein catabolism results from:

- A really big protein meal
- Severe stress (myocardial infarction, high fever, etc.)
- Upper GI bleeding (blood being digested and absorbed)

In acute renal failure, BUN increases around 20 mg/dL each day (*estimates vary; range of increase is 10-50 mg/dL daily).

Decreased BUN results from:

- Lack of protein (celiac disease, some patients with nephrotic syndrome)
- Severe liver disease (end-stage cirrhosis, yellow atrophy, really bad hepatitis, halothane or acetaminophen toxicity, enzyme defects)
- Over hydration (iatrogenic, psychogenic water-drinking)

- ***Creatinine:*** This breakdown product of creatine phosphate is released from skeletal muscle at a steady rate. (Only a small amount comes from meat in the diet.) Serum creatine correlates quite well with the percent of the body that is skeletal muscle. It is filtered by the glomerulus, and a small amount is also secreted into the glomerular filtrate by the proximal tubule (hence at low GFR's, the usual reciprocal relationship breaks down and creatinine tends to underestimate how low the GFR has gotten).

  If the urine volume goes up, the serum creatinine does go down slightly.

  Creatinine is generally considered a somewhat more sensitive and specific test of renal function than BUN.

  Normal serum creatinine is 0.6-1.5 mg/dL (53-133 micromoles/L).

Increased creatinine is due to any cause of impaired kidney function listed above, a lot of meat in the diet, or a very large muscle mass (bodybuilders, anabolic steroid users, giants and acromegaly patients).

- A few drugs block the tubular secretion of creatinine, and will increase serum creatinine levels even though they have not damaged the kidney. This will be important if, and only if, the GFR is already very low. Remember probenecid, cimetidine, triamterene, trimethoprim, and amiloride.
- In massive rhabdomyolysis / crush injury, there is so much creatine released that the creatinine will probably rise.
- Athletes taking oral creatine may have slightly increases in serum creatinine levels for the next day or so, but the effect is slight and unlikely to take a person above the normal range

Decreased creatinine has little significance

- A few medicines can falsely elevate the picrate Jaffe creatinine assay. High bilirubin levels can falsely lower serum creatinine values by some of the newer methods.

- ***Creatinine clearance:*** Creatinine Clearance is widely used to approximate glomerular filtration rate

  Clearance = (conc. in urine) × (urine volume)/(conc. in plasma).

  Creatinine clearance is not a perfect measure of GFR, because some is not filtered and some is secreted into the proximal tubule. These fractions tend to cancel each other out in health, but when GFR drops below 30 mL/min, tubular secretion approaches or even exceeds the amount filtered at the glomerulus

  Reference range for creatinine clearance is 90-120 mL/min for young adults; values tend to fall by around 0.5 mL/year over age 20, worse for hypertensives

Other renal function tests

- ***N-acetyl-beta-D-glucosaminidase***: ("glucosaminidase", NAG) is a lysosomal enzyme (MW 140,000) found in serum and urine. Urinary NAG is a proposed marker for tubular disease, especially subtle industrial poisoning, acute pyelonephritis, early acute tubular necrosis, and early transplant rejection.

- ***The long ammonium chloride test*** checks for renal tubular acidosis type I (i.e., inability of the distal tubule to excrete a load of fixed acid). Ammonium chloride is administered orally and a person with "RTA I" supposedly will not be able to acidify the urine as low as pH 5.4.

- ***Adenosine Deaminase Binding Protein*** is an enzyme from the brush borders of the proximal tubule. Like NAG, its presence in urine indicates tubular disease.

- ***Urinary alkaline phosphatase*** in urine comes from the proximal tubular brush border.
- ***Beta-2 microglobulin (beta-2-m)*** is the short chain of the HLA class I proteins. In health, it is freely filtered by the glomerulus, and fully reabsorbed by the proximal tubule.
- ***Serum beta-2-m*** has been suggested as a measure of glomerular filtration rate, similar to creatinine. Obviously this isn't a good idea for patients with tissue necrosis, lymphomas, etc.
- ***Urine beta-2-m*** has found widespread acceptance as an research tool. It appears if levels in the serum and glomerular filtrate exceed what the proximal tubule can reabsorb (more than 4.5 mg/L) or if there is renal tubular disease. It is very sensitive as an indicator of the latter.

Tubular Functions

- *Urinary amino acids* and *maximum concentrating ability* are sensitive screens for tubular damage.
- *Isotope scans* exist to compare the function of the kidneys
- *Positron emission tomography* is the latest way of measuring renal blood flow.

Specific Gravity of Urine

Checking urine specific gravity provides very important information about tubular function and hydration.

Normal people (people who drink low quantity of fluids) have fairly concentrated urine (SG greater than 1.010). The same is true of patients in prerenal azotemia (high urinary specific gravity, low or zero urinary sodium). Patients with tubular disease ("renal azotemia", i.e., acute tubular necrosis, really bad bilateral pyelonephritis or interstitia nephritis, or on diuretics, or with end-stage kidney) will have isosthenuria. Patients getting lots of fluid by IV, or with diabetes insipidus, or enthusiastic water-drinkers (asthmatics, crazies) will have low urine specific gravity.

Uric Acid

This breakdown product of purine metabolism is filtered by the glomeruli and both reabsorbed and secreted by the renal tubules. Serum levels are highly variable from day to day.

Indications for ordering this test include suspected gout and suspect uric acid nephropathy. However, it is generally measured as part of an automated chemistry profile.

Increased serum uric acid is often seen in:

- renal failure
- gout (remember all patients with gout have hyperuricemia, but most patients with hyperuricemia do not have symptomatic gout)
- liver-and-sweetbread gourmets
- increased breakdown of nucleoprotein (burns, crush injuries, very severe hemolytic anemia, plasma cell myeloma, myeloproliferative disorders, and especially leukemias under treatment)
- lead poisoning
- patients receiving thiazide diuretics or high doses of aspirin
- Idiopathic (relatives of gout victims, etc.)

Low uric acid levels are of no concern.

20.9 Pulmonary Function Tests

Pulmonary function tests are a group of tests that measure how well the lungs take in and release air and how well they move oxygen into the blood.

Lung function tests are done to:

- Determine the cause of breathing problems.
- Diagnose certain lung diseases, such as asthma or chronic obstructive pulmonary disease (COPD).
- Evaluate a person's lung function before surgery.
- Monitor the lung function of a person who is regularly exposed to substances such as asbestos that can damage the lungs.
- Monitor the effectiveness of treatment for lung diseases.

Spirometry is the first lung function test done. It measures how much and how quickly the air is moved out of the lungs. By measuring how much air is exhaled, and how quickly, spirometry can evaluate a broad range of lung diseases.

Lung volume measures the amount of air in the lungs without forcibly blowing out. Some lung diseases (such as emphysema and chronic bronchitis) can make the lungs contain too much air. Other lung diseases (such as fibrosis of the lungs and asbestosis) make the lungs scarred and smaller so that they contain too little air.

By testing the diffusion capacity (also called the DLCO) we can estimate how well the lungs move oxygen from the air into the bloodstream.

Normal values are based upon age, height, ethnicity, and sex. Normal results are expressed as a percentage. A value is usually considered abnormal if it is less than 80% of your predicted value. Abnormal results usually mean that the individual may have some chest or lung disease. The tests can diagnose lung diseases, measure the severity of lung problems, and check to see how well treatment for a lung disease is working.

Other tests such as residual volume, gas diffusion tests, body plethysmography, inhalation challenge tests, and exercise stress tests may also be done to determine lung function.

Common lung function values measured with spirometry are

- ***Forced vital capacity (FVC):*** This measures the amount of air you can exhale with force after you inhale as deeply as possible.
- ***Forced expiratory volume (FEV):*** This measures the amount of air you can exhale with force in one breath. The amount of air you exhale may be measured at 1 second (FEV1), 2 seconds (FEV2), or 3 seconds (FEV3). FEV1 divided by FVC can also be determined.
- ***Forced expiratory flow 25% to 75%:*** This measures the air flow halfway through an exhale (FVC).
- ***Peak expiratory flow (PEF):*** This measure's how quickly you can exhale. It is usually measured at the same time as your forced vital capacity (FVC).
- ***Maximum voluntary ventilation (MVV):*** This measures the greatest amount of air you can breathe in and out during one minute.
- ***Slow vital capacity (SVC):*** This measures the amount of air you can slowly exhale after you inhale as deeply as possible.
- ***Total lung capacity (TLC):*** This measures the amount of air in your lungs after you inhale as deeply as possible.
- ***Functional residual capacity (FRC):*** This measures the amount of air in your lungs at the end of a normal exhaled breath.
- ***Expiratory reserve volume (ERV):*** This measures the difference between the amount of air in your lungs after a normal exhale (FRC) and the amount after you exhale with force (RV).

Gas diffusion tests

Gas diffusion tests measure the amount of oxygen and other gases that cross the lungs' air sacs (alveoli) per minute. These tests evaluate how well gases are being absorbed into the blood from lungs. Gas diffusion tests include:

- ***Arterial blood gases,*** which determine the amount of oxygen and carbon dioxide in the bloodstream.
- Carbon monoxide diffusing capacity (also called transfer factor, or TF), which measures how well the lungs transfer a small amount of carbon monoxide (CO) into the blood. Two different methods are used for this test. If the single-breath or breath-holding method is used, the individual will take a breath of air containing a very small amount of carbon monoxide from a container while measurements are taken. In the steady-state method, the individual will breathe air containing a very small amount of carbon monoxide from a container. The amount of carbon monoxide in the breath exhaled is then measured.

Body plethysmography may be used to measure

- ***Total lung capacity (TLC)*** is the total amount of air the lungs can hold. For this test, the individual will sit inside an airtight booth called a plethysmograph and breathe through a mouthpiece while pressure and air flow measurements are collected.
- ***Residual volume (RV)*** is the amount of air that remains in the lungs after exhalation as completely as possible. For this test, the individual will sit inside the plethysmograph booth and breathe a known amount of a gas (either 100% oxygen or a certain amount of helium in air). The test measures how the concentration of the gases in the booth changes.

Inhalation challenge tests

Inhalation challenge tests are done to measure the response of your airways to substances (allergens) that may be causing asthma or wheezing. The tests also may determine the effect of chemicals such as histamine or methacholine on your airways. These tests are also called provocation studies.

During inhalation testing, increasing amounts of an allergen are inhaled through a nebulizer, a device that uses a face mask or mouthpiece to deliver the allergen in a fine mist (aerosol). Alternatively, increasing amounts of a substance (histamine or methacholine) may be inhaled through the nebulizer. Before and after inhaling the substance, spirometry readings are taken to evaluate lung function.

Exercise stress tests

Exercise stress tests evaluate the effect of exercise on lung function tests. Spirometry readings are done after exercise and then again at rest.

Lung function results are measured directly in some tests and are calculated in others. No single test can determine all of the lung function values, so more than one type of test may be done. Some of the tests may be repeated after you inhale medicine that enlarges your airways (bronchodilator).

Table 20.2 Lung function values in obstructive disease.

Lung function test	Result as predicted for age, height, sex, weight, or race
Forced vital capacity (FVC)	Normal or lower than predicted value
Forced expiratory volume (FEV1)	Lower
FEV1 divided by FVC	Lower
Forced expiratory flow 25% to 75%	Lower
Peak expiratory flow (PEF)	Lower
Maximum voluntary ventilation (MVV)	Lower
Slow vital capacity (SVC)	Normal or lower
Total lung capacity (TLC) (V_T)	Normal or higher
Functional residual capacity (FRC)	Higher
Residual volume (RV)	Higher
Expiratory reserve volume (ERV)	Normal or lower
RV divided by TLC ratio	Higher

20.10 Thyroid Function Tests

Thyroid function tests (TFTs) is a collective term for blood tests used to check the function of the thyroid.

A TFT panel may include:

- Circulating concentrations of:
  - Total Hormones
    - thyroid-stimulating hormone (TSH, thyrotropin)
    - thyroxine (T_4),
    - triiodothyronine (T_3)

- Free hormones (direct measurements)
    - Free T_4
    - Free T_3
- Carrier proteins
    - Thyroid binding globulin
    - Transthyretin
    - Albumin

- Measures of protein binding of thyroid hormones
    - T_{uptake}
    - Thyroid hormone binding ratio (THBR)
    - Thyroxine-binding index (TBI)
- Calculated indices of free hormones
    - Free T4 index
    - Free T3 index

TFTs may be requested if a patient is thought to suffer from *hyperthyroidism* (overactive thyroid) or *hypothyroidism* (under active thyroid), or to monitor the effectiveness of either thyroid-suppression or hormone replacement therapy. It is also requested routinely in conditions linked to thyroid disease, such as atrial fibrillation.

The glands essentially that are involved in thyroid function are

- Thyroid
- Parathyroid

Thyroid: The thyroid gland influences body growth, metabolism, and the storage of iodine. Body growth and metabolism are controlled by two hormones, thyroxine and triiodothyronine. The iodine absorbed from the intestinal tract is removed from the plasma by this gland. The inorganic iodine is converted to organic iodide when it is incorporated into the nucleus of the amino acid tyrosine to form monoiodotyrosine. Diiodotyrosine is formed when a second iodine atom is incorporated. Thyroxine (T_4) is formed when diiodotyrosine condenses with itself. If diiodotyrosine condenses with monoiodotyrosine, triiodothyronine (T_3) is formed. Diseases of the thyroid may or may not affect hormone production. The over production of hormone is called hyperthyroidism. Abnormal conditions not associated with hormone production include goiters and acute and chronic thyroiditis.

Thyroid function is best ascertained by the use of several tests: free thyroxine (T_F); protein-bound iodine (PBI); blood cholesterol; triiodothyronine (T_3) test on red blood cell uptake or resin; radioactive iodine thyroid uptake; butanol-extractable iodine (BEI); and T_4 by column chromatography.

Parathyroid: The parathyroid hormone is responsible for regulating the concentrations of serum calcium and phosphorus levels. In the blood there is a reciprocal relationship between serum calcium and phosphorus. When one has a low serum concentration, the other exists in a high serum level. Hypoparathyroidism is characterized by low serum calcium and high serum phosphorus levels. A low level of serum phosphorus with increased levels of serum calcium, and an increased excretion of calcium in the urine are found in hyperparathyroidism. Sulkowitch's test is a commonly used method for urine calcium determination, and was discussed in the section on urine tests.

Table 20.3 Common Thyroid function tests, values and interpretation

Name of the Test	Normal Range	Interpretation
"TSH" Test -- Thyroid Stimulating Hormone / Serum thyrotropin	0.4 to 6 0.3 to 3.0 (as of 2003)	Less than .4 can indicate possible hyperthyroidism. Over 6 are considered indicative of hypothyroidism. **Note:** the American Association of Clinical Endocrinologists has revised these guidelines as of early 2003, narrowing the range to .3 to 3.0. Many labs and practitioners are not, however, aware of these revised guidelines.)
Total T4 / Serum thyroxine	4.5 to 12.5	Less than 4.5 can be indicative of an under functioning thyroid when TSH is also elevated. Over 12.5 can indicate hyperthyroidism. Low T4 with low TSH can sometimes indicate a pituitary problem.
Free T4 / Free Thyroxine - FT4	0.7 to 2.0	Less than 0.7 is considered indicative of possible hypothyroidism.
T3 / Serum Triiodothyronine	80 to 220	Less than 80 can indicate hypothyroidism.

Table 20.4 Some common lab values.

Albumin	3.2 - 5 g/dl	
Alkaline phosphatase (Adults: 25-60)	33 - 131 IU/L	
Adults > 61 years	51 - 153 IU/L	
Ammonia	20 - 70 mcg/dl	
Bilirubin, direct	0 - 0.3 mg/dl	
Bilirubin, total	0.1 - 1.2 mg/dl	
Blood Gases		
	Arterial	Venous
Ph	7.35 - 7.45	7.32 - 7.42
pCO_2	35 - 45	38 - 52
pO_2	70 - 100	28 - 48
HCO_3	19 - 25	19 - 25
O_2 Sat %	90 - 95	40 - 70
BUN	7 - 20 mg/dl	
Complete blood count (CBC)		
	Male	Female
Hemoglobin (g/dl)	13.5 - 16.5	12.0 - 15.0
Haematocrit (%)	41 - 50	36 - 44
RBC's (x 10^6/ml)	4.5 - 5.5	4.0 - 4.9
RDW (RBC distribution width)	< 14.5	
MCV	80 – 100	
MCH	26 – 34	
MCHC %	31 – 37	
Platelet count	100,000 to 450,000	
Creatinine kinase (CK) isoenzymes		
CK-BB	0%	
CK-MB (cardiac)	0 - 3.9%	
CK-MM	96 - 100%	
Creatine phosphokinase (CPK)	8 - 150 IU/L	
Creatinine (mg/dl)	0.5 - 1.4	
Electrolytes		
Calcium	8.8 - 10.3 mg/dL	
Calcium, ionized	2.24 - 2.46 meq/L	
Chloride	95 - 107 mEq/L	
Magnesium	1.6 - 2.4 mEq/L	
Phosphate	2.5 - 4.5 mg/dL	

Table 20.4 *Contd...*

Potassium	3.5 - 5.2 mEq/L
Sodium	135 - 147 mEq/L
Ferritin (ng/ml)	13 – 300
Folate (ng/dl)	3.6 – 20
Glucose, fasting (mg/dl)	60 – 110
Glucose (2 hours postprandial) (mg/dl)	Up to 140
Hemoglobin A_{1c}	6-8
Iron (mcg/dl)	65 – 150
Lactic acid (meq/L)	0.7 - 2.1
LDH (lactic dehydrogenase)	56 - 194 IU/L
Lipoproteins and triglycerides	
Cholesterol, total	< 200 mg/dl
HDL cholesterol	30 - 70 mg/dl
LDL cholesterol	65 - 180 mg/dl
Triglycerides	45 - 155 mg/dl (< 160)
Osmolality	289 - 308 mOsm/kg
SGOT (AST)	< 35 IU/L (20-48)
SGPT (ALT)	<35 IU/L
Thyroid Function tests	
Free T3	2.3-4.2 pg/ml
Serum T3	70-200 ng/dl
Free T4	0.5-2.1 ng/dl
Serum T4	4.0-12.0 mcg/dl
TSH	0.25-4.30 microunits/ml
Total iron binding capacity (TIBC)	250 - 420 mcg/dl
Transferrin	> 200 mg/dl
Uric acid (male)	2.0 - 8.0 mg/dl
(female)	2.0 - 7.5 mg/dl
WBC + differential	
WBC (cells/ml)	4,500 - 10,000
Segmented neutrophils	54 - 62%
Band forms	3 - 5% (above 8% indicates left shift)
Basophils	0 - 1 (0 - 0.75%)
Eosinophils	0 - 3 (1 - 3%)
Lymphocytes	24 - 44 (25 - 33%)
Monocytes	3 - 6 (3 - 7%)

Table 20.5 Some important lab values and their interpretation.

Lab	Normal value	Comments
Albumin	3.5 - 5.0 mg/dl	**Decreased:** cystic fibrosis, chronic glomerulonephritis, alcoholic cirrhosis, Hodgkin's disease, malnutrition, nephrotic syndrome, multiple myeloma, inflammatory bowel disease, leukemia, collagen-vascular diseases
Aldosterone	upright: 4-31 ng/dl	**Increased:** hyperaldosterism (primary or secondary). **Decreased:** adrenal insufficiency, panhypopituitarism.
Amylase	30-100 U/liter	**Increased:** acute pancreatitis, pancreatic duct obstruction, alcohol ingestion, mumps, parotitidis, renal disease, cholecystitis, peptic ulcers, intestinal obstruction, mesenteric thrombosis, postoperative abdominal surgery. **Decreased:** Liver damage, pancreatic destruction (pancreatitis, cystic fibrosis)
Bilirubin	Total: 0.2 - 1.2 mg/dl; direct: <0.3 mg/dl	**Increased total:** hepatic damage (hepatitis, toxins, cirrhosis), biliary obstruction, hemolysis, fasting. **Increased direct** (conjugated): biliary obstruction / cholestasis, drug induced cholestasis.
BUN	7-20 mg/dl	**Increased:** renal failure, pre-renal azotemia, shock, volume depletion, post renal (obstruction), GI bleeding, stress, drugs (aminoglycosides, vanco etc). **Decreased:** starvation, liver failure, pregnancy, infancy, nephrotic syndrome, and over hydration.
Calcium	8.8 – 10.3 mg/dl	**Increased:** primary hyperthyroidism, parathyroid hormone secreting tumors, vitamin D excess, metastatic bone tumors, chronic renal failure, milk-alkali syndrome, osteoporosis, thiazide drugs, pagets disease, multiple myeloma, and sarcoidosis. **Decreased:** hypoparathyroidism, insufficient vitamin D, hypomagnesaemia, renal tubular acidosis, hypoalbuminemia, chronic renal failure (phosphate retention), acute pancreatitis
C02 (total)	23-30 meq/l	**Increased:** respiratory acidosis, compensation for metabolic acidosis, severe vomiting, primary aldosteronism, volume contraction, emphysema **Decreased:** Respiratory alkalosis, starvation, DKA, lactic acidosis, alcoholic ketoacidosis, severe diarrhea, renal failure, drugs (salicylates etc), dehydration.
Chloride	95-107 meq/l	**Increased:** diarrhea, renal tubular acidosis, mineral corticoid deficiency, hyper alimentation, medications (acetazolamide, ammonium chloride) **Decreased:** mineral corticoid excess, vomiting, diabetes mellitus with ketoacidosis
Creatinine	0.5 - 1.4 mg/dl	**Increased:** renal failure including prerenal, drug-induced (aminoglycosides, vancomycin, others), acromegaly. **Decreased:** loss of muscle mass, pregnancy.
Ferritin	13 - 300 ng/ml	**Decreased:** iron deficiency anemia (earliest sign)

Lab	Normal value	Comments
Iron binding capacity (TIBC)	250-420 mcg/dl	**Increased:** acute and chronic blood loss, iron deficiency anemia, hepatitis, and oral contraceptives. **Decreased:** anemia of infection and chronic diseases, cirrhosis, nephrosis, haemochromatosis
Magnesium	1.6 - 2.6 mg/dl	**Increased:** renal failure, hypothyroidism, severe dehydration, lithium intoxication, antacids, Addison's disease. **Decreased:** hyperthyroidism, aldosteronism, diuretics, malabsorption, hyperalimentation, nasogastric suctioning, chronic dialysis, renal tubular acidosis, drugs (aminoglycosides, cisplatin, ampho B), and hungry bone syndrome, and hypophosphatemia, intracellular shifts with respiratory or metabolic acidosis.
Osmolality	278 – 298 mOsm/kg	**Increased:** hypernatremia, hyperglycemia, water loss (diuretics, diabetes), alcohol ingestion, ethylene glycol ingestion, and mannitol. **Decreased:** hyponatremia, diuretics, Addison's disease, SIADH.
Phosphorus	2.5 - 4.5 mg/dl	**Increased:** hypoparathyroidism, excess vitamin D, secondary hyperparathyroidism, renal failure, bone disease, Addison's disease. **Decreased:** hyperparathyroidism, alcoholism, diabetes, hyperalimentation, acidosis, hypomagnesaemia, diuretics, vitamin D deficiency, and phosphate-binding antacids.
Transferrin	200-400 mg/dl	**Increased:** iron deficiency anemia. **Decreased:** acute and chronic inflammatory states, poor nutritional status, and chronic liver disease.
Uric acid	Male: 3 - 8 mg/dl. female: 2-7 mg/dl	**Increased:** gout, renal failure, drugs (diuretics, others), hypothyroidism, chemotherapy, parathyroid diseases, lactic acidosis. **Decreased:** drugs (allopurinol, probenecid, others), Wilson's disease, Fanconi's syndrome.

APPENDIX 1

ROUTES OF ADMINISTRATION

Term	Site
Oral peroral (per os[1])	Mouth gastrointestinal tract via mouth
Sublingual	Under the tongue
Parentral	Other than the gastrointestinal tract (by injection)
Intravenous	Vein
Intra-arterial	Artery
Intracardiac	Heart
Intraspinal or intrathecal	Spine
Intraosseous	Bone
Intra-articular	Joint
Intrasynovial	Joint-fluid area
Intracutaneous or intradermal	Skin
Subcutaneous	Beneath the skin
Intramuscular	Muscle
Epicutaneous (topical)	Skin surface
Transdermal	Skin surface
Conjunctival	Conjunctiva
Intraocular	Eye
Intranasal	Nose
Aural	Ear
Intrarespiratory	Lung
Rectal	Rectum
Vaginal	Vagina
Urethral	Urethra

[1]The abbreviation "p.o." is commonly employed on prescriptions to indicate to be swallowed.

Reference: Ansel HC, et al. Pharm. Dosage Forms and Drug Delivery Systems, 6th Ed., 1995.

APPENDIX 2

POISON / OVERDOSE ANTIDOTES

POISON	ANTIDOTE	ADULT DOSAGE	COMMENTS
Acetaminophen	N-Acetylcysteine	140mg/kg initial dose	Most effective within 16 hrs
Arsenic	(See Mercury)		
Atropine	Physostigmine	Initial dose 0.5-2mg (IV)	Can produce convulsions, bradycardia
Benzodiazepines	Flumazenil	1.5-10mg IV for reversing	Lower doses are used in coma and sedation, anesthesia reversal.
Carbon monoxide	Oxygen		
Cyanide	Amyl nitrite; then	Pearls every 2 min	Methemoglobin cyanide complex.
	Sodium nitrite	10ml of 3% solution over 3 min (IV). 0.33ml (10mg 3% sol) / kg initially for children	Causes hypotension. Dosage assumes normal hemoglobin.
	Sodium thiosulfate	25% solution – 50 ml	Forms harmless sodium thiocyanate.
Digoxin Digitoxin	Digoxin Immune Fab	Calculated fromw total digoxin in patient's body. 38mg binds with approx. 0 .5mg of digoxin.	Administred IV over 30 min. using 0.22 M filter. Bolus has also been given.

Contd...

POISON	ANTIDOTE	ADULT DOSAGE	COMMENTS
Ethylene glycol	(See Methyl alcohol)		
Gold	(See Mercury)		
Heparin	Protamine	1-1.5 mg IV for every 100 units of heparin, if given within the first few minutes. The dose should be reduced depending on the time of heparin admin.	Coagulation tests are performed 5-15 minutes after protamine admin. 10mg/ml solution is injected slowly over 1-3 min. The drug has also been given continuous IV infusion.
Iron	Deferoxamine	Initial dose:40-90mg/kg IM not to exceed 1 gm.	Forms excretable ferrioxamine complexes.
Lead	Edetate calcium disodium	5ml of 20% ampoule/250ml in D5W over 1 hour.	Dilute to less than 3% solution. Calcium displaced by lead, to form stable complexes.
	Succimer	Children: Start dosage at 10mg/kg or 350mg/m^2q 8 h x 5 days, then q 12h for 14 days. (Total 19 days)	Patient who received EDTA with or without BAL may use Succimer for subsequent treatment after an interval of 4 weeks. Concomitant use not recommended.
Mercury Arsenic Gold compounds	BAL (British antilewisite)	5mg/kg (IM) as soon as possible.	Forms stable non-excretable cyclic compounds.
Methyl alcohol	Ethyl alcohol in conjunction with dialysis	1mL/kg of 100% ethanol initially in glucose solution; maintain blood level of 100 mg/100ml.	Competes for genase; prevents formation of formic acid, oxalates.
Nitrites	Methylene blue	0.2ml/kg of 1% solution (IV) over 5 min.	Often exchange transfusion is needed for severe methemoglobinemia.

Contd…

POISON	ANTIDOTE	ADULT DOSAGE	COMMENTS
Opiates Darvon Lomotil	Naloxone	0.4-0.8mg (IV) 0.01 mg/kg (IV)-Children	Naloxone does not cause respiratory depression.
Organophosphates	Atropine	Initial dose:0.5-2mg(IV) Children:0.05mg/kg (IV) initially.	Atropine blocks acetylcholine. Up to 5mg (IV) every 15 minutes may be necessary in critical adults.
	Pralidoxime (Protopam)	Initial dose: 1 gm IV children: 25-50mg/kg IV	Pralidoxime breaks alkyl phosphate cholinesterase bond. Up to 500 mg every hour may be necessary in the critical adult.

Reference: Emergency Medicine, American College of Emergency Physicians

APPENDIX 3

SUGGESTED GUIDELINES FOR THERAPEUTIC DRUG CONCENTRATION MONITORING

	DESIRED SERUM LEVEL
ACETAMINOPHEN : (Oral) - overdose : at least 4 hours post ingestion.	10-20mcg/ml
AMIKACIN: - (IV peak): 30 minutes after completion of infusion. - (IM peak): 60 minutes after dose administered. - (IV/IM trough) : 30 – 60 minutes prior to next dose.	20-30 mcg/ml <10mcg/ml
CARBAMAZEPINE: (Oral) - sample just before next dose (trough).	4-12 mcg/ml
CYCLOSPORIN A: (IV, Oral) - sample just before next dose (trough).	250-900ng/ml whole blood 50-300ng/ml plasma
DIGOXIN: (IV, Oral) - sample just before next dose (trough) - if peak desired, at least 4 hours after IV dose and 6 hours after PO dose administered.	1-2ng/ml

Contd...

DISOPYRAMIDE: (Oral) - sample just before next dose (trough). - if peak desired, at least 2 to 2.5 hours after dose administered.	 2-6mcg/ml
ETHOSUXIMIDE: (Oral) - sample just before next dose (trough) - if peak desired, at least 2.5 to 4 hours after dose administered.	 40-100mcg/ml
GENTAMICIN: - (IV peak): 30 minutes after completion of infusion. - (IM peak): 60 minutes after dose administered. - (IV/IM trough): 30-60 minutes prior to next dose.	 4-8mcg/ml < 2mcg/ml
HEPARIN: - blood sample for PTT at least 6 hours after infusion rate changed.	 1.2-1.5 times control 1.5-2 times control
LIDOCAINE: - (IV infusion): sample anytime after steady-state achieved. May take sample 4-8 hours after start of maintenance infusion.	 1-5mcg/ml
METHOTREXATE: (IV) - blood sample during infusion, at 48 hours, and every 24 hours until level drops below concentration where patient considered to be rescued.	 Variable Plasma concentrations exceeding 1×10^{-8} to 1×10^{-7} molar for 48 hrs or more are associated with toxicity.
NAPA [n-acetyl-procainamide]: (Oral) - sample just before next dose (trough).	 10-20 mcg/ml
PHENOBARBITAL: (Oral and Parenteral) - sample just before next dose (trough). - if peak desired, at least 1 hour after dose administered.	 10-30mcg/ml Up to 40 mcg/ml in children.

Contd...

PHENYTOIN: (Oral and Parenteral) - sample just before next dose (trough). - If peak desired after loading dose, at least 2-4 hours after completion of loading dose.	10-20mcg/ml
PRIMIDONE: (Oral) - sample just before next dose (trough).	5-12mcg/ml
PROCAINAMIDE: (Oral and Parenteral) - sample just before next dose (trough). - if peak desired, at least 2.5 hours after PO (plain) dose, 4 hours after PO (sustained release), and 2 hours after beginning of maintenance infusion.	4-8mcg/ml
QUINIDINE: (Oral) - sample just before next dose (trough). - if peak desired, at least 1.5 hours after PO (sulfate) dose, and 4 hours after PO (gluconate) dose.	2-5mcg/ml
THEOPHYLLINE: (Oral) - sample just before next dose (trough). - if peak desired, at least 2 hours after PO (sulfate) dose, and 4 hours after PO (sustained released) dose. - (IV infusion): sample anytime after reaching steady state. May take sample 30 minutes after IV loading dose, then 14-20 hours after the start of a maintenance infusion.	10-20mcg/ml
TOBRAMYCIN: - (IV peak): 30 minutes after completion of infusion. - (IM peak): 60 minutes after dose administered. - (IV/IM trough): 30-60 minutes prior to next dose.	4-8mcg/ml < 2mcg/ml
VALPROIC ACID: (Oral) - sample just before next dose (trough). - if peak desired, at least 2-3 hours after dose.	50-100 mcg/ml

Contd...

VANCOMYCIN:	
- (IV peak) : 30 minutes after completion of infusion.	40-50 mcg/ml
- (IV trough) : 30-60 minutes prior to next dose.	<10mcg/ml

***References*:**

1. WINTER M.E. Basic Clinical Pharmacokinetics: 2nd ed Applied Therapeutics, 1988
2. MIODVEL H.J. Therapeutic Drug Monitoring. Hospital Pharmacy, 24:614-631; 1989
3. American Society of Hospital Pharmacists AHFS Drug Information, 1990

APPENDIX 4

COMMON LATIN ABBREVIATIONS USED IN PRESCRIPTIONS

Latin Phrase	Abbreviation	English Meaning
Ana	aa.	Of cach
Ante	a.	Before
Ante Cibos	a.c.	Before meal
Aqua	aq.	Water
Aqua distillate	aq.dist.	Distilled water
Auris	aur.	Ear
Auris utrae	a.u.	Each ear
Auris dextra	a.d.	Right ear
Aris laeva	a.l.	Left ear
Bis	b.	Twice
Bis in die	b.i.d	Twice a day
Cibus	c.	Food
Collutorium	collut.	A mouth wash
Collyrium	collyr.	An eye wash
Compositus	comp.	Compounded
Cum	c.	With
Et	et	And
Fortis	fort.	Strong
Gutta	gtt.	Drop

Latin Phrase	Abbreviation	English Meaning
Hora Somni	h.s.	At bedtime
Liquor	liq.	Solution
Mistura	mist.	Mixture
Nox, Nocte	noct.	Night
Oculus	o.	Eye
Oculus dexter	o.d.	Right eye
Oculus laevus	o.l	Left eye
Oculus sinister	o.s.	Left eye
Oculi uterque	o.u	Both eyes
Per Os	p.o.	By mouth
Post Cibos	p.c.	After meals (after eating)
Pro re nata	p.r.n	When necessary (as needed)
Pulvis	pulv.	Powder
Quaque, quisque	q.	each, every
Quaque die	q.d	every day
Quantum satis/ Quantum sufficiat	q.s.	As much as is sufficient
Quarter in die	q.i.d	Four times a day
Semi, Semis	ss.	A half
Statim	stat	Immediately
Ter in die	t.i.d./t.d.	Three times a day
Unguentum	ung.	Ointment

APPENDIX 5

CONVERSION TABLES

WEIGHTS MEASURE

Avoirdupois Weight

1 pound (lb) = 16 ounces (oz) = 256 drams = 7000 grains (gr)

1 ounce …. ….. = 16 drams = 437.5 grains

Apothecary Weight

1 pound (lb) = 2 ounces (oz) = 96 drams = 288 scruples = 5760 grains

1 ounce …. = 8 drams = 24 scruples = 480 grains

Metric System

1 kilogram (kg) = 1000 grams (gm) 1 gram = 1000 milligrams (mg)

1 milligram (mg) = 1000 micrograms (mcg) 1 microgram = 1000 nanograms(ngm)

Conversion

1 kilogram = 2.2 avoirdupois pounds… …. … = 2.68 apothecary's pound

1 pound avoirdupois = 454 grams

1 pound apothecaries = 373 gram

1 ounce avoirdupois = 28.3 gram

1 ounce apothecaries = 31.1 gram

1 gram = 15.43 grains (avoirdupois / apothecaries)

1 grain = 64.8 milligrams

LINEAR MEASURE

Conversion

1 kilometer = 0.621372 mile

1 meter = 39.37 inches

1 inch = 2.54 cm

VOLUME MEASURE

Apothecaries (USA)			Metric
1 Gallon….. ….. ….	= 4 quarts …	= 8 pints … …. ….	= 3.785 liters
1 Pint …. …… …..	= 16 fl oz ….	= 128 fl drams …..	= 473 ml
1 fluid ounce ….	= 8 fl drams …	= 480 minims …. …	= 29.6 ml

British Imperial			Metric
1 Gallon …. ….	= 8 pints …. …..	= 160 fl oz …. ….	= 4.546 liters
1 Pint ….. …..	= 20 fl oz … …..	= 128 fl drams….	= 568 ml
1 fluid ounce …	= 8 fl drams …..	= 480 minims …..	= 28.4 ml

HOUSEHOLD MEASURES

1 ml … … …. = 15 to 20 drops

1 teaspoonful .. … = 5 ml

1 tablespoonful… = 15ml

1 glassful …. …. = 240 ml … …. = 8 fl ounces

TEMPERATURE EQUIVALENTS

Centigrade Degrees	Fahrenheit Degrees	Centigrade Degrees	Fahrenheit Degrees
0	32	35	95
2	35.6	37	98.6
8	46.4	38	100.5
22	71.6	39	102.2
25	77	100	212

To convert Centigrade to Fahrenheit: $F = (C x 9/5) + 32$

To covert Fahrenheit to Centigrade: $C = (F - 32) \times 5/9$

MILLIEQUIVALENTS AND MILLIMOLES

Element	Milliequivalent (mEq)		Milli mole (mMol)		Milligram (mg)
Calcium (Ca)	1	=	0.5	=	20
Chloride (Cl)	1	=	1	=	35.5
Magnesium (Mg)	1	=	0.5	=	12
Phosphorous (P)	---		1	=	31
Potassium (K)	1	=	1	=	39
Sodium (Na)	1	=	1	=	23

APPENDIX 6

ELEMENTAL CONTENT OF SOME SALTS

Salt	mEq/gram	Elemental content per gram
Ammonium chloride	18.7 mEq of Cl	.....
Calcium carbonate	20.0 mEq of Ca	400 mg of Ca
Calcium chloride	13.6 mEq of Ca	272 mg of Ca
Calcium glubionate	3.3 mEq of Ca	65 mg of Ca
Calcium gluconate	4.5 mEq of Ca	90 mg of Ca
Ferrous fumarate	.....	330 mg of Fe
Ferrous gluconate	.....	116 mg of Fe
Ferrous sulfate	.....	200 mg of Fe
Magnesium sulfate 7 H_2O	8.12 mEq of Mg	97.4 mg of Mg
Potassium acetate	10.2 mEq of K	398 mg of K
Potassium chloride	13.4 mEq of K	523 mg of K
Potassium phosphate	7.3 mEq of K and	285 mg of K and
(monobasic)	7.3 mMol of P	226 mg of P
Potassium phosphate	11.5 mEq of K and	449 mg of K and
(diabasic)	5.7 mMol of P	177 mg of P
Sodium acetate	7.3 mEq of Na	168 mg of Na
Sodium bicarbonate	11.9 mEq of Na	274 mg of Na
Sodium chloride	17.1 mEq of Na	393 mg of Na

Salt	mEq/gram	Elemental content per gram
Sodium lactate	8.9 mEq of Na	205 mg of Na
Sodium phosphate H_2O	7.2 mEq of Na and	166 mg of Na and
(monobasic)	7.2 mMol of P	223 mg of P
Sodium phosphate	14.1 mEq of Na and	550 mg of Na and
(dibasic)	7 mMol of P	217 mg of P
Zinc sulfate $7H_2O$	.....	227 mg of Zn

APPENDIX 7

CREATININE CLEARANCE (Cl_{CR}) ESTIMATION IN PATIENTS WITH STABLE RENAL FUNCTION

Children: 1-18 years

***Traub method*:** units = mg/dl

(Traub SL, Johnson CE. *Am J Hosp Pharm,* 1980, 37: 195-201)

$$Cl_{cr} = \frac{0.48 \times \text{height(cm)} \times \text{BSA}(m^2)}{\text{serum creatinine(mg / dl)} \times 1.73}$$

BSA – Body Surface Area

Adults: 18 years and older

1. ***Cockroft and Gault method*:** units = ml/min

   (Cockroft DW and Gault MH. *Nephron* 1976, 16:31-41)

   Male: $Cl_{cr} = \frac{(140 - \text{age in years}) \times \text{IBW (kg)}}{72 \times \text{serum creatinine(mg / dl)}}$

   Female: $Cl_{cr} = Cl_{cr}\ (\text{male}) \times 0.85$

   Note: The use of the patient's ideal body weight (IBW) is recommended for the above formula except when the patient's actual body weight is less than ideal. Use of the IBW is especially important in obese patients.

2. ***Jelliffe method***: units = $ml/min/1.73m^2$

(Jelliffe RW. *Ann Intern Med,* 1973, 79: 604)

Male: $Cl_{cr} = \dfrac{98 - 0.8\,(\text{age in yrs} - 20)}{\text{serum creatinine (mg/dl)}}$

Female: $Cl_{cr} = Cl_{cr}\,(\text{male}) \times 0.90$

Reference: Taketomo CK, et al. Pediatric Dosage Handbook, 2nd Ed, 1993-94

APPENDIX 8

IDEAL BODY WEIGHT

Children

1. 1-18 years

$$\text{IBW (in kg)} = \frac{\text{height}^2\,(\text{cm}) \times 1.65}{1000}$$

2. 5 feet and taller

   Male: IBW = 39 + (2.27 x height in inches over 5 feet)

   Female: IBW = 42.2 + (2.27 x height in inches over 5 feet)

References: Traub Sl, Johnson CE. *Am J Hosp Pharm, 1980,* 37:195-201
Taketomo CK, et al. Pediatric Dosage Handbook, 2nd Ed, 1993-94

Adults:

18 years and older

Male: IBW (in kg) = 50 + (2.3 × height in inches over 5 feet)

Female: IBW (in kg) = 45.5 + (2.3 × height in inches over 5 feet)

References: Evans WE, et al. Applied Pharmacokinetics, 3rd Ed, 1992
Taketomo Ck, et al. Pediatric Dosage Handbook, 2nd Ed, 1993-94

APPENDIX 9

HEIGHT WEIGHT CHART

Standard Height and Weight for Indian Men and Women

	Men	Women
Height (Feet & Meters)	**Weight (kgs)**	**Weight (kgs)**
5'-0" (1.523 m)	50.8 - 54.4	50.8 - 54.4
5'-1" (1.548 m)	51.7 - 55.3	51.7 - 55.3
5'-2" (1.574 m)	56.3 - 60.3	53.1 - 56.7
5'-3" (1.599 m)	57.6 - 61.7	54.4 - 58.1
5'-4" (1.624 m)	58.9 - 63.5	56.3 - 59.9
5'-5" (1.650 m)	60.8 - 65.3	57.6 - 61.2
5'-6" (1.675 m)	62.2 - 66.7	58.9 - 63.5
5'-7" (1.700 m)	64.0 - 68.5	60.8 - 65.3
5'-8" (1.726 m)	65.8 - 70.8	62.2 - 66.7
5'-9" (1.751 m)	67.6 - 72.6	64.0 - 68.5
5'-10" (1.777 m)	69.4 - 74.4	65.8 - 70.3
5'-11" (1.802 m)	71.2 - 76.2	67.1 - 71.7
6'-0" (1.827 m)	73.0 - 78.5	68.5 - 73.9
6'-1" (1.853 m)	73.3 - 80.7	73.3 - 80.7
6'-2" (1.878 m)	77.6 - 83.5	77.6 - 83.5
6'-3" (1.904 m)	79.8 - 85.9	79.8 - 85.9

Height and Weight Chart for Indian Boys and Girls

Boys			Girls	
Height (Cm)	**Weight (Kg)**	**Age**	**Height (Cm)**	**Weight (Kg)**
47.1	2.6	Birth	46.7	2.6
59.1	5.3	3 months	58.4	5.0
64.7	6.7	6 Months	63.7	6.2
68.2	7.4	9 Months	67.0	6.9
73.9	8.4	1 Year +	72.5	7.8
81.6	10.1	2 Years +	80.1	9.6
88.9	11.8	3 Years +	87.2	11.2
96.0	13.5	4 Years +	94.5	12.9
102.1	14.8	5 Years +	101.4	14.5
108.5	16.3	6 Years +	107.4	16.0
113.9	18.0	7 Years+	112.8	17.6
119.3	19.7	8 Years +	118.2	19.4
123.7	21.5	9 Years +	122.9	21.3
124.4	23.5	10 Years +	123.4	23.6

APPENDIX 10

DRUG AND FOOD INTERACTIONS

The following is the list of drugs whose bioavailability or concentration may ***increase*** significantly when given concurrently with food. Interaction can be prevented by avoiding concurrent administration. It will be advisable to administer the drug one hour before or two hours after meals.

Drug Name	Food Type	Comments
Cefuroxime	Food or diary food	
Cyclosporine	Food	
Cyclosporine	Grapefruit juice	May cause drug toxicity (renal dysfunction)
Diltiazem	Food	
Erythromycin	Food	Altered drug serum levels
Griseofulvin	Food	
Isoniazid	Tyramine food	May increase blood pressure
Isotretinoin	Food	
Labetalol	Food	
Lithium	Food	
Mebendazole	Food	
Methoxsalen	Food	
Morphine	Food	
Nitrofurantoin	Food	
Oral Contraceptives	Caffeine	CNS stimulation
Propranolol	Food	
Selegiline	Tyramine food	May increase blood pressure
Theophylline	Caffeine	
Theophylline	Food	Altered drug serum levels (May increase or decrease)

The following is the list of drugs whose bioavailability or concentration may **decrease** significantly when given concurrently with food. Interaction can be prevented by avoiding concurrent administration. It will be advisable to administer the drug one hour before or two hours after meals.

Ampicillin	Food	
Astemizole	Food	
Cefaclor	Food	
Ciprofloxacin	Diary Food	
Didanosine	Food	
Digoxin	Food	
Estramustine	Diary food	
Furosemide	Food	
Hydralazine	Enteral nutrition of food	
Iron	Diary food	
Isoniazid	Food	
Levothyroxine	Food	
Methotrexate	Food	
Mesalamine	Food	
Misoprostol	Food	
Nifedipine	Food	Drug concentration may increase or decrease
Nifedipine	Grapefruit juice	May cause severe hypotension, myocardial ischemia, increase vascular side effects.
Norfloxacin	Diary food	
Penicillamine	Food	
Phenytoin	Enternal nutrition	Decreased therapeutic effect (May have very significant effect on patient)
Tetracycline	Food	
Warfarin	Food high in Vitamin K	
Zidovudine	Food	

References: Pharma CIS™, the new clinical integration system for drug utilization review™ from red book database services

APPENDIX 11

DRUGS IN G-6-PD DEFICIENCY

Drugs and chemicals that should be avoided in persons with G-6-PD deficiency

Acetanilide	Phenazopyridine
Cotrimoxazole	Phenylhydrazine
Dapsone	Primaquine
Doxorubicin	Sulfacetamide
Furazolidone	Sulfamethoxazole
Methylene blue	Sulfanilamide
Nalidixic acid	Sulfapyridine
Naphthalene	Sulfasalazine
Niridazole	Sulfoxone
Nitrofurantoin	Thiasolsulfones
Pamaquine	Toluidine Blue
Pentaquine	Trinitrotoluene

Drugs which can probably safely be given in normal therapeutic doses to G-6-PD deficient subjects without Nonspherocytic Hemolytic Anemia

Acetaminophen	Phenylbutazone
Acetophenetidin (Phenacetin)	Phenytoin
Acetylsalicylic Acid (Aspirin)	Probenecid
Aminopyrine	Procainamide Hydrochloride

Antazoline
Antipyrine
Ascorbic Acid (Vitamin C)
Benzhexol (Artane)
Chloramphenicol
Chlorguanidine (Paludrine)
Chloroquine
Colchicine
Diphenhydramine
Isoniazid
L-Dopa
Menadione Sodium Bisulfite
Menapthone
P-Aminobenzoic Acid
Pyrimethamine
Quinacrine
Quinidine
Quinine
Streptomycin
Sulfacytine
Sulfadiazine
Sulfaguanidine
Sulfamerazine
Sulfamethoxypyridazine
Sulfisoxazole
Trimethoprim
Tripelennamine
Vitamin K

APPENDIX 12

EQUIVALENT GLUCOCORTICOID ORAL DOSAGES

The approximate equivalent glucocorticoid oral dosages established by various laboratory assays are:

Drug	Equivalent Dose
Cortisone	25 mg
Hydrocortisone	20 mg
Prednisolone	5 mg
Prednisone	5 mg
Methylprednisolone	4 mg
Triamcinolone	4 mg
Dexamethasone	0.750 mg
Betamethasone	0.6 mg

Equivalent dosages are general approximations and may not apply to all diseases or routes of administration (especially oral inhalation, IM or intrasynovial injections).

Reference: AHFS Drug Information 1997

APPENDIX 13

OPIOID EQUIANALGESIC DOSES

Drug	IM / SQ [a]	PO / PR [a] / Transdermal
Butorphanol[b]	3.0mg	
Codeine	60 mg	180mg; 120 mg PR
Fentanyl	0.15 mg	0.05mg/hr transdermal[c]
Hydromorphone	2mg	8mg; 6mg PR
Meperidine	100mg	200mg
Morphine	10mg	60 mg (30mg[d]); 30 mg PR
Nalbuphine [b]	20 mg	
Oxycodone		20mg
Pentazocine[b]	60mg	200mg

Note: Equivalent doses are provided only as a guide; individual patient variations may exist.

(a) IM = Intramuscular, PO = Oral, PR = Rectal, SQ = Subcutaneous

(b) Mixed agonist/antagonist analgesics can precipitate opioids withdrawal symptoms in patients who are dependent upon opioid agonists.

(c) Equivalent transdermal dose is based upon an average intravenous dosing interval of 3 hr.

(d) Equianalgesic dose is based upon single dose studies. With repeated administration, the equivalent dose may be much lower, in parentheses.

Reference: Young LY, Koda-Kimble MA. Applied Therapeutics: The Clinical Use of Drugs; 6th Ed, 1995.

APPENDIX 14

COMPLETE IMMUNISATION SCHEDULE (AS GIVEN BY IMA)

Recommended Immunization Schedule followed in India				
Sl No.	**Age**	**Disease**	**Vaccination**	**Remarks**
1	At Birth	Hepatitis B	Hepatitis B Vaccine –I	
2	At Birth	Polio	Oral PV 0 Dose	
3	Birth To 6 Wk	Tuberculosis	BCG	
4	4 -6 Weeks	Hepatitis B	Hepatitis B Vaccine –II	
5	6 Weeks	Diphtheria Pertusis Tetanus Polio	DPT-I Oral PV –I	
6	10 Weeks	Diphtheria Pertusis Tetanus Polio Hepatitis B	DPT-II Oral PV-II Hepatitis B Vaccine III*	*Delhi Government Recommendation
7	14 Weeks	Diphtheria Pertusis Tetanus Polio	DPT-III OPV- III Hepatitis B Vaccine IV*	*Delhi Government Recommendation
8	24 Weeks	Hepatitis B	Hepatitis B Vaccine III*	*IAP Recommendation
9	9 -12 months	Polio Measles	OPV-IV Measles	

Contd...

Sl No.	Age	Disease	Vaccination	Remarks
10	15-18 Months	Mumps Measles Rubella	MMR*	
11	18 Months	Diphtheria Pertusis Tetanus Polio	DPT –Booster I OPV –V	*Recommended By Delhi Government & IAP Only
12	24 Months	Typhoid	Typhoid*	*IAP Recommendation
13	4-5 Yr	Diphtheria Pertusis Tetanus Polio	DPT Booster – II OPV –VI	
Other available Vaccines				
14	6 Weeks	H Influenza B	HIB	*IAP Recommendation
15	10 Weeks	H Influenza B	HIB	
16	14 Weeks	H Influenza B	HIB	*IAP Recommendation
17	18 Months	H Influenza B	HIB	*IAP Recommendation
18	24 Months	Hepatitis A	H A Vaccine-I	Suggested Vaccination
19	30 Months	Hepatitis A	H A Vaccine –II	Suggested Vaccination
20	12 Months	Chickenpox	Varicella Vaccine	Suggested Vaccination
21	24 Months	Meningococcal A&C	Meningococcal Vaccine	Suggested Vaccination
22	12 Months	Pneumococcal	Pneumococcal Vaccine	In Special Circumstances
23	12 Months	Influenza	Influenza Vaccine	In Special Circumstances
On going Vaccines				
24	10 Years	Tetanus	TT	Every Five Years
25	5 Years	Typhoid	Typhoid	Every Three Years
26	5 Years	Meningococcal A&C	Meningococcal Vaccine	Every Three Years
27	Nid's & Snid's	Polio Eradication	Pulse Polio	As per Government Directives

Reference: Website www.babycareindia.com

APPENDIX 15

COMMON LAB VALUES WITH INTERPRETATION

1. Haematology Values

- ***HAEMATOCRIT (HCT)***

    Normal Adult Female Range: 37 - 47%

    Optimal Adult Female Reading: 42%

    Normal Adult Male Range : 40 - 54%

    Optimal Adult Male Reading : 47

    Normal Newborn Range: 50 - 62%

    Optimal Newborn Reading: 56

- ***HAEMOGLOBIN (HGB)***

    Normal Adult Female Range: 12 - 16 g/dl

    Optimal Adult Female Reading: 14 g/dl

    Normal Adult Male Range: 14 - 18 g/dl

    Optimal Adult Male Reading: 16 g/dl

    Normal Newborn Range: 14 - 20 g/dl

    Optimal Newborn Reading: 17 g/dl

- ***MCH (Mean Corpuscular Haemoglobin)***

    Normal Adult Range: 27 - 33 pg

    Optimal Adult Reading: 30

- ***MCV (Mean Corpuscular Volume)***

    Normal Adult Range: 80 - 100 cu microns

    Optimal Adult Reading: 90

- ***MCHC (Mean Corpuscular Hemoglobin Concentration)***

  Normal Adult Range: 32 - 36 %

  Optimal Adult Reading: 34

- ***R.B.C. (Red Blood Cell Count)***

  Normal Adult Female Range: 3.9 - 5.2 million/ cu mm
  Optimal Adult Female Reading: 4.55
  Normal Adult Male Range: 4.2 - 5.6 million/ cu mm
  Optimal Adult Male Reading: 4.9
  New Born: 4.5 – 6.0 million/cu mm
  Children (varies with age): 4.0 – 5.0 million/ cu mm

- ***W.B.C. (White Blood Cell Count)***

  Normal Adult Range: 3.8 - 10.8 thousands/ cu mm

  Optimal Adult Reading: 7.3

  Children (varies with age): 8.0 – 21.0 thousands/ cu mm

- ***PLATELET COUNT***

  Normal Adult Range: 130 - 400 thousands/ cu mm

  Optimal Adult Reading: 265

- **NEUTROPHILS and NEUTROPHIL COUNT** - this is the main defender of the body against infection and antigens.

  High levels may indicate an active infection.

  Normal Adult Range: 48 - 73 %

  Optimal Adult Reading: 60.5

  Normal Children's Range: 30 - 60 %

  Optimal Children's Reading: 45

- **LYMPHOCYTES and LYMPHOCYTE COUNT** – Elevated levels may indicate an active viral infections such as measles, rubella, chickenpox, or infectious mononucleosis

  Normal Adult Range: 18 - 48 %

  Optimal Adult Reading: 33

  Normal Children's Range: 25 - 50 %

  Optimal Children's Reading: 37.5

- **MONOCYTES and MONOCYTE COUNT** - Elevated levels are seen in tissue breakdown or chronic infections, carcinomas, leukemia (monocytic) or lymphomas.

  Normal Adult Range: 0 - 9 %

  Optimal Adult Reading: 4.5

- **EOSINOPHILS and EOSINOPHIL COUNT** - Elevated levels may indicate an allergic reactions or parasites.

  Normal Adult Range: 0 - 5 %

  Optimal Adult Reading: 2.5

- **BASOPHILS and BASOPHIL COUNT** - Basophilic activity is not fully understood but it is known to carry histamine, heparin and serotonin.

  High levels are found in allergic reactions.

  Normal Adult Range: 0 - 2 %

  Optimal Adult Reading: 1

2. Electrolyte Values

- **SODIUM** - Sodium is the most abundant cation in the blood and its chief base. It functions in the body to maintain osmotic pressure, acid-base balance and to transmit nerve impulses.

  Normal Adult Range: 135-146 mEq/L

  Optimal Adult Reading: 140.5

- **POTASSIUM** - Potassium is the major intracellular cation.

  Very low value: Cardiac arrhythmia

  Normal Range: 3.5 - 5.5 mEq/L

  Optimal Adult Reading: 4.5

- **CHLORIDE** - Elevated levels are related to acidosis as well as too much water crossing the cell membrane. Decreased levels with decreased serum albumin may indicate water deficiency crossing the cell membrane (edema).

  Normal Adult Range: 95-112 mEq/L

  Optimal Adult Reading: 103

- **CO_2 (Carbon dioxide)** - The CO_2 level is related to the respiratory exchange of carbon dioxide in the lungs and is part of the bodies buffering system. Generally when used with the other electrolytes, it is a good indicator of acidosis and alkalinity.

  Normal Adult Range: 22-32 mEq/L

  Optimal Adult Reading: 27

Normal Children Range - 20 - 28 mEq/L

Optimal Children Reading: 24

- **CALCIUM** - involved in bone metabolism, protein absorption, fat transfer muscular contraction, transmission of nerve impulses, blood clotting and cardiac function. Regulated by parathyroid.

  Normal Adult Range: 8.5-10.3 mEq/dl

  Optimal Adult Reading: 9.4

- **PHOSPHOROUS** - Generally inverse with Calcium.

  Normal Adult Range: 2.5 - 4.5 mEq/dl

  Optimal Adult Reading: 3.5

  Normal Children Range: 3 - 6 mEq/dl

  Optimal Children Range: 4.5

- **ANION GAP** (Sodium + Potassium - CO2 + Chloride) - An increased measurement is associated with metabolic acidosis due to the overproduction of acids (a state of alkalinity is in effect). Decreased levels may indicate metabolic alkalosis due to the overproduction of alkaloids (a state of acidosis is in effect).

  Normal Adult Range: 4 - 14 (calculated)

  Optimal Adult Reading: 9

- **CALCIUM/PHOSPHORUS Ratio**

  Normal Adult Range: 2.3 - 3.3 (calculated)

  Optimal Adult Reading: 2.8

  Normal Children's range: 1.3 - 3.3 (calculated)

  Optimal Children's Reading: 2.3

- **SODIUM/POTASSIUM**

  Normal Adult Range: 26 - 38 (calculated)

  Optimal Adult Reading: 32

3. Hepatic Enzymes

- **AST (Serum Glutamic-Oxaloacetic Transaminase - SGOT)** - found primarily in the liver, heart, kidney, pancreas, and muscles. Seen in tissue damage, especially heart and liver.

  Normal Adult Range: 0 - 42 U/L

  Optimal Adult Reading: 21

- **ALT (Serum Glutamic-Pyruvic Transaminase - SGPT) -** Decreased SGPT in combination with increased cholesterol levels is seen in cases of a congested liver. Increased levels are seen in mononucleosis, alcoholism, liver damage, kidney infection, chemical pollutants or myocardial infarction.

    Normal Adult Range: 0 - 48 U/L

    Optimal Adult Reading: 24

- **ALKALINE PHOSPHATASE** - Used extensively as a tumor marker. Elevated reading present in bone injury, pregnancy, or skeletal growth. Low levels are sometimes found in hypoadrenia, protein deficiency, malnutrition and a number of vitamin deficiencies

    Normal Adult Range: 20 - 125 U/L

    Optimal Adult Reading: 72.5

    Normal Children Range: 40 - 400 U/L

    Optimal Children Reading: 220

- **GGT (Gamma-Glutamyl Transpeptidase)** - Elevated levels may be found in liver disease, alcoholism, bile-duct obstruction, cholestitis, drug abuse, and in some cases excessive magnesium ingestion. Decreased levels can be found in hypothyroidism, hypothalamic malfunction and low levels of magnesium.

    Normal Adult Female Range: 0 - 45 U/L

    Optimal Female Reading: 22.5

    Normal Adult Male Range: 0 - 65 U/L

    Optimal Male Reading: 32.5

- **LDH (Lactic Acid Dehydrogenase) -** Increases are usually found in cellular death and/or leakage from the cell or in some cases it can be useful in confirming myocardial or pulmonary infarction (only in relation to other tests). Decreased levels of the enzyme may be seen in cases of malnutrition, hypoglycemia, adrenal exhaustion or low tissue or organ activity.

    Normal Adult Range: 0 - 250 U/L

    Optimal Adult Reading: 125

- **BILIRUBIN, TOTAL -** Elevated in liver disease, mononucleosis, hemolytic anemia, low levels of exposure to the sun, and toxic effects to some drugs, decreased levels are seen in people with an inefficient liver, excessive fat digestion, and possibly a diet low in nitrogen bearing foods

    Normal Adult Range: 0 - 1.3 mg/dl

    Optimal Adult Reading: 65

4. Renal Related

- **B.U.N. (Blood Urea Nitrogen) -** Increases can be caused by excessive protein intake, kidney damage, certain drugs, low fluid intake, intestinal bleeding, exercise or heart failure. Decreased levels may be due to a poor diet, malabsorption, liver damage or low nitrogen intake.

  Normal Adult Range: 7 - 25 mg/dl,

  Optimal Adult Reading: 16

- **CREATININE -** Low levels are sometimes seen in kidney damage, protein starvation, liver disease or pregnancy. Elevated levels are sometimes seen in kidney disease due to the kidneys job of excreting creatinine, muscle degeneration, and some drugs involved in impairment of kidney function.

  Normal Adult Range: 7 - 1.4 mg/dl

  Optimal Adult Reading: 1.05

- **URIC ACID -** High levels are noted in gout, infections, kidney disease, alcoholism, high protein diets, and with toxemia in pregnancy. Low levels may be indicative of kidney disease, malabsorption, poor diet, liver damage or an overly acidic kidney.

  Normal Adult Female Range: 2.5 - 7.5 mg/dl

  Optimal Adult Female Reading: 5.0

  Normal Adult Male Range: 3.5 - 7.5 mg/dl

  Optimal Adult Male Reading: 5.5

- **BUN/CREATININE** - This calculation is a good measurement of kidney and liver function.

  Normal Adult Range: 6 -25 (calculated)

  Optimal Adult Reading: 15.5

- **PROTEIN, TOTAL** - Decreased levels may be due to poor nutrition, liver disease, malabsorption, diarrhea, or severe burns. Increased levels are seen in lupus, liver disease, chronic infections, alcoholism, leukemia, tuberculosis amongst many others.

  Normal Adult Range: 6.0 -8.5 g/dl

  Optimal Adult Reading: 7.25

- **ALBUMIN** - major constituent of serum protein (usually over 50%). **High levels are seen in liver disease (rarely), shock, dehydration, or multiple myeloma. Lower**

levels are seen in poor diets, diarrhea, fever, infection, liver disease, inadequate iron intake, third-degree burns and edemas or hypocalcaemia.

Normal Adult Range: 3.2 - 5.0 g/dl

Optimal Adult Reading: 4.1

- **GLOBULIN** - Globulins have many diverse functions such as, the carrier of some hormones, lipids, metals, and antibodies (IgA, IgG, IgM, and IgE). Elevated levels are seen with chronic infections, liver disease, rheumatoid arthritis, myelomas, and lupus. Lower levels in immune compromised patients, poor dietary habits, malabsorption and liver or kidney disease.

  Normal Adult Range: 2.2 - 4.2 g/dl (calculated)

  Optimal Adult Reading: 3.2

- **A/G RATIO (Albumin/Globulin Ratio)**

  Normal Adult Range: 0.8 - 2.0 (calculated)

  Optimal Adult Reading: 1.9

5. Lipids

- **CHOLESTEROL - High density lipoproteins (HDL) is desired as opposed to the low density lipoproteins (LDL). Elevated cholesterol has been seen in artherosclerosis, diabetes, hypothyroidism and pregnancy. Low levels are seen in depression, malnutrition, liver insufficiency, malignancies, anemia and infection.**

  Normal Adult Range: 120 - 240 mg/dl

  Optimal Adult Reading: 180

- **LDL (Low Density Lipoprotein)** - studies correlate the association between high levels of LDL and arterial atherosclerosis

  Normal Adult Range: 62 - 130 mg/dl

  Optimal Adult Reading: 81 mg/dl

- **HDL (High Density Lipoprotein)** - A high level of HDL is an indication of a healthy metabolic system if there is no sign of liver disease or intoxication.

  Normal Adult Range: 35 - 135 mg/dl

  Optimal Adult Reading: +85 mg/dl

- **TRIGLYCERIDES** - Increased levels may be present in atherosclerosis, hypothyroidism, liver disease, pancreatitis, myocardial infarction, metabolic disorders, toxemia, and nephrotic syndrome. Decreased levels may be present in chronic obstructive pulmonary disease, brain infarction, hyperthyroidism, malnutrition, and malabsorption.

Normal Adult Range: 0 - 200 mg/dl

Optimal Adult Reading: 100

- **CHOLESTEROL/LDL RATIO**

  Normal Adult Range: 1 – 6

  Optimal Adult Reading: 3.5

6. Thyroid

- **THYROXINE (T4)** - Increased levels are found in hyperthyroidism, acute thyroiditis, and hepatitis. Low levels can be found in Cretinism, hypothyroidism, cirrhosis of liver , malnutrition, and chronic thyroiditis.

  Normal Adult Range: 4 - 12 µg/dl

  Optimal Adult Reading: 8 µg/dl

- **T_3-UPTAKE** - Increased levels are found in hyperthyroidism, severe liver disease, metastatic malignancy, and pulmonary insufficiency. Decreased levels are found in hypothyroidism, normal pregnancy, and hyperestrogenis status.

  Normal Adult Range: 27 - 47%

  Optimal Adult Reading: 37 %

- **FREE T_4 INDEX (T7)**

  Normal Adult Range: 4 – 12

  Optimal Adult Reading: 8

- **THYROID-STIMULATING HORMONE (TSH)** - produced by the anterior pituitary gland, causes the release and distribution of stored thyroid hormones. When T_4 and T_3 are too high, TSH secretion decreases, when T_4 and T_3 are low, TSH secretion increases.

  Normal Adult Range: 5 - 6 mil U/L

  AACE (2003) target level: 0.3 to 3.04

7. Cardiac

- **Creatine phosphokinase (CK)** - Levels rise 4 to 8 hours after an acute MI, peaking at 16 to 30 hours and returning to baseline within 4 days

  25-200 U/L

  32-150 U/L

- **CK-MB CK isoenzyme** - It begins to increase 6 to 10 hours after an acute MI, peaks in 24 hours, and remains elevated for up to 72 hours.

  < 12 IU/L if total CK is <400 IU/L

  < 3.5% of total CK if total CK is >400 IU/L

- **(LDH) Lactate dehydrogenase** - Total LDH will begin to rise 2 to 5 days after an MI; the elevation can last 10 days.

  140-280 U/L

  LDH-1 and LDH-2 LDH isoenzymes - Compare LDH 1 and LDH 2 levels. Normally, the LDH-1 value will be less than the LDH-2. In the acute MI, however, the LDH 2 remains constant, while LDH 1 rises. When the LDH 1 is higher than LDH 2, the LDH is said to be flipped, which is highly suggestive of an MI. A flipped pattern appears 12-24 hours post MI and persists for 48 hours.

  LDH-1 18%-33%

  LDH-2 28%-40%

  SGOT - will begin to rise in 8-12 hours and peak in 18-30 hours - 10-42 U/L

  Myoglobin - early and sensitive diagnosis of myocardial infarction in the emergency department. This small haem protein becomes abnormal within 1 to 2 hours of necrosis, peaks in 4-8 hours, and drops to normal in about 12 hours.

  0 < 1

- **Troponin Complex** - Peaks in 10-24 hours, begins to fall off after 1-2 weeks.

  < 0.4

APPENDIX 16

USEFUL RESOURCES FOR COMMONLY REQUESTED DRUG INFORMATION

Type of Inquiry	Tertiary Resources	Secondary Resources
Adverse events	ClinAlert 2000, Meyler's Side Effects of Drugs, Textbook of Adverse Drug Reactions AHFS Drug Information, Clinical Pharmacology, DRUGDEX, Drug Facts and Comparisons, Drug Information Handbook, Handbook. Hand-book of clinical Drug Data, Martindale: The Complete Drug Reference, Physicians' Desk Reference, Mosby's GenRx, STAT!-Ref, USPDI Volume 1	Reactions Weekly, ClinAlert Embase, Index Medicus, International Pharmaceutical Abstracts, lowa Drug Information System, Medline
Alcohol-free/sugar-free Products	American Drug Index, Red Book, Drug Facts and Comparisons DRUGDEX, Handbook of Non-Prescription Drugs	-
Bioequivalency ratings	Approved Bioequivalency Codes, USPDI Volume 3, Mosby's GenRx, PDR Generics	Lexis-Nexis
Chemical data (molecular weight, solubility, pKa,etc)	Merck Index, Remington's, Martindale's: The Complete Drug Reference	International Pharmaceutical Abstracts
Cost	Red Book, Mosby's GenRx PDRGenerics, Price Chek PC, Facts and comparisons (Cost Index)	Lexis-Nexis, Pharmacoeconomics, InPharma, International Pharmaceutical Abstracts

Type of Inquiry	Tertiary Resources	Secondary Resources
Disease state information	Cecil Textbook of Medicine, Harrison's, The Merck Manual, Scientific American Medicine, STAT!-Ref Applied Therapeutics, Clinical Pharmacy and Therapeutics, Conn's Current Therapy, Current Medical Diagnosis and Treatment, Non-Prescription Drug Therapy, Pharmacotherapy, Handbook of Non-prescription Drugs	Index Medicus, lowa Drug Information System, MEDLINE, Lexis-Nexis, Embase, InPharma, International Pharmacetical Abstracts, Journal Watch
Dosage guidelines (general)	AHFS Drug Information, DRUGDEX, Drug Facts and Comparisons, Physicians' Desk Reference, Mosby's GenRx, STAT!-Ref, USPDI Volume 1 Clinical Pharmacology, Drug Information Handbook, Handbook Of Clinical Drug Data, Martindale: The Complete Drug Reference, Handbook of Nonprescription Drugs, Physicians' Desk Reference for Non-Prescription Drugs, PDR Generics, Applied Therapeutics, Conn's Current Therapy, Pharmacotherapy	Index Medicus, InPharma, International Pharmaceutical Abstracts, lowa Drug Information System, MEDLINE, Lexis-Nexis Embase
Dosage guidelines (hepatic failure)	Geriatric Dosage Handbook, Merck Manual of Geriatrics, AFS Drug Information, DRUGDEX Drug Facts and Comparisons, Drug Information Handbook, Handbook of Clinical Drug Data, Physicians' Desk Reference, Mosby's GenRx, STAT!-Ref, USPDI volume 1, Applied Therapeutics, Textbook of Therapeutic, Conn's Current Therapy, Pharmacotherapy	Embase, Index Medicus, InPharma, International Pharmaceutical Abstracts, lowa Drug Information System, MEDLINE, Lexis-Nexis

Type of Inquiry	Tertiary Resources	Secondary Resources
Dosage guidelines (pediatrics)	Harriet Lane Handbook, Pediatric Dosage Handbook, Problems in Pediatric Drug Therapy, Drug Information Handbook, AHFS Drug Information, DRUGDEX, Drug Facts and Comparisons, Handbook of Clinical Drug data, Physicians' Desk Reference, Mosby's GenRx, STAT!-Ref, USPDI Volume 1, Applied Therapeutics, Textbook of Therapeutics, Conn's Current Therapy, Pharmacotherapy.	Paediatrics Today Embase, Index Medicus, InPharma, International Pharmaceutical Abstracts, Iowa Drug Information System, MEDLINE, Lexis-Nexis
Dosage guidelines (renal failure)	Geriatric Dosage Handbook, Drug Prescribing in Renal Failure, Dosing Guidelines for Adults, Pocket Reference to Renal Dialysis, Scientific American Medicine, Drug Information Handbook, DRUGDEX, AHFS Drug Information, Drug Facts and Comparisons, Handbook of Clinical Drug Data, Physicians' Desk Reference, Mosby's GenRx, STAT!-Ref, USPDI Volume 1, Applied Therapeutics, Textbook of Therapeutics, Conn's Current Therapy, Pharmacotherapy	Embase, Index Medicus, InPharma, International Pharmaceutical Abstracts, Iowa Drug Information System, MEDLINE, Lexis-Nexis
Drug administration	AHFS Drug Information, DRUGDEX, Drug Information Handbook Clinical Pharmacology, Drug Facts And Comparisons, Handbook of Clinical Drug Data, Martindale: The Complete Drug Reference, Physicians' Desk Reference, Mosby's GenRx, PDR Generics, STAT!-Ref,USPDI Volume1	Embase, Index Medicus, International Pharmaceutical Abstracts, Iowa Drug Information System, MEDLINE, STAT!-Ref, Lexis-Nexis

Type of Inquiry	Tertiary Resources	Secondary Resources
Drug information centers	Red Book	
Drug interactions	Drug Interaction Facts, Drug Interactions and Updates, Drug-REAX, Evaluation of Drug Interactions	ClinAlert, Reactions, International Pharmaceutical Abstracts
	MediSpan Drug Therapy Screening Medicus,IowaSystem, Clinical reference Library, AHFS Drug Information, Clinical Pharmacology, DRUGDEX, Drug Facts and Comparisons, Drug Information Handbook, Handbook Of Clinical Drug Data, Martindale: The Complete Drug Reference, Physicians' Desk Reference, Mosby's GenRx, STAT!-Ref USPDI Volume 1	Embase,Index Drug Information System, MEDLINE, Lexis-Nexis
Drug use in pregnancy and lactation	Drugs in Pregnancy and Lactation, Reprorisk, DRUGDEX AHFS Drug Information, Drug Facts and Comparisons, Drug Information Handbook, Handbook of Clinical Drug Data, Physicians' Desk Reference, Mosby's GenRx, STAT!-Ref, USPDI Volume 1, PDR Generics	Reactions, Lexis-Nexis Embase, Index Medicus, lowa Drug Information System, MEDLINE, International Pharmaceutical Abstracts
Extemporaneous compounding	Extemporaneous Ophthalmic Preparations, Stability of Compounded Formulations, Handbook of Extemporaneous Compounding, Pediatric Formulations, Remington's Pharmaceutical Sciences, AHFS Drug information, DRUGDEX	International Pharmaceutical Abstracts, lowa Drug Information System MEDLINE, Embase, Index Medicus
Herbal and homeopathic Medications	A Clinical Guide to Chinese Herbs and Formulae, The Honest Herbal, Information Sourcebook of Herbal Medicine, PDR Herbal, Natural Medicines Comprehensive Database, Professional's Handbook of Complementary and Alternative Medicine, Review of Natural Products, POISINDEX, Martindale: The Complete Drug Reference, Commission E Monographs, PDR for Herbal Medicine, Therapeutic Use of Phytochemicals Herbs of Choice, F-D-C Tan Sheets	International Pharmaceutical Abstracts, lowa Drug Information System, Reactions, ClinAlert, Lexis-Nexis, Embase , Index Medicus,MEDLINE

Type of Inquiry	Tertiary Resources	Secondary Resources
Identification (domestic products)	American Drug Index, POISINDEX, Drug Facts and comparisons Red Book, Clinical Pharmacology, UPS Dictionary of USAN & Inter-National Names, AHFS Drug Information, DRUGDEX, Drug Information Handbook, Handbook of Clinical Drug Data, Physicians' Desk Reference for Non-Prescription Drugs, STAT!-Ref, PDR Generics	Embase, Index Medicus, InPharma, International Pharmaceutical Abstracts, lowa Drug Information System, MEDLINE, Lexis-Nexis
Identification (foreign products)	British National Formulary, Diccionario de Especialidades Farmaceuticas, European Drug Index, Index Nominum, Martindale: The Complete Drug Reference	Embase, Inpharma, International Pharmaceutical Abstracts Index Medicus, lowa Drug Information System, MEDLINE, Lexis-Nexis
Identification (imprint code)	IDENTIDEX, PDR, PDR Generics, Mosby's GenRx, Ident-A-Drug Reference, Clinical Reference Library	-
Identification (street drug)	IDENTIDEX, POISINDEX	-
Indications(approved only)	Physicians' Desk Reference, Mosby's GenRx, PDR Generics	Lexis-Nexis
Indications (approved and unapproved)	AHFS Drug Information, DRUGDEX, Martindale: The Complete Drug Reference, PDR Generics Clinical Pharmacology, Drug Facts and comparisons, Drug Information Handbook, Handbook of Clinical Drug Data, STAT!-Ref, USPDI Volume 1	Embase, Index Medicus, InPharma, Iowa Drug Information System, Clinical MEDLINE, International Pharmaceutical Abstracts, Lexis-Nexis
Investigational drugs	DRUGDEX, Martindale: The Complete Drug Reference, USP Dictionary of Drug Names, Handbook of Clinical Drug Data, Drug Facts and Comparisons	Embase, Index Medicus, Inpharma, lowa Drug Information System, MEDLINE, International Pharmaceutical Abstracts, Lexis-Nexis

Type of Inquiry	Tertiary Resources	Secondary Resources
Laboratory tests	Clinical Guide to Laboratory Tests, Laboratory Test Handbook, Laboratory Tests and Diagnostic Procedures, STAT!-Ref	Embase, Index Medicus, MEDLINE Reactions, Lexis-Nexis, lowa Drug Information Services, International Pharmaceutical Abstracts
	Cecil Textbook of Medicine, Harrison's Principles of Internal Medicine, The Merck Manual, Scientific American Medicine	
Manufacturer Information (foreign)	European Drug Index, Index Nominum, Martindale: The Complete Drug Reference, Merck Index, other foreign pharmacopeias	-
Manufacturer information (domestic)	American Drug Index, Red Book. POISINDEX, Drug Facts and Comparisons, Physicians' Desk Reference, Mosby's GenRx, PDR Generics, USP Dictionary	-
Over-the –counter drugs	Handbook of Nonprescription Drugs, Nonprescription Products: Formulations and Features, Physicians' Desk Reference for Non-Prescription Drugs, Drug System Facts and Comparisons, DRUGDEX, POISINDEX, USPDI Volume 1	Lexis-Nexis Embase, Index Medicus, InPharma, International Pharmaceutical Abstracts, lowa Drug Information MEDLINE
Patient counseling	Aftercare, Medication Teaching Manual, Patient Counseling Handbook, Patient Drug Facts, USPDI Volume 2 AHFS Drug Information, DRUGDEX, Drug Facts and Comparisons, Drug Information Handbook, Handbook of Clinical Drug Data, Physicians' Desk Reference, Physicians GenRx, Dr.Scheueler's Home Medical Advisor	Lexis-Nexis
Pharmaceutical Calculations	Remingtons' Pharmaceutical Sciences Redbook, Handbook of Clinical Drug Data, A Practical Guide to Contemporary Pharmacy Practice	-

Type of Inquiry	Tertiary Resources	Secondary Resources
Pharmaceutical Organizations (state and national)	Red Book	
Pharmacy law	Pharmacy Law Digest, Individual state law books	Lexis-Nexis, International Pharmaceutical Abstracts
Physical assessment	Physical Assessment: A Guide for Evaluating Drug Therapy	
Pharmacokinetics	Applied Pharmacokinetics: Principles of Therapeutic Drug Monitoring, Basic Clinical Pharmacokinetics, AHFS Drug Information, DRUGDEX, Drug Facts and Comparisons, Drug Information Handbook, Handbook of Clinical Drug Data, Reference, Physicians' Desk Reference, Mosby's GenRx, USPDI Volume 1, PDR Generics	International Pharmaceutical Abstracts Embase, Index Medicus, lowa Drug Information System, MEDLINE, InPharma
Pharmacology	Goodman and Gilman's Pharmacologic Basis of Therapeutics, Human Pharmacology: Molecular to Clinical, Principles of Pharmacology, Basic Concepts & Clinical Applications AHFS Drug Information, DRUGDEX, Drug Facts and Comparisons, Drug Information Handbook, Handbook of Clinical Drug Data, Martindale: The Complete Drug Reference, Physicians GenRx, STAT!-Ref, USPDI Volume1	lowa Drug Information System, Embase, Index Medicus, MEDLINE, InPharma, International Pharmaceutical Abstracts
Poison control centers	Red Book, Mosby's GenRx, Poisoning & Toxicology Handbook, PDR Generics	
Stability/compatibility	Guide to Parenteral Admixtures, Handbook on Injectable Drugs AHFS Drug Information, DRUGDEX, STAT!-Ref	International Pharmaceutical Abstracts Index Medicus, lowa Drug Information System, MEDLINE

Type of Inquiry	Tertiary Resources	Secondary Resources
Toxicology/poisoning	Clinical Management of Poisoning and Drug Overdose, Ellenhorn's Medical Toxicology, POISINDEX, Poisoning & Toxicology Handbook, Principles of Clinical Toxicology, Goldfrank's Toxicologic Emergencies AHFS Drug Information, DRUGDEX, STAT!-Ref	Reactions Embase, Index Medicus, International Pharmaceutical Abstracts, lowa Drug Information System, MEDLINE
Veterinary	The Merck Veterinary Manual, Small Animal Medicine Therapeutics, Veterinary Drug Therapy, Verterinary Pharmaceuticals and Biologicals (VPB), DRUGDEX, POISINDEX, USP-DI Vol.1	Biosis, Embase, MEDLINE

APPENDIX 17

GUIDELINES FOR I.V ADMINISTRATION OF POTASSIUM CHLORIDE

General Guidelines

KCl must not be administrated undiluted

IV push is contraindicated

Slow IV infusion is recommended

Extreme care must be taken to avoid extravasation

KCl must be administered using an infusion pump

Solutions used for fluid challenge must not contain KCl

Nurses must be aware of medications incompatible with KCl

1. Maintenance IV KCl

A. Adults

20-40mEq KCl/liter at 120ml/hour (not greater than 10-20eEq/hour) via peripheral line

Maximum of 60mEq/liter via peripheral line

KCl>60 mEq/liter must be administered via a central line.

KCl>60mEq/liter, patient must be in a monitored setting.

Maximum of 80mEq/liter of fluid.

B. Pediatrics

KCl infusion rate range of 0.3-1 mEq/kg/hour. The dose should not exceed 1mEq/kg/hr, up to a maximum of 20 mEq/hour.

>0.5mEq/kg/hour requires cardiac monitoring.

2. Intermittent Infusion

All intermittent KCl infusions must be administered via infusion pump to patients on cardiorespiratory monitoring.

A. Adults

Administer intermittent infusions via or central line.

10-20 mEq KCl in 100ml fluid over one to two hours.

Maximum of 20 mEq/hour (may be repeated).

B. Pediatrics

Intermittent infusions may be administered via a central or peripheral IV.

KCl infusion rate range of 0.3-1 mEq/kg/hour. The dose should not exceed 1mEq/kg/hr, up to a maximum of 20 mEq/hour over 1-2 hours.

>0.5mEq/hour requires cardiac monitoring.

Maximum peripheral IV solution concentration : £40mlEq/liter.

References:

I.V. Medications 10th edition (1994) Recommendations

Hazinski 1992 2nd edition "Nursing Care of the Critically ill Child"

Trissel Handbook on Injectable Drugs; 7th Ed.

AHFS DI 1994

ASHP Guidelines for Administration of Intravenous Medications to Pediatric Patients; 1993

APPENDIX 18

NURSING GUIDELINES FOR ADMINISTERING DRUGS VIA I.V PUSH

NURSING GUIDELINES FOR ADMINISTERING DRUGS VIA IV PUSH

NOTE: 1 The appearance of a medication in these guidelines does not imply that IV push is the only route of administration or even the route of choice. The user is encouraged to consult additional references for other acceptable routes of administration.

2 The statement **"DO NOT GIVE IV PUSH"** beside a drug entity does not imply that the medication must be given IM, SC etc. Some medications may be administered by IV infusion even though they cannot be given IV push. Again, the reader is encouraged to consult additional references.

DRUG NAME & CONCENTRATION	DILUTION REQUIRED FOR IV PUSH	RATE OF ADMINISTRATION	PRECAUTIONS COMMENTS /STABILITY
Acetazolamide Na 500 mg vial	Dilute with 5 ml SWI to provide concentration of 100 mg/ml	500mg or fraction thereof over 1 minute	Contraindicated in severe renal or hepatic disease, electrolyte imbalance. Use within 24 hours after reconstitution.
Acetylcysteine 200 mg/ml, 10 ml amp	**DO NOT GIVE IV PUSH**		
Acyclovir 250mg vial	**DO NOT GIVE IV PUSH**		
Adenosine 3 mg/ml, 2 ml vial	None	Give over 1-2 seconds. Follow with rapid saline flush.	Monitor ECG.
Alprostadil 0.5 mg/ml amp	**DO NOT GIVE IV PUSH**		
Amikacin 250 mg/ml, 2 ml vial	**DO NOT GIVE IV PUSH**		
Aminophylline Injection 250 mg/10ml	None. However, slow IV infusion is preferable	Not to exceed 25 mg/minute	Monitor vital signs, Incompatible with most other drugs.

Contd...

Amiodarone HCl 50 mg/ml, 3 ml	Dilute with D_5W to provide 15 mg/ml in emergencies only. Slow IV infusion in 250 ml D_5W is preferable	Not to exceed 150 mg/min in emergencies only	Monitor vital signs. Incompatible with NS.
Amoxicillin/Clavulanic acid 600 mg vial	Dilute 600 mg in 10 ml SWI or 1.2 gm in 20 ml SWI	Slowly over 3-4 minutes	Use immediately after reconstitution.
Amphotericin B 50 mg vial	**DO NOT GIVE IV PUSH**		
Ampicillin Sodium 500 mg	Dilute with 5ml SWI or BWI to provide 100 mg/ml	Over 3-5 minutes for doses up to 500 mg and 10-15 minutes for larger doses	Hypersensitivity reactions possible. Use reconstituted vial within 1 hr.

DRUG NAME & CONCENTRATION AVAILABLE	DILUTION REQUIRED FOR IV PUSH	RATE OF ADMINISTRATION	PRECAUTIONS COMMENTS/STABILITY
Ampicillin Sodium 500 mg)	Dilute with 5 ml SWI or BWI to provide 100 mg/ml	Over 3-5 minutes for doses up to 500mg and 10-15 minutes for larger doses	Hypersensitivity reactions possible Use reconstituted vial with 1 hr.
Amrinone Lactate 5 mg/ml, 20 ml amp	None. IV push used only for loading and supplemental bolus doses	Give over 2-3 minutes	Do not dilute with dextrose solutions Safe use in children not established. Protect from light.
Ascorbic Acid 100 mg/ml, 5 ml amp	None	Give 100mg or a fraction thereof over 1 minute	
Atracurium Besylate 10 mg/ml, 5ml amp	None	Give over 30-60 seconds	Safe use in children less than 1 month not established. Constant monitoring required.
Atropine (various) 0.1 mg/ml, 5 ml prefilled syringe 0.6 mg/ml amp	None	Give 1 mg or fraction thereof over 1 minute	Monitor vital signs. Caution with asthma, acute MI.
Aztreonam 1 gm vial	Dilute with 6-10 ml SWI	Slowly over 3-5 minutes	Observe for vein irritation and hypersensitivity. Use in children not established.
Benztropine Meslate 1 mg/ml, 2ml amp	None	Give 1 mg or fraction thereof over 1 minute	IV route seldom used. Manufacturer states that there is no clinically important difference in onset between IM or IV routes. Contraindicated in children less than 3 years.
Betamethasone Sodium Phosphate/Acetate 6 mg/ml amp	**DO NOT GIVE IV PUSH**		

Contd...

DRUG NAME & CONCENTRATION AVAILABLE	DILUTION REQUIRED FOR IV PUSH	RATE OF ADMINISTRATION	PRECAUTIONS COMMENTS/STABILITY
Bretylium Tosylate 50 mg/ml, 10ml amp	Use undiluted only in life-threatening ventricular fibrillation.	Administer over approximately 1 minute	Constant monitoring of ECG and vital signs. Not high incidence of nausea and vomiting.
Butorphanol Tartrate 2 mg/ml vial	None	Over 3-5 minutes	Monitor vital signs and respiratory depression. Use in children less than 18 years of age not established.
Calcitonin Salmon Synthetic 100 IU/ml	**DO NOT GIVE IV PUSH**		
Calcium Chloride 100mg/ml, 10ml pre-filled syringe	None	0.5-1 ml per minute	Avoid extravasation. Monitor BP, ECG. Observe closely in digitalized patients.
Calcium Sandoz equivalent to 100 mg/ml calcium Gluconate, 10ml amp	None	1-2 ml per minute	Avoid extravasation. Monitor BP, ECG. Observe closely in digitalized patients.
Carboprost Tromethamine 0.25 mg/ml	**DO NOT GIVE IV PUSH**		
Cefazolin Sodium 500 mg	Dilute with 10 ml SWI to provide 50 mg/ml	Give slowly over 3-5 minutes	Observe for hypersensitivity
Cefotaxime Inj. 1 g	Dilute with 10ml SWI to provide 100 mg/ml	Give slowly over 3-5 minutes	Observe for vein irritation and hypersensitivity
Cefoxitin 1 g	Dilute with 10 ml SWI to provide 100 mg/ml	Give slowly over 3-5 minutes	Observe for vein irriation and hypersensitivity
Ceflazidine 1 g	Dilute with 10 ml SW to provide 100 mg/ml	Give slowly over 3-5 minutes	Observe for vein irritation and hypersensitivity
Ceftriaxone 1g	Dilute with SWI to provide 100 mg/ml	Give slowly over 2-4 minutes. As this method is currently not approved by US FDA, recommend an infusion.	Observe for vein irritation and hypersensitivity
Cefuroxime 750 mg	Dilute with 8 ml SWI to provide 90 mg/ml	Give slowly over 3-5 minutes.	Use in children less than 3 months not established.
Chloramphenicol Sodium Succinate 1.2 g	Dilute with 11 ml SWI to provide 90mg/ml	Give over 1 minute	
Chlorpromazine 25 mg/ml, 2 ml amp	Dilute with NS to concentration of 1 mg/ml	Do not exceed 1 mg/min (adult)/ 0.5 mg/min (ped)	Use in children less than 6 months not established.
Cholecalciferol 300,000 U/ml amp	**DO NOT GIVE IV PUSH**		

Contd...

DRUG NAME & CONCENTRATION AVAILABLE	DILUTION REQUIRED FOR IV PUSH	RATE OF ADMINISTRATION	PRECAUTIONS COMMENTS/STABILITY
Chorionic gonadotropin 5000 w/amp	**DO NOT GIVE IV PUSH**		
Clindamycin 300 mg/2ml. ampule	**DO NOT GIVE IV PUSH**		
Codeine Phosphate inj 30 mg/2ml perfilled syringe	None	Give very slowly 0.5 mg/min	Usually given IM or subcutaneously. Intravenous injection rarely used.
Corticotropin 40 units / vial	**DO NOT GIVE IV PUSH**		
Cosyntropin 0.25 mg amp	Reconstitute with 1.1 ml NS to provide 0.25 mg/ml	Give over 2 minutes	
Cosyntropin Zinc Phodphsyr 1 mg/ml amp	**DO NOT GIVE IV PUSH**		
Cotrimoxazole 80 mg TRIMETHOPRIM & 400 mg Sulfamethoxazole/ 5ml	**DO NOT GIVE IV PUSH**		
Cyclosporine 50 mg/ml, 5 ml amp	**DO NOT GIVE IV PUSH**		
Dantrolene Sodium 20 mg vial	Add 60 ml SWI to produce 0.33 mg/ml SHARE UNTIL CLEAR	Give by rapid IV injection	Use within 6 hours of reconstitution.
Defeoxamine Mesylate 500 mg vial	**DO NOT GIVE IV PUSH**		
Desmopressin 4 mcg/ml amp	None	Give over 30 seconds	
Dexamethasone Sodium Phosphate 4 mg/ml, 2 ml vial	None	Give slowly over 1-several minutes	
Dextrose 50%, 50ml vial pre-filled syringe	None	Give slowly, 3ml per minute	
Diazepam 5 mg/ml, 2ml amp	None	Adults: 2-5 mg per minute. Children? 1 month: Slowly over 3 minutes, not exceeding 0.25 mg/kg into large vein.	Avoid administration into small vein.
Diazoxide 15 mg/ml, 20 ml amp	None	Rapid IV injection over 30 seconds or less into established peripheral line	Patient should be in recumbent postion. Avoid extravasation as alkaline solution is very irritating

Contd...

DRUG NAME & CONCENTRATION AVAILABLE	DILUTION REQUIRED FOR IV PUSH	RATE OF ADMINISTRATION	PRECAUTIONS COMMENTS/STABILITY
Diclofenac 25 mg/ml, 3ml amp	**DO NOT GIVE IV PUSH**		
Digoxin 0.25 mg/ml, 2ml amp, Pediatric 0.1 mg/ml amp	None	Give over at least 5 minutes	Before administering take apical pulse nothing the rate, rhythm and quality.
Digoxin Immune FAB 40 mg/vial	Dilute with 4ml SWI to provide 10 mg./ml For small doses (<2 mg), dilute with 36 ml NS for 1 mg/ml.	Rapid IV injection only if cardiac arrest is imminent. Infusion is preferred.	Sensitivity testing recommended in patients at increased risk of hypersensitivity reaction.
Dihydroergotamine Mesylate 1 mg/ml amp	None	1 mg over seconds	Use in children not established
Dimenhydrinate 50mg/ml, 1 ml amp	Dilute 50 mg with 10ml of NS	Give 50 mg or fraction thereof over 2 minutes	IV dose in pediatrics has not been established
Dimercaprol 3 ml amp	**DO NOT GIVE IV PUSH**		
Diphenhydramine HCI 10 mg/ml, 30 ml vial 50mg/ml vial 50 mg/ml amp	None	Give 25 mg or fraction thereof over 1 minute	Avoid extravasation Contraindicated in infants and neonates.
Dobutamine Hydricgkirude 250mg vial	**DO NOT GIVE IV PUSH**		
Dopamine Hydrochloride 40 mg.ml, 5ml syringe	**DO NOT GIVE IV PUSH**		
Doxapram HCI 20 mg/ml, 20ml vial	None	Slow IV injection	Incompatible with alkaline solutions. Contains benzyl alcohol.Do not use in neonates. Safe use in children not less than 12 years not established.
Doxycycline Hyclate 10mg vial	**DO NOT GIVE IV PUSH**		
Droperidol injection 2.5mg/ml, 2ml amp	None	Give 10 mg or fraction thereof over 30-60 seconds	Safe use in children less than 2 years not established.
Edetate Calcium Disodium 200mg/ml, 5ml amp	**DO NOT GIVE IV PUSH**		
Edrophonium Chloride 10 mg/ml amp	None	Give over 30-45 seconds	Monitor vital signs
Ephedrine Sulphate 50 mg/ml, 1 ml amp	None	Give 10 mg or fraction thereof over 30-60 seconds	Patients receiving parenteral ephedrine must be constantly monitored.

Contd...

DRUG NAME & CONCENTRATION AVAILABLE	DILUTION REQUIRED FOR IV PUSH	RATE OF ADMINISTRATION	PRECAUTIONS COMMENTS/STABILITY
Epinephrine 1:10,000 10 ml (1mg) pre-filled syringe 1:1000, 1 mg/ml, 30 ml vial	1:1000 must be diluted with 10 ml NS	Give over minute.	Do not use if discoloured, Patients receiving parenteral epinephrine must be constantly monitored.
Erthromycin Lactobionate 500mg vial	**DO NOT GIVE IV PUSH**		
Esmolol Hydrochloride 250mg/ml, 10ml amp	**DO NOT GIVE IV PUSH**		
Estradiol Hydrochloride 250 mg/ml, 10 ml amp	**DO NOT GIVE IV PUSH**		
Estogens, Conjugated 25 mg vial)	Reconstitute with diluent provided. Agitate gently.	Give 5mg/min	Rapid IV injection may cause skin flushing.
Ethacynate Sodium 50 mg vial	Reconstitute with 50 ml D_5W, NS to produce 1 mg/ml	Give over several minutes	Safe use in children has not been established. Use within 24 hours of reconstitution.
Factor VIII 250 units/500 units	Reconstitute according to manufacturer's directions and with diluent supplied.	For preparation greater than 34 AHFU/ml do not exceed 2 ml per minute. Less than 34 AHFU ml 10, 20 ml	Check pulse rate. Use within 3 hr after reconstitution.
Flumazenil mg/ml, 3ml amp	None	Rapid IV injection over 15-30 seconds	Administer through a freely flowing IV infusion into large vein. Avoid extravasation.
Flupentixol decanoate 20mg/ml amp	**DO NOT GIVE IV PUSH**		
Fluphenazine deconate 20 mg/ml amp	**DO NOT GIVE IV PUSH**		
Furosemide 10mg/ml 2ml and 10ml amps	None	Give 20 mg or fraction thereof over 1 minute	Ototoxicity seen with>4 mg/min in patients with impaired renal function. Protect from light.Injections with a yellow colour should not be used.
Gentamicin Sulfate 40 mg/ml, 2ml vial	**DO NOT GIVE IV PUSH**		

Contd...

DRUG NAME & CONCENTRATION AVAILABLE	DILUTION REQUIRED FOR IV PUSH	RATE OF ADMINISTRATION	PRECAUTIONS COMMENTS/STABILITY
Glucagon Injection 1 mg (1unit) vial	Reconstitute with 1ml diluent provided	Give over 1 minute	Flush line with D_5W NOT NS.
Glycopyrolate 0.2 mg/ml, 1 ml vial	None	Give 0.2 mg or fraction thereof over 1-2 minutes	Use with caution in patients with glaucoma or asthma. Safe use in children less than 12 years not established, except in conjunction with anesthesia.
Gold Sodium Thiomalate 50 mg/ml amp	**DO NOT GIVE IV PUSH**		
Gonadorelin Hydrochloride 0.1 mg/vial	Reconstitute with 1 ml diluent provided	Giver over 15-30 seconds	Reconstitute immediately before administration
Growth Hormone Human 4 IU or 12 IU/vial	**DO NOT GIVE IV PUSH**		
Haloperidol 5 mg/ml amp	**DO NOT GIVE IV PUSH**		
Heparin Sodium 1000 u/ml amp & 5000 unit/ml, vial	None	Give over 60 seconds	Solutions of heparin which contain benzyl alcohol as preservative should not be used in neonates.
Hydralazine HCI 20 mg/ml diluent	None	Give 10 mg or fraction thereof over 1 minute	Monitor blood pressure frequently
Hydrocortisone Hydrochloride 2 mg/ml amp	Dilute in at least 5 ml SWI, NS	Give 2 mg over 3-5 minutes	Monitor for respiratory depression.
Hydroxyprogresterone Caproate 250 mg/ml amp	**DO NOT GIVE IV PUSH**		
Hydroxyzine Hydrochloride 50 mg/ml, 2 ml,	**DO NOT GIVE IV PUSH**		
Hyoscine-N-Butyl bromide, 20 mg/ml amp	Dilute with SWI	Give slowly	
Imipenem-Cilastatin 500mg Imipenem & 500 mg Cilastatin per vial	**DO NOT GIVE IV PUSH**		
Indomethacin 1 mg/vial	Dilute with 1 ml of preservative free NS or SWI	Give over 5-10 seconds	Avoid extravasation. Do not use diluents containing benzyl alcohol.

Contd...

DRUG NAME & CONCENTRATION AVAILABLE	DILUTION REQUIRED FOR IV PUSH	RATE OF ADMINISTRATION	PRECAUTIONS COMMENTS/STABILITY
Insulin Regular 100 u/ml, 10 ml vial	None	Give each 50 units or fraction thereof over1 minute	Use only in patients with circulatory collapse, diabetic ketoacidosis or hyperkalemia. Only regular insulin is given IV.
Iron Dextran 50 mg/ml, 2ml ampule	May give undiluted if not greater than 100 mg	Do not exceed 50 mg per minute	
Isoproteribik HCI inj 1:5000, 10 ml syringe	Dilute 1 ml of 1:5000 solution to 10 ml NS or D_5W to provide 20 mcg/ml	Give slowly	Avoid simultaneous administration of epinephrine. Use only in extreme emergencies. Patients must be constantly monitored.
Labetalol, 5mg/ml, 20ml vial	None	Give over 2 minutes	Monitor BP. Safe use in children not established.
Leuprolide Acetate 1 mg/0.2ml, 2.8 ml, vial, 7.5 mg/syring	**DO NOT GIVE IV PUSH**		
Levothyroxine Sodium 0.5 mg/ml	Add 5 ml NS without preservatives to produce 0.1 mg/ml	Give 0.1 mg or a fraction thereof over 1 minute	Reconstitute immediately before administration.
Lidocaine, 20 mg/ml, 5ml syringe	None	Give 50 mg or fraction thereof over 1 minute	ECG monitoring required. Solutions containing 200mg/ml of lidocaine are not for direct IV use.
Lorazepam Injection 3mg/ml, 1ml tubex	Must be diluted with equal volume SWI, NS or D_5W	Do not exceed 2 mg per minute	Dilute immediately prior to injection.
Magnesium Sulphate 10%, 20 ml amp 50%, 2ml amp	Concentration of 20% or less should be used	Do not exceed 1.5ml of a 10% solution (or equivalent) per minute	Constant monitoring required. In life threatening arrhythmias, up to 4 gm may be administered over 30 seconds with caution.
Medroxyprogesterone Acetate 100mg/ml, 5 ml vial	**DO NOT GIVE IV PUSH**		
Menotropins 75 IV FSH and IV LH/amp	**DO NOT GIVE IV PUSH**		
Meperidine HCI, 25, 50, 75 & 100mg/ml amp	Dilute to 10 mg/ml with NS or SWI	Do not exceed 25 mg/min. Slower injection preferred.	Monitor for respiratory depression. High incidence of side effects associated with IV use.
Metaraminol Bitartrate 10 mg/ml, 10 ml vial	None	Give 5 mg over at least 1 minute	Direct IV in severe shock only. Constant monitoring. Avoid extravasation.
Methylene Blue inj 1%, 10ml amp	None	Give slowly over several minutes	Avoid extravasation and do not use in G_6PD patients.

Contd...

DRUG NAME & CONCENTRATION AVAILABLE	DILUTION REQUIRED FOR IV PUSH	RATE OF ADMINISTRATION	PRECAUTIONS COMMENTS/STABILITY
Methylergonomine Maleate 0.2mg/ml amp	Undiluted or diluted to 5ml NS	Give 0.2 mg over 1 minute	Do not use if discoloured or containing visible particles. IV use only in life threatening emergencies.
Methylprednisolone Acetate 40mg/ml vial	**DO NOT GIVE IV PUSH**		
Methylprednisolone Sodium Succinate 125 mg vial	Reconstitute with diluent provided	Give over one to several minutes	Use within 48 hours after reconstitution. Diluent contains benzyl alcohol. Do not use in children
Metoclopramide 5mg/ml, 2 ml amp	None	Doses of 10mg or less may be given over 1-2 minutes	
Metronidazole 5 mg/ml, 100 ml container	**DO NOT GIVE IV PUSH**		
Midazolam Injection 15 mg/3ml amp	To facilitate slow intravenous injection, may dilute with NS D_5W to concentration of 0.25 mg/ml	For conscious sedation, give over 2 or more minutes. For anesthesia induction give over 20-30 seconds.	Monitor for respiratory depression. Safe use in children less than 18 years of age not established.
Morphine Sulphate, 15mg/ml, 1ml syringe	Dilute dose in 4 or 5 ml SWI	Give over 4-5 minutes	Monitor for respiratory depression.
Morrhuate Sodium 50mg/ml, 30ml vial	None	Specialized references should be consulted for procedures and techniques of administration	Avoid extravasation. Use only a clear solution.
Naficllin Sodium, 1 g vial	Dilute with 15-30 ml SWI/NS	Give over 5-10 minutes preferably into tubing of running intravenous solution	Safe use for IV in neonates and infants is not established.
Nalbuphine Hydrochloride 10mg/ml, 2 ml ampoule	None	10 mg over 3-5 minutes	Safe in children less than 18 years not established. However, there is documentation of 0.2-0.3 mg/kg doses in pediatric patients>10 months being used safely.
Naloxone, 0.02 mg/ml, 2ml amp, 0.4 mg/ml 1ml amp	None	Give rapidly at 2-3 minute intervals until desired narcotic reversal is achieved.	IV route is recommended in emergency situations.

Contd...

DRUG NAME & CONCENTRATION AVAILABLE	DILUTION REQUIRED FOR IV PUSH	RATE OF ADMINISTRATION	PRECAUTIONS COMMENTS/STABILITY
Neostigmine Methyl-sulphate, 0.5ml/1ml amp, 2.5 mg/ml, 5ml vial,	None	Give 0.5 mg or fraction thereof over 1 minute	Injection is available in various concentrations. Read label carefully
Nitroglycerin 5 mg/ml, 5ml vial	**DO NOT GIVE IV PUSH**		
Nitroprusside Sodium 50 mg/vial	**DO NOT GIVE IV PUSH**		
Norephinephrine 1:1000 1 ml/mg, 4ml ampoule	**DO NOT GIVE IV PUSH**		
Ondansetron HCI 2 mg/ml	Must be diluted with 50 ml NS D_5 W	Give over 15 minutes	Safe use in children less than 3 years of age not established
Oxytocin 10u/ml amp	**DO NOT GIVE IV PUSH**		
Pancuronium Bromide 2mg/ml, 2ml amp	None	Give over 30-90 seconds	Initial test dose 0.02 mg/kg recommended in neonates. Constant monitoring required.
Papaverine Hydrochloride 30 mg/ml, 2ml amp	Undiluted or diluted in equal volume SWI	Give slowly over 1-2 minutes	Monitor vital signs.
Penicillin G Sodium 1, 000, 000 u/vial	**DO NOT GIVE IV PUSH**		
Pentazocine Lactate 30mg/ml, 1 ml amp	May give undiluted or diluted with 1 ml SWI for each 5 mg	5 mg over 60 seconds	Safe use in children less than 12 years not established.
Phenobarbial Sodium 20 mg/ml, 2 ml vial & 200 mg/ml vial	None	Do not exceed 60 mg/min in adults and 30 mg/min. in infants and children.	Avoid extravasation, may case tissue damage. Observe for respiratory depression.
Phentolamine Mesylate 10 mg/ml, 1 ml amp	Dilute with 1 ml SWI	Give over 60 seconds	Use reconstituted solution immediately. Patient should be in supine position.
Phenytoin Sodium 50 mg/ml, 5 ml vial	None	Do not exceed 50 mg/min in adults and 1-3 mg/kg/min in neonates.	Flush with NS after injection to reduce venous irritation.

Contd...

DRUG NAME & CONCENTRATION AVAILABLE	DILUTION REQUIRED FOR IV PUSH	RATE OF ADMINISTRATION	PRECAUTIONS COMMENTS/STABILITY
Physostigmine Salicylate 1 mg/ml 2 ml ampule	None	Do not exceed 1 mg per minute in adults and 0.5 mg/minute in children	
Phytonadione 10 mg/ml, ml amp	None	Do not exceed 1 mg/min	IM and subcutaneous routes are preferred.
Polymixin B Sulfate *500,000 Units/vial*	**DO NOT GIVE IV PUSH**		
Potassium Acetate 2mEq/ml, 20ml vial	**DO NOT GIVE IV PUSH**		
Potassium Chloride 2mEq/ml, 10 ml vial	**DO NOT GIVE IV PUSH**		
Potassium Phosphate 4.4mM of Phosphate/ml, 15 ml vial	**DO NOT GIVE IV PUSH**		
Pralidoxime chloride 1 gm vial	Dilute with 20ml NS to produce 50mg/ml	Over at least 5 minutes	IV influsion is preferable.
Procanamide 100 mg/ml, 10ml vial	Dilute each 100 mg with 10ml D_5 W/SWI to facilitate control of dosage rate	Do not exceed 25 to 50 mg/minute	Monitor BP and ECG
Prochlorperazine 12.5 mg/ml, 2 amp	Dilute with D_5W/NS, to concentration of 1mg/ml	Do not exceed 5 mg/min. 1mg/min preferable	Use in children less than 2 years of age or weighing less than 9 kg has not been established.
Promethazine 25 mg/ml, 2 ml ampule	May give undiluted if concentration is no greater than 25 mg/ml	Do not exceed 25 mg per minute and administer through the tubing of a freely flowing IV infusion set	Avoid extravasation
Propranolol 1 mg/ml amp	May give undiluted or dilute in 10ml D_5W	Do not exceed 1 mg/min	Monitor ECG.
Protamine sulphate 50 mg protamine activity / 5 ml amp	Reconstitute 50 mg with 5 ml SWI	Give over 1-3 mins	Not more than 50 mg in any 10 minute period
Protirelin 0.5 mg amp	None	Give over 15-30 seconds	Monitor blood pressure
Pyridoxine Hydrochloride 150 mg/ml 2 ml amp	None	50 mg or fraction thereof over 60 seconds	

Contd...

DRUG NAME & CONCENTRATION AVAILABLE	DILUTION REQUIRED FOR IV PUSH	RATE OF ADMINISTRATION	PRECAUTIONS COMMENTS/STABILITY
Quinidine Gluconate 80 mg/ml 10ml vial	**DO NOT GIVE IV PUSH**		
Ranitidine 25 mg/ml, 2 ml ampule	Dilute 50 mg with NS to total volume of 20 ml	Do not exceed 4 ml/minute	
Recombinant Human Erythropoietin (*EPREX*) 4000 U/ml	None	Give as bolus dose	
Ritodrine 10 mg/ml, 5 ampule	**DO NOT GIVE IV PUSH**		
Sodium Acetate 2mEq/ml, 20 ml vial	**DO NOT GIVE IV PUSH**		
Sodium Bicarbonate 8.4%, 1mEq/ml, 50 ml vial and syringe	None	Rapid IV injection Slow IV injection in pediatrics	Avoid extravasation, use 4.2% solution in children less than 2 years of age.
Sodium Nitrite 30mg/ml, 10 ml amp	None	300 mg over <5 mins for cyanide poisoning (10mg/kg initially for children)	Hypotension if injected too rapidly
Sodium Phosphate 4mEq Na and 3mMPO$_4$/ml, 15 ml vial	**DO NOT GIVE IV PUSH**		
Sodium Thiosulphate 250 mg/ml, 50 ml vial	None	Slow IV injection (12.5g over 10 mins for cyanide poisoning) 1.65 mg/kg for children	
Succinylcholine Chloride 20 mg/ml, 10ml vial	None	Give over 10 – 30 seconds	Constant monitoring required.
Testosterone Enanthate 250 mg/ml amp	**DO NOT GIVE IV PUSH**		
Thiamine Hydrochloride 50 mg/ml, 2 ml amp	None	Give 100 mg over 5 minutes	
Ticarcillin and Clavulanate Potassium	**DO NOT GIVE IV PUSH**		
Tolazoline Hydrochloride 25 mg/ml, 4ml amp	May be diluted in D_5W, NS, LR	Give over 10-15 minutes via scalp vein in neonates	Monitor vital signs, pulmonary artery pressure and pulmonary capillary wedge pressure.
Tranexamic Acid, 100 mg/ml, 5 ml	None	Slow IV injection of 5-10 ml at rate of 1 ml/min	

Contd...

DRUG NAME & CONCENTRATION AVAILABLE	DILUTION REQUIRED FOR IV PUSH	RATE OF ADMINISTRATION	PRECAUTIONS COMMENTS/STABILITY
Traimcinolone Acetonide Diacetate 10mg/ml, 5 ml vial 40 mg/ml via, 25 mg/ml, 5ml vial	**DO NOT GIVE IV PUSH**		
Trimethaphan Camsylate 50 mg/ml, 10 ml amp	**DO NOT GIVE IV PUSH**		
Tubocurarine Chloride 15 mg/ 1.5ml	None	Give slowly over 60-90 seconds	Solution should not be used if more than faintly discoloured. Constant monitoring required.
Urofolitropin 75 IU FSH/amp	**DO NOT GIVE IV PUSH**		
Vancomycin 500 mg/vial	**DO NOT GIVE IV PUSH**		
Vasopressin Synthetic 20 u/ml amp	**DO NOT GIVE IV PUSH**		
Vecuronium Bromide Powder 10 mg with diluent	Reconstitute with SWI to provide solution containing 1 mg/ml	Give by rapid IV injection	Safe use in children less than 7 weeks of age has not been established. Constant monitoring required.
Verapamil 2-5 mg/ml, 2ml amp	May be given undiluted or dilute in 5 ml SWI	Give slow IV push over a period of not less than two minutes. In geriatric patients, not less than 3 minutes.	Monitor ECG and blood pressure.
Vitamin B complex 2 ml amp	None	Give slow IV injection	
Zinc Chloride 1 mg/ Zn/ml, 10 ml vial	**DO NOT GIVE IV PUSH**		

KEY :

BWI Bacteriostatic Water for Injection
SWI Sterile Water for Injection
D_5W Dextrose 5% in Water
NS Normal Saline (0.9% Sodium Chloride)
LR Lactated Ringers

References:

I.V. Medications 10th edition (1994) Recommendations

Hazinski 1992 2nd edition "Nursing Care of the Critically ill Child"

Trissel Handbook on Injectable Drugs; 7th Ed.

AHFS DI 1994

ASHP Guidelines for Administration of Intravenous Medications to Pediatric Patients; 1993

APPENDIX 19

USEFUL PHARMACY WEBSITES

Associations

- AAPS – www.aaps.org

  Information on officers, activities and membership from the American Association of Pharmaceutical Scientists.

- ABPI -- www.abpi.org.uk/_private/welcome/default.htm

  Information from the Association of the British Pharmaceutical Industry for companies producing prescription medicines.

- ACSDMC – www.wizard.pharm.wayne.edu

  American Chemical Society Division of Medicinal Chemistry is an organization for scientists involved in drug research and development.

- Action Programme on Essential Drugs - www.who.int/dap/DAP_Homepage.html

  Information on this World Health Organization program supporting and coordinating comprehensive national drug policies.

- American Clinical Pharmacy – www.accp.com

  College for promoting clinical pharmacy practice, research and education. With news, an events calendar and membership details.

- American Assoc. of Colleges of Pharmacy – www.aacp.org

  American body representing the interests of pharmaceutical educators and education. With activity details and a software library.

- Board of Pharmaceutical Specialties -- www.bpsweb.org

  BPS recognizes specialties in pharmacy and provides advanced practice specialty certification for qualifying pharmacists.

- CPFI – www-cpfi.pharmacy.uiowa.edu

  Christian Pharmacists Fellowship International, an interdenominational ministry of individuals working in pharmaceutical service and practice.

- CSPS Home Page – www.ualberta.ca/~csps/

  Canadian Society for Pharmaceutical Sciences is a organization established to foster research. Includes journal articles and links.

- California Pharmacists Association – www.cpha.com

  Publications, education, legislative information and a calendar of events, from this group serving the pharmacy profession.

- Canadian Pharmaceutical Association -- www.cdnpharm.ca

  National advocacy and professional organization, providing programs, publications, news and benefits to members.

- Compounding Pharmacists – www.iacprx.org

  International Academy of Compounding Pharmacists, a professional body with members in the US, Canada, Australia and Chile.

- Controlled Release Society – www.crsadmhdq.org

  International society focusing on the advancement of science and technology of drug delivery systems.

- Division for Drug Affairs -- www.rfv.pharmasoft.se

  Swedish National Social Insurance Board's division dealing with drug pricing and reimbursement program issues.

- Food and Drug Administration – www.fda.gov:80/default.htm

  News, publications and research reports, with links to other sites. Includes the Center for Drug Evaluation and Research.

- Guild of Hospital Pharmacists -- www.netlink.co.uk/users/stmarys/

  Information from this UK advocacy and professional organization, part of the Manufacturing, Science and Finance Union.

- Infectious Disease Pharmacists -- 165.6.9.23

  Society updates, grant information, job listings and newsletters from this American society for professionals.

- Kappa Psi International – www.kappa-psi.org

  Pharmaceutical society promoting pharmacy education and research. Includes information on activities, member directory and job listings.

- NDMA – www.ndmainfo.org

  Hosted by the Nonprescription Drug Manufacturers Association.With news, information on the industry, facts and figures, and info on OTC issues.

- National Pharmaceutical Association – www.npa.co.uk

  Organization of Britain's community and retail pharmacies. Information on services, publications and membership benefits.

- Pharmaceutical Society of Australia – www.psa.org.au

  The Pharmaceutical Society of Australia (PSA) is the national professional organization for pharmacists in Australia.

- Pharmacy Guild of Australia – www.guild.org.au

  The Pharmacy Guild of Australia was established in 1928, bringing together several small retail pharmacy organizations then operating in the various States.

- PharmWeb – www.pharmweb.net

  Guide to pharmacy and related resources on the Internet. Includes jobs, forums and directories of individuals and organizations.

- Phi Delta Chi – www.angelfire.com/biz/pdcfraternity/index.html

  Phi Delta Chi Pharmacy Fraternity, founded on November 2, 1883 at the University of Michigan in Ann Arbor, is an association formed to advance the science of pharmacy and its allied interests and to foster and promote a fraternal spirit among its members.

- Professional Compounding Centers-- www.pccarx.com

  American association provides information for the compounding pharmacist to help in fulfilling unique patient needs.

Databases

- World Wide Web Pharmaguide - http://www.geocities.com/pharmalinks/

  Directory of pharmaceutical companies and institutions, with information on products and services, research, industry and government.

- LookSmart Spotlight Site – Pharmacology –

  pharmacology.miningco.com/index.htm?COB=looksmart

  Get facts on legal drugs, trials, and treating specific ailments. Search databases geared toward consumers and professionals. From The Mining Co.

- Virtual Pharmacy - Martindale's –

  wwwsci.lib.uci.edu/~martindale/Pharmacy.html

  Huge site with pharmacy, pharmacology, clinical pharmacology and toxicology information. Features journals, student resources and databases.

- AIDS - HIV – ÆGIS -- www.aegis.com

  Considered the largest AIDS/HIV database in the world. Free Access to AIDSLINE, the AIDS news database, and an online library.

- Animal Drug Database -- www.fda.gov/cvm/

  Searchable listing provides facts and figures on all animal drug products approved by the FDA.

- Antimicrobial Use Guidelines –

  http://www.medsch.wisc.edu/clinsci/amcg/amc.html

  Guidelines for the selection of antimicrobials and their cost-effective use in hospitals. With advice to maximize patient care.

- Bio Online -- www.bio.com/bio.html

  Directory of pharmaceutical and biotechnology companies and institutes, with information on products and services, research, industry and government.

- Center for Molecular Modeling -- cmm.info.nih.gov/modeling/

  Guides, tutorials, articles, software and research tools for molecular modeling, from this center which works with NIH on research.

- Chemical Abstracts Service -- info.cas.org/welcome.html

  Provides scientific information and other online resources for chemists, chemical engineers and educators.

- Cutaneous Drug Reactions –

  gopher://gopher.dartmouth.edu/11/Research/BioSci/CDRD

  Easy-to-use database of drug reactions that have skin manifestations. Includes reaction incidence and journal references.

- Drug Data Base -- chrom.tutms.tut.ac.jp/JINNO/DRUGDATA/00database.html

  Drugs listed by name or function, with details of their chemical composition, physical properties and UV spectrum.

- Drug Database- PharmInfoNet -- pharminfo.com/drugdb/db_mnu.html

  Information from this database includes recent announcements and warnings about side effects of drugs, written mainly for professionals.

- Drug Discrimination -- www.dd-database.org

  Searchable bibliography of abstracts, journal articles, and books on this method for studying the effects of drugs.

- Drug InfoNet -- http://www.druginfonet.com

  Information resource for consumers and professionals on health care and pharmaceutical-related businesses.

- General Pharmaceutical Topics -- www.newspage.com/browse/

  Daily news on topics such as drug manufacturing and development. With searchable database of past articles.

- HIV Medication Guide -- www.jag.on.ca/hiv/

  Up-to-date information on HIV medications including drug interactions, education pamphlets, and tools to improve adherence.

- HotMolecBase -- bioinformatics.weizmann.ac.il/hotmolecbase/

  Information about proteins and other biologically active molecules that play a role in disease or have medical applications.

- Informed Online -- www.infomed.org/index-e.html

  Swiss publishing house publishes detailed information on what they consider the 100 most important prescribed drugs.

- Internet Medical Bookstore -- www.fimb.com/whoweare.html

  Online medical text sales. Catalog contains over 24,000 entries covering medical, dental, nursing, and allied sciences.

- Merck Manual -- www.merck.com/pubs/mmanual/

  Manual of diagnosis and therapy covering most disorders, describing symptoms, common clinical procedures, and drug treatment.

- NCI Drug Information System – http://dtp.nci.nih.gov/epnrd/3dis.html

  National Cancer Institute provides this collection of 3D structures for over 400,000 drugs.

- PediWeb -- solar.rtd.utk.edu/~esmith/pedi.html

  Journal reviews, news, original articles and links to pediatric pharmacology resources, for parents and professionals.

- PhRMA -- www.phrma.org

  Organization representing America's pharmaceutical research companies provides details of drug development, industry news,and health guides.

- PharmInfoNet Index -- pharminfo.com/idx_toc.html#drug

  Extensive list of publications, discussion groups, disease centers and pharmacy products and services. Includes a drug database.

- PharmWeb -- http://www.pharmweb.net/

  Extensive directory of most aspects of pharmacology. Search their yellow pages for publications and discussion groups.

- Pharmaceutical Information Network -- pharminfo.com/pin_hp.html

  Drug information, discussion groups, a virtual drugstore, and online publications for both consumers and professionals.

- Pharmaceutical Newsgroup Archive –

  www.bio.net/hypermail/PHARMACEUTICAL-BIOTECHNOLOGY/

  Search this newsgroup archive by keyword or phrase for information on pharmaceuticals and biotechnology.

- Pharmacokinetics & Pharmacodynamics -- www.boomer.org/pkin/

  Information and resources about these two disciplines studying the dynamics of drug and metabolite levels in the body.

- Pharmacology Departments World-Wide –

  www.kfunigraz.ac.at/ekpwww/linkinst.html

  Austria's Graz University provides this exhaustive directory of pharmacology departments from around the world.

- Pharmacy Archive -- pharminfo.com/drugdb/smp_mnu.html

  Archive of threads from the sci.med.pharmacy newsgroup, with an index of the trade and generic names of drugs.

- Pharmacy Sites -- www.exit109.com/~zaweb/pjp/pharm.htm

  This guide to pharmacy resources on the Internet gives a description of links and includes mailing lists.

- Regulatory Affairs Information --www.medmarket.com/tenants/rainfo/rainfo.htm

  Find any regulatory body, organization, meeting, document or guideline in this extensive directory. Covers regulated product industries.

- Rx-List Internet Drug Index -- www.rxlist.com

  First stop for finding informative reports about almost any drug. Lists over 4,000 drugs and common side effects.

- Schools of Pharmacy -- www.li.net/~edhayes/rxschool.html

  US pharmacy schools listed by state. With their address, telephone numbers and Internet links.

- The Drug Development Homepage -- members.tripod.com/~ChristopherMarrs/

  Internet resource for drug development and outsourcing information for pharmaceutical professionals.

- Virtual Pharmacy Center -- www-sci.lib.uci.edu/HSG/Pharmacy.html

  Find medical dictionaries, journals, pharmacy and pharmacological resources and related information in this huge directory.

- World Wide Drugs -- community.net/~neils/new.html

  This comprehensive resource includes a pharmaceutical drug directory, links, news and access to related information.

- Worldwide Healthcare Forums -- www.healthcareforums.com

  Created to facilitate interaction among healthcare professionals on specific topics which includes discussion of cases, research and other relevant issues.

Continuing Education

- The Pharmacy Stand -- www.arcwebserv.com/pharm/

  Weekly pharmacy articles by registered pharmacists, advice about careers, tips, and a useful database of links for students doing research.

- Applied Pharmacokinetics -- www.usc.edu/hsc/lab_apk/

  Information, software and event details pertaining to pharmacokinetic systems and individualized drug therapy.

- Calcium Channel Blockers -- www.cc.emory.edu/WHSC/MED/CME/CCB/

  Information regarding the use of calcium channel blockers in the treatment of hypertension. From Emory University.

- Course in Pharmacokinetics – http://157.142.72.143/gaps/pkbio/pkbio.html

  Online course pharmacokinetics and biopharmaceutics, covering drug administration, data analysis, and modeling systems.

- Cutaneous Drug Reactions –

  gopher.dartmouth.edu:70/11/Research/BioSci/CDRD

  Database of drug reactions that have skin manifestations, organized alphabetically by the drug's generic name. Maintained by Jerome Z. Litt, MD.

- Drugs and Devices -- www.hsph.harvard.edu/Organizations/DDIL/ddilhpge.html

  Review articles, resources and general information on pharmacoepidemiology from Harvard University.

- EthnoMedicinals -- Walden.MO.NET:80/~tonytork/

  Information on the use of herbs and other natural products in biochemistry, pharmacology, and traditional medicine.

- Francom's Pharmacy Page -- hometown.aol.com/mefrancom/index.html

  Information for the compounding pharmacist with formulae and supplier list. With a range of downloadable shareware for pharmacists.

- Glaxo Wellcome Guide -- www.glaxowellcome.co.uk/science/phguide/

  Quick reference guide to the important terms and concepts of pharmacology, including sections on receptor binding and neurotransmitter systems.

- Helix -- www.helix.com

  Healthcare Education Learning & Information Exchange is sponsored by Glaxo and has resources for professionals and patients.

- Medicom -- medicaled.com

  Offers pharmacists free continuing CE credits via online and teleconference courses.

- Pharmacokinetics & Pharmacodynamics -- www.boomer.org/pkin/

  Information and resources about these two disciplines studying the dynamics, over time, of drug and metabolite levels in the body.

- Professional Compounding Centers -- www.thecompounders.com

  American association provides information for the compounding pharmacist to help in fulfilling unique patient needs.

- Searching the Internet -- www.drugs.indiana.edu/pubs/newsline/searching.html

  Concise articles offering strategies for locating accurate and scientifically accepted information on pharmaceuticals.

- Self Assessment in Pharmacology – www.university.com/ISAP/

  Designed to make studying pharmacology and looking up drug information easier. Access is free to all educational users.

- Virtual En-psych-lopedia -- uhs.bsd.uchicago.edu/dr-bob/tips/tips.html

  Information for both patients and professionals on a range of psychopharmacological medications, including their uses and side effects.

- Virtual Pharmacy - Martindale's – wwwsci.lib.uci.edu/~martindale/Pharmacy.html

  Huge site with pharmacy, pharmacology, clinical pharmacology and toxicology information. Features journals, student resources and databases.

- WWW Virtual Library: Medicine -- www.ohsu.edu/cliniweb/wwwvl/

  Searchable index of biosciences, a list of biomedical sites, and a history of science, technology, and medicine.

Patient Education

- AltiMed -- www.altimed.com

  Canadian pharmacist's guide to the Net. Includes product info, monthly topics for discussion, forum, disease advice, and links.

- Antibiotic Information -- www.hovione.com

  Useful information about the antibiotic (doxycycline). Includes advice for patient and doctor, information about side-effects and bibliography.

- Ask the Pharmacist -- www.wilmington.net/dees/

  Post your medication questions to Mr. Frank Purdy or view the frequently asked questions already answered.

- Council on Family Health -- www.cfhinfo.org/home_b.html

  Non-profit organization dedicated to educating consumers about the proper use of nonprescription and prescription medicines. With ten step guide.

- Drug Emporium Online -- www.drugemporium.com/rx-f.htm

  RxAnswerLine provides personal and confidential answers to all questions about prescriptions and over-the-counter medications.

- Drug Information -- www.pharmacy.ab.umd.edu/~umdi/umdi.html

  Your questions about pharmaceuticals to the University of Maryland Drug Information Service are answered within three days.

- EthnoMedicinals – Walden.MO.NET:80/~tonytork/

  Information on the use of herbs and other natural products in biochemistry, pharmacology, and traditional medicine.

- FDA Food and Drug Interactions – http://vm.cfsan.fda.gov/~lrd/fdinter.html

  From the US Food and Drug Administration with information that explains how certain foods may interact with some groups of medications.

- Helix -- www.helix.com

  Healthcare Education Learning & Information Exchange is sponsored by Glaxo and has resources for professionals and patients.

- LookSmart Spotlight Site – Pharmacology –

  pharmacology.miningco.com/index.htm?COB=looksmart

  Get facts on legal drugs, trials, and treating specific ailments.Search databases geared toward consumers and professionals. From The Mining Co.

- Medicine Program -- www.ims-1.com/%7Efreemed/

  Information on a privately sponsored program which provides prescription medicine free-of-charge to individuals in need.

- Pharmaceutical Chemistry Group -- www.pharma.ethz.ch

  Introduction to pharmaceutical chemistry, research into immunological therapeutics and computer aided drug design from Swiss institute.

- Rx-List Internet Drug Index -- www.rxlist.com

  First stop for finding informative reports about almost any drug. Lists over 4,000 drugs and common side effects.

- Searching the Internet -- www.drugs.indiana.edu/pubs/newsline/searching.html

  Concise articles offering strategies for locating accurate and scientifically accepted information on pharmaceuticals.

- Taking Your Medicine -- www.hmri.com/managingyourhealth/guides/tym.html

  Instructions about dose, route, and taking of medications. Includes a list of questions you should ask you pharmacist or doctor.

- Top 200 Prescriptions -- www.rxlist.com/top200.htm

  List of the 200 most popular US pharmaceuticals. Includes brand name, manufacturer, and generic name.

- Virtual En-psych-lopedia -- uhs.bsd.uchicago.edu/dr-bob/tips/tips.html

  Information for both patients and professionals on a range of psychopharmacological medications, including their uses and side effects.

Undergraduate Education

- Antibiotics Guideline -- www.usc.edu/hsc/lab_apk/

  Introduction to antibiotics, including their mechanism of action, resistance and host-antibiotic-microbe interactions.

- Applied Pharmacokinetics -- www.usc.edu/hsc/lab_apk/

  Information, software and event details pertaining to pharmacokinetic systems and individualized drug therapy.

- Course in Pharmacokinetics -- 157.142.72.143/gaps/pkbio/pkbio.html

  Online education in pharmacokinetics and biopharmaceutics, covering drug administration, data analysis and modeling systems.

- Drugs and Devices -- www.hsph.harvard.edu/Organizations/DDIL/ddilhpge.html

  Review articles, resources and general information on pharmacoepidemiology from Harvard University.

- Glaxo Wellcome Guide –

  www.interchg.ubc.ca/interchgv2/lockdown/notice.html/mainmenu.html

  Quick reference guide to the important terms and concepts of pharmacology, including receptor binding and neurotransmitter systems.

- Infra-red Spectroscopy –

  www.interchg.ubc.ca/interchgv2/lockdown/notice.html/mainmenu.html

  Intended for undergraduate students, this online tutorial focuses on infra-red spectroscopy in drug analysis.

- Net Pharmacology -- lysine.pharm.utah.edu

  Online lecture in cardiovascular pharmacology from the University of Utah. With a cardiology glossary, and 3D drug structure images.

- Pharmacology and Toxicology -- www.pharm.ukans.edu/pharmtox/index.html

  Resources from the University of Kansas Department of Pharmacology and Toxicology, one of the premier programs in the country.

- Phase Technologies -- www.phase-technologies.com/html/vol._1_no._6.html

  Discussion of the use of the Pirani gauge in monitoring and controlling the lyophilization process

- Psychopharmacology –

  http://indy.radiology.uiowa.edu/Providers/Lectures/Conferences/CPS/TOC.html

  From the University of Iowa comes this online textbook on the use of drugs in the treatment of a range of mental disorders.

- Searching the Internet -- www.drugs.indiana.edu/pubs/newsline/searching.html

  Concise articles offering strategies for locating accurate and scientifically accepted information on pharmaceuticals.

- Self Assessment in Pharmacology – wwwusers.cs.umn.edu/~isap/welcome.html

  Designed to make studying pharmacology and looking up drug information easier. Access is free to all educational users.

- Virtual Pharmacy - Martindale's –

  wwwsci.lib.uci.edu/~martindale/Pharmacy.html

  Huge site with pharmacy, pharmacology, clinical pharmacology and toxicology information. Features journals, student resources and databases.

News and Journals

- AVICENNA -- www.avicenna.com

  Comprehensive medical information resource for all medical professionals. Register for free Medline abstract searches.

- Medical Sciences Bulletin -- pharminfo.com/pubs/msb/msbmnu.html

  Articles on pharmaceutical research and product reviews of new drugs. Published by the Pharmaceutical Information Associates.

- Williams & Wilkins -- www.wwilkins.com

  Stock a wide range of publications for medical professionals which can be ordered online.

- Adverse Drug Reactions -- www.oup.co.uk/drugsj/contents/

  Table of contents and abstracts from this journal which focuses on adverse drug reactions and acute poisoning.

- Alimentary Pharm. & Therapeutics –

  www.blacksci.co.uk/products/journals/apt.htm

  Details and table of contents from this journal specializing in the effects of drugs on the gastrointestinal tract, gall bladder and pancreas.

- Antiviral Agents Bulletin -- www.bioinfo.com/biotech/antiviral.html

  Summaries from recent editions covering antiviral drug and vaccine developments, with emphasis on HIV-infection and AIDS-related therapeutics.

- CJPP -- www.cisti.nrc.ca/cisti/journals/cjpp.html

  Canadian Journal of Physiology & Pharmacology published in full text in Adobe Acrobat portable document format (PDF files).

- CSPS -- www.ualberta.ca/~csps/

  Canadian Society for Pharmaceutical Sciences is a organization established to foster research. Includes journal articles and links.

- Clinical Drug Investigation –

  www.medscape.com/adis/CDI/public/journal.CDI.html

  Free electronic version of the journal of the same title. Aim is rapid publication of original drug research info.

- Clinical Psychopharmacology – www.apa.org/journals/pha.html

  Abstracts from the current issue of Experimental and Clinical Psychopharmacology. With subscription details.

- Doctor's Guide – www.pslgroup.com/NEWDRUGS.HTM

  Articles on approved new drugs and new indications for previously available drugs, plus medical news and Internet sites.

- Drug Approvals List -- www.fda.gov/cder/da/da.htm

  Listing of new drug approvals from the Food and Drug Administration, recording drug name, use and applicant.

- Drug Benefit Trends -- www.medscape.com/SCP/DBT/public/journal.DBT.html

  Publication for managed health care professionals who control pharmacy service and drug benefits. With selected articles and subscription details.

- Drug Wise Online -- home.vicnet.net.au/~drugwise/drugwise.htm

  Online newsletter on psychotropic and therapeutic drugs, with reviews of international literature summarizing drug developments and research.

- Drug, Equipment and Procedure News -- www.angelfire.com/newterms/

  Information on new drugs, equipment, and procedures is regularly presented. For medical transcriptionists and other professionals.

- Essential Drugs Monitor -- www.who.int/dap/edm.html

  Selected articles from this World Health Organization journal containing features on national drug policies and public education.

- Financial Times Healthcare -- www.fthealthcare.com

  International publisher of global business intelligence and information on the healthcare, biotechnology and pharmaceutical industries.

- IAVI Report -- www.iavi.org

  Report is unique in its coverage of issues surrounding HIV vaccine research and development.

- IJPPP -- www.psycom.net/ijppp.html

  International Journal of Psychopathology, Psychopharmacology, and Psychotherapy. Full text of case reports, research and reviews.

- Japanese Journal of Pharmacology -- www.soc.nacsis.ac.jp/tjps/jjp/

  Published by the Japanese Pharmacological Society contains the tables of contents and abstracts from the past year's issues.

- Journal of Pharmaceutical Care -- http://198.79.220.3:80/pharmacy/jpc/

  Details of this new electronic journal which focuses on issues pertaining to pharmaceutical care. With editorial guidelines.

- Lippincott-Raven Publishers -- www.lrpub.com

  Extensive catalog of medical texts with informative reviews of each and online ordering. Covers electronic media, books and journals.

- Mosby -- www.1.mosby.com/Mosby/index.html

  Catalog of new publications from Mosby, the world's leading publisher of books, journals and serial publications in the health sciences.

- Oncology Pharmacy Practice -- www.cpb.uokhsc.edu/pkin/jopp.html

  Information on a new international journal dedicated to educating pharmacists about the care of cancer patients.

- Pharmacy Online -- www.priory.com/pharmol.htm

  Features papers, articles, letters and educational material, edited by Dr. M. Partridge Director of Pharmacy in a UK hospital. With search.

- Pharmacy Times -- members.aol.com/pharmtimes/index.html

  Updated weekly this forum for pharmacists provides news, feature articles, career information and product reviews.

- Standard -- www.usp.org/standard/9901.htm

  Official newsletter from the United States Pharmacopoeia provides details of new drug regulations and standards plus member news.

- Uncover Web -- uncweb.carl.org

  Fee-based article retrieval service lists over 17,000 periodicals. Use the free search and pay for articles of interest to be faxed.

- Virtual Pharmacy - Martindale's –

  wwwsci.lib.uci.edu/~martindale/Pharmacy.html

  Huge site with pharmacy, pharmacology, clinical pharmacology and toxicology information. Features journals, student resources and databases.

- World Pharma Web -- www.worldpharmaweb.com

  Pharmaceutical industry news service has stories from around the world updated daily, plus contact information.

Regulatory Issues

- Drug Development & Approval -- www.allp.com/drug_dev.htm

  Alliance Pharmaceutical Corporation explains the rigorous process of drug testing, development and approval.

- Drug Evaluation & Research Center -- www.fda.gov/cder/

  Find out information about new drugs, clinical trials and the process of regulation from the Food and Drug Administration.

- Doctor's Guide to New Drugs – www.pslgroup.com/NEWDRUGS.HTM

  Articles on approved new drugs or new indications for previously available drugs, with latest medical news and Internet sites.

- Dot Pharmacy -- www.dotpharmacy.co.uk

  Professional pharmacist and druggist publication with articles on pharmaceuticals, pharmacist practices and general events affecting this industry.

- Drug Information -- www.pharmacy.ab.umd.edu/~umdi/umdi.html

  your questions about pharmaceuticals to the University of Maryland Drug Information Service answered within three days.

- Drug Publications Menu -- http://pharminfo.com/pubs/pubs_mnu.html

  Articles focusing on new drugs and drug therapies. Includes the Medical Sciences Bulletin and the Electronic Highlights Bulletin.

- FDA Drug Approvals 1997 -- www.micromedex.com/cmdx-c/hcs-cfda.htm

  Summary of drugs approved by the Food and Drug Administration for this year. Includes dosage information and clinical applications.

- FDA Drug Approvals List -- www.fda.gov/cder/da/da.htm

  Details of original new drug applications under consideration by the Food & Drug Administration. Updated monthly.

- FDA News -- www.fda.gov/opacom/hpnews.html

  Newsletter offering the latest news from the Food and Drug Administration, with reports on the latest products approved.

- Government & Regulatory Bodies –

  www.pharmweb.net/pwmirror/pwk/pharmwebk.html

  Listing of international pharmaceutical regulatory bodies including the US Food and Drug Administration.

- New Drug Approvals - Mining Company –

  http://pharmacology.tqn.com/library/newdr98/blindxa.htm

  Starting point for a search for information about newly-approved or newly-released medicines in the United States.

- Regulatory Affairs -- www.medmarket.com/tenants/rainfo/rainfo.htm

  find any regulatory body, organization, meeting, document or guideline in this extensive directory. Covers regulated product industries.

  Source : Website www.pharmainfo.net compiled by Mr. Laxminarayana Adepu

SELECTED REFERENCES

1. A method of estimating the probability of adverse drug reactions – Naronjo CA, Busto U, Sellers EM, Sandor P, Ruiz I, Roberts EA et al – *Clin Pharmacol Ther* 1981; 30: 239-45.
2. Adverse drug reactions: definitions, diagnosis, and management – Edwards IR, Aronson JK, Uppsala Monitoring Centre, WHO Collaborating Centre for International drug monitoring, Sweden.
3. Adverse drug reactions: Types and Treatment options – Marc A.Riedl, and Adrian M.Casillas – University of California, Los Angeles, California.
4. Adverse drug reactions in the community health setting:Approaches to recognizing, counseling, and reporting – Jones JK – *Fam Comm Health* 1982; 5(2):58-67
5. Adverse drug reaction reporting, problems and solutions – Hoffman RP – *FDA Med Bull* 1993; 23: insert.
6. Adverse drug events, adverse drug reactions and medication errors – frequently asked questions – VA Center for Medication Safety and VHA Pharmacy Benefits Management Strategic Healthcare group and The Medical Advisory Panel, November 2006.
7. Adverse drug effects – Lamy PP – *Clin Ger Med* 1990; 6: 293-307
8. American Society of Health System Pharmacists. Suggested definitions and relationships among medication misadventures, medication errors, adverse drug events, and adverse drug reactions. *Am J Health-Syst Pharm* 1998; 55:165-6
9. ASHP guidelines on a standardized method for pharmaceutical care – *American Journal of Health system Pharmacists* – 1996; 53:1713-1716
10. ASHP guidelines on preventing medication errors in hospitals - *Am J Hosp Pharm* 1993;50:305-14
11. Clinical Pharmacy: Reflections and Forecasts- *The annals of Pharmacotherapy* – Feb 2007, Vol.41.

12. Computer assisted instruction for responding to drug information requests – Host TR, Krkwood CF – Paper presented at the 22nd Annual ASHP Midyear Clinical Meeting. December 1987; Atlanta. Abstract.
13. Cognitive processes in medication errors – Grasha AF, O'Neill M – *US Pharm 1*996; 21: 96-109.
14. Cost effectiveness of Total Parenteral Nutrition – Patrick L.Twomey, *Journal of Parenteral Enteral Nutrition*, 9: 3-10; 1985
15. Cytochrome P450 – Their impact on drug treatment – *Hospital Pharmacy*, June 2002, Vol.9
16. Drug distribution in milk – *The Australian Prescriber* – 1997 Vol.20.
17. Drug information resources – Price KO, Goldwire MA – *Am Pharm* 1994; NS34:30-9
18. Drug Interactions : what you should know – Council on Family Health website www.cfhinfo.org
19. Drug Interactions – *The annals of Pharmacotherapy* – March *2006, Vol.40*
20. Editorial - The Clinical Pharmacist – *The annals of Pharmacotherapy* – Feb 2007, Vol.41
21. Effectiveness of a pharmacist – acquired medication history in promoting patient safety – *American Journal of Health System Pharmacy* – posted online 01/02/2003.
22. Errors in pharmacy practice – Abood RR – *US Pharm* 1996;21:122-32.
23. Evolvement of Clinical Pharmacy – *The annals of Pharmacotherapy* – January 2007, Vol.41
24. Frequency, type and clinical importance of medication history errors at admission to hospital: a systematic review – *CMAJ* – Aug 2005, 173 (5).
25. Handbook of institutional pharmacy practice. Baltimore: Williams & Wilkins; 1986.pp 249-54
26. How to evaluate reports of clinical trials – Weintraub M – *P & T* 1990 Dec:1463-76.
27. How to read clinical journals: I. Why to read them and how to start reading them critically – Department of Clinical Epidemiology and Biostatistics, McMaster University of Health Sciences - *CMAJ* 1981; 124:555-8
28. Institute for Safe Medication Practices. The "five rights". 1999 August 17 (Available from: www.ismp.org/MSAarticles/FiveRights.html).

29. Medication errors : Picking up the pieces – Coleman IC – *Drug Topics* 1999;143:83-92

30. Patient interviewing: Health and Medication history – Susan C.Lakey, Online Power point Presentation

31. Recommendations from the American College of Physicians – Mazza JJ – *Ann Intern Med* 1994; 120:699-720.

32. Review of Literature: Oral patient counseling by Pharmacists – Beardsley, RS. Proceedings of the National Symposium on oral counseling by Pharmacists about prescription medicines; September 1997, Lansdowne, Virginia.

33. Selected topics in drug information access and practice: an update – Baker DE, Smith GH, Abate MA – *Ann Pharmacotherapy* 1994; 28:1389-94

34. Systematic approach to drug information requests – Watababe AS, McCart G – *Am J Hosp Pharm* 1975; 32(12):1282-5

35. Theory and analysis of typical errors in a medical setting – Senders JW – *Hosp Pharm* 1993; 28:505-8

36. The Physician-Pharmacist interface in the clinical practice of pharmacy – *The annals of Pharmacotherapy* – December 2006, Vol.40

37. Toward the operational identification of adverse dug reactions – Karch FE, Lasagna L – *Clin Pharmacol Ther* 1977; 21:247-54

38. Website - College of Pharmacy, University of Arizona www.pharmacy.arizona.edu

39. Website – Pharmacists board of Queensland www.pharmacyboard.qld.gov.au

40. Website – Drug Information and Research Centre - www.dirc.ca

INDEX

A

D

E

F

G

P

Q

R

S

T